A GUIDE FOR THE STATIS.___ _____ ____ _____

Selected Readings for Clinical Researchers

Do statistics-heavy research papers give you a headache. Are you baffled by bias, confused by correlation, or flummoxed by F-tests? *A Guide for the Statistically Perplexed* is here to help! This book, designed for students, clinicians, and researchers, covers basic statistical and research techniques while drawing attention to many common problem areas.

Inspired to write this book in reaction to mistakes he encountered in actual research papers, David L. Streiner explains complex statistical concepts in lucid, jargon-free language. Using his trademark sense of humour and light-hearted style, he explains how to present data (or, conversely, how *not* to), and outlines statistical techniques and more advanced procedures. To help readers detect problems with research design and interpretation, Streiner details important 'CRAP' (convoluted reasoning or anti-intellectual pomposity) indicators to look out for. Even those with little or no background in statistics, measurement theory, or research will gain a new understanding and appreciation of these topics from this lively and accessible guide.

DAVID L. STREINER is a professor emeritus in the Department of Psychiatry and Behavioural Neurosciences and the Department of Clinical Epidemiology and Biostatistics at McMaster University and a professor in the Department of Psychiatry at the University of Toronto. He is senior scientific editor of *Health Reports*.

A Guide for the Statistically Perplexed

Selected Readings for Clinical Researchers

DAVID L. STREINER

UNIVERSITY OF TORONTO PRESS
Toronto Buffalo London

© Canadian Psychiatric Association 2013
Published by University of Toronto Press
Toronto Buffalo London
www.utppublishing.com
Printed in the U.S.A.

ISBN 978-1-4426-1353-9

Printed on acid free paper.

Library and Archives Canada Cataloguing in Publication

Streiner, David L.
A guide for the statistically perplexed : selected readings for clinical
researchers / David L. Streiner.

Includes bibliographical references and index.
ISBN 978-1-4426-1353-9

1. Medical statistics.   2. Medicine–Research–Statistical methods.   I. Title.

RA409.S77 2012   610.72'7   C2012-906124-7

University of Toronto Press acknowledges the financial assistance to its publishing
program of the Canada Council for the Arts and the Ontario Arts Council.

Canada Council Conseil des Arts
for the Arts   du Canada

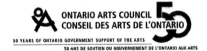
ONTARIO ARTS COUNCIL
CONSEIL DES ARTS DE L'ONTARIO
50 YEARS OF ONTARIO GOVERNMENT SUPPORT OF THE ARTS
50 ANS DE SOUTIEN DU GOUVERNEMENT DE L'ONTARIO AUX ARTS

University of Toronto Press acknowledges the financial support of the Government
of Canada through the Canada Book Fund for its publishing activities.

Contents

Part Three: Research Methods

Part Four: Measurement

Introduction

I should begin this introduction with apologies to Moses Maimonides, from whom I stole the idea for the title; his *Guide for the Perplexed* has been a basic reader for those struggling to understand the Bible. However, since the Rambam (as he is known to generations of Talmudic scholars) died in 1204, I don't think that there will be any injunctions from his lawyers raising issues of infringement of copyright. In fact, though, the title is a very appropriate one, given the genesis of this book. When Dr. Eddie Kingstone was editor of the *Canadian Journal of Psychiatry*, he asked me to serve as the statistical consultant for the journal. After reviewing just a few of the manuscripts, it became obvious to me that perplexity would be a welcome trait among many aspiring authors, because it presupposes that the people are aware of some doubt or puzzlement in their minds. Rather, I was struck by what seemed to me to be a blithe ignorance of some of the basic tools of statistics and measurement theory, such as the difference between the standard error and the standard deviation, how to combine results in a meta-analysis, or what distinguishes a useful scale from a useless one.

I offered to write a few "tutorial" type of articles, to address issues in papers that I was asked to review. After a while, though, these articles took on a life of their own and began appearing with almost monotonous regularity. A number of people, in particular Dr. Roger Bland, encouraged me to put them together in book form and this is the result. But a word of warning is necessary. This collection of articles did not start out to be a book, and it did not end up being an introductory book on statistics. You will not learn the basics in here, such as types of numbers (e.g., nominal, ordinal, interval, and ratio), and many of the most widely used tests, such as *t*-tests, analysis of variance, or correlations, aren't mentioned at all. (If you want a basic textbook, I can't think of any better ones to recommend than *PDQ Statistics* as a very basic introduction; or *Biostatistics: The Bare Essentials* for a more thorough treatment. Oh, by the way, did I mention that both of them were written by Dr. Geoff Norman and me?) Rather, it is a compilation of my take on where many people get things wrong. So, the reader should know the basics of statistics, but not much more.

A secondary purpose, and one that's been a major theme in my 43 years of teaching in medical schools, is to make physicians think more like psychologists. It's not that psychologists think in better ways than physicians in general; it's just that we think differently. When it comes to measuring things and using statistical tests, though, my parochial bias is that our ways *are* better. Physicians tend to chop continuous variables into categories, dividing beautifully continuous variables such as blood pressure or body mass index into "normal" versus "abnormal," or "below normal," "normal," and "above normal," and then rely on statistics based on counting the number of people in each group. Psychologists see this as a tremendous waste of information; we much prefer to keep continua as continua whenever possible, and to emphasize statistics that deal with amounts rather than counts. Also, all psychologists, irrespective of their area of specialization, get a firm background in statistical methods, research design, and psychometrics (the science – or art – of measuring things). The result is that psychological articles use some very useful and powerful techniques, such as path analysis, structural equation modelling, and item response theory, that are only now beginning to find their way into medical journals. So, another aim of my articles has been to introduce some of these techniques on an intuitive, understanding level, rather than to delve into the arcane mathematics. You will find no advanced math in this book, and relatively few equations; the emphasis is on *what* these techniques can do, rather than *how* they do them.

A final note on these chapters. The series began over 20 years ago, and some of the articles were woefully out of date; these have been brought up to date. Also, in the reference section of each chapter, I have cited more recent editions of texts, whenever I could find them. As an added bonus, I've added a section to each chapter called "To Read Further" which, as the name implies, tells you where to go to read up on the topic in greater depth.

So, sit back, relax, and become a bit less perplexed.

David L. Streiner
Hamilton, Ontario

Acknowledgments

I would like to thank the people who were instrumental in bringing this book to fruition. Dr. Eddie Kingstone was the editor of the *Canadian Journal of Psychiatry* when this series of articles began. They were somewhat of a departure from the usual style of the journal at that time; authors didn't use the first person singular, write in the active voice, or sprinkle their text with irreverent (and sometimes irrelevant) asides, off-the-wall examples, and somewhat groan-inducing puns. Eddie allowed me to do all of that, and more, and encouraged me to write more.

Dr. Roger Bland was a big fan of the series from the beginning, and encouraged me for a number of years to gather the articles together and put them out as a book. His enthusiasm and support were instrumental in motivating me to do just that.

Virginia St. Denis, the Director of Scientific Publications at the *Canadian Journal of Psychiatry*, deserves the largest share of my thanks. She kept the idea for the book alive when everyone else (including me) had given up hope of finding a publisher, and she worked diligently to get the old files into a form that I could use.

Finally, to my co-authors – Drs. Paula Goering, Betty Lin, Anne Rhodes, and John Cairney – many thanks for all the help in areas I knew nothing about.

PART ONE

Introductory Statistics

1 Do You See What I Mean?
Indices of Central Tendency

DAVID L. STREINER, PH.D.

Canadian Journal of Psychiatry, 2000, 45, 833–836

A recent headline in a leading Canadian paper stated, with unfeigned horror, that one-half of the hospitals in Toronto were below average. Needless to say, this brings to mind Garrison Keillor's fabled town of Lake Wobegon, where "all the women are strong, all the men are good-looking, and all the children are above average." It also illustrates how difficult it is to come to grips with the seemingly simple concept of "average." The purpose of this chapter is threefold: to try to explain the difference between the lay and the statistical concepts of average, to review the more common indices of average, and to introduce some lesser-known but very useful ways of calculating averages.

The Lay and Statistical Definitions

To the statistician, "average" has a very definite meaning: a number, determined through some arithmetic operations, that best describes the middle – or "central tendency" – of a group of numbers. So, if two statisticians are given the same set of numbers and told to compute the same measure of central tendency, they will come up with identical answers (assuming they make no computational errors along the way – a tenuous assumption, at best). This number will divide the original group of numbers roughly in half, although as we'll see, "half" can refer to the number of numbers, or to the "weight" of the numbers, or to some other criterion. In any case, we would be very surprised if all of the numbers fell above or below this index of central tendency; it then wouldn't be central. To the lay person, though, "average" has a very different meaning, implying an "ordinary standard" (Barber, 1998) or "good enough." In this light, neither the headline nor Keillor's description is so surprising; both actually reflect a psychological truth: people may believe that all (or none) of the hospitals meet their standards for adequate care, irrespective of the fact that some hospitals are better than others, and all of the children in Lake Wobegon are doing more, or better, than just "good enough" work.

The difficulty arises when we confuse these meanings of "average." Using the statistical definition, one-half of the physicians graduating each year are below average. Even if we were to extend medical school by another five years to cram more facts into their already overstuffed brains and raise the mean score on their qualifying exams by 50 points, one-half of the students would fall below this new mean. This is an inescapable fact of the strict definition of "average," and no amount of training (or cheating) will get around it. If, on the other hand, we mean "average" as "meeting acceptable standards," then it is quite conceivable that all of the graduates are above this criterion (it is equally possible, logically, that all are below it). The difference is best illustrated by the mathematical dictum that people have, on average, fewer than two legs. Since nobody has more than two legs, the amputation of even one leg reduces the average in the population to something less than two legs. The major problem occurs when a study defines "average" using statistical criteria but interprets it according to lay criteria, or vice versa.

The Usual Suspects: Mean, Median, and Mode

When we use the terms "mean" or "average" statistically, what occurs to most people (including statisticians) is to add all of the numbers and divide by the number of numbers, n; in statistical notation:

$$\text{Arithmetic Mean} = \frac{\sum X_i}{n}, \tag{1}$$

where Σ (the Greek capital letter sigma) means "to sum." Strictly speaking, this is called the *arithmetic mean* (AM), to differentiate it from some other means we'll discuss later, and is often referred to by the cognoscenti as "X-bar." Because many word processors have difficulty producing $\bar{X}$ (X with a bar over it), a new symbol to denote the mean has been introduced: M, which adequately accommodates the machines invented to serve us.

If the distribution of the numbers is symmetrical, then the number of numbers above and below the mean is equal. But, more generally, the mean is the average of the "weight" or magnitude of the numbers. That is, the mean of 4, 5, and 9 is 6. In this case, 4 is two units below 6, and 5 is one unit below, balancing the 9, which is three units above. As we'll see, this can be a disadvantage of the AM in some situations.

In some instances, numbers are used to indicate ranks of objects or people rather than absolute amounts; the statistical term for these data is ordinal, reflecting the fact that the numbers put the observations in rank order. We cannot assume, however, that the distances between successive ranks are equal. For example, breast cancer is usually staged as I, II, III, and IV, but the amount of disease progression from stage I to stage II is not necessarily the same as between stages II and III or between III and IV. Consequently, it doesn't make sense to talk of the "average" stage of cancer of 100 women. For these data, we use a different index of central tendency, called the *median*. The median is the number (or rank) such that 50% of the cases fall above it and 50% below.

In Statistics 101 we learn that we use the mean when the data have equal intervals between successive numbers (interval or ratio data – let's not worry about the distinction) and the median for ordinal data. Now that we've learned the rules, we can break them. If the data deviate from symmetry to a large degree (that is, they are skewed, with a much longer tail at one end of the distribution than at the other), then the mean may give a misleading representation of the "average." For example, if nine physicians each nets $100,000 yearly and a tenth earns $300,000, then the average is $120,000, which is 20% greater than the average for 90% of the sample. In this case, the median is a more accurate reflection of the central tendency than is the mean. The take-home message is that when the data are highly skewed, use the median.

Conversely, most of the scales used in psychiatry to measure affective states, such as the Beck Depression Inventory (BDI; Beck, Steer & Brown, 1996) or the State-Trait Anxiety Inventory (Spielberger, Gorsuch, Lushene, Vagg, & Jacobs, 1983), represent, in fact, ordinal data. That is, we cannot assume that the increase in the underlying depression reflected in a difference in BDI score from 5 to 10 is the same as the difference between 20 and 25. Most of the time, the measure of central tendency used with these scales is the mean, and unless the data are highly skewed, this choice is appropriate. So when, with ordinal data, can we switch from using the median (cancer staging) to the mean (the BDI)?

The answer is a definite "we don't know." A rule of thumb is that if the scale yields more than 10 possible numbers, it's fairly safe to use the mean. Indeed, the mean is often used with Likert scales (which rank responses: for example, strongly agree, agree, neutral, disagree, strongly disagree) that have 5 or 7 points, as long as the distribution of scores is relatively normal or flat. The reason people prefer the mean to the median is that much more can be done with it; many more statistical tests use the mean than use the median, so we can perform more sophisticated analyses.

Last (and definitely least), the *mode* is used with nominal (that is, named) data, such as sex, diagnosis, race, eye colour, political affiliation, and the like, where there is no rank ordering among the categories (sexists and racists to the contrary, notwithstanding). The mode is simply the most frequently used category and suffers from three major problems. First, it is very unstable; unless one category is clearly dominant, adding new subjects to the sample can shift the mode from one category to another quite unpredictably. Second, two or more categories often have nearly equal numbers of subjects, so that assigning primacy of place to just one of them is artificial. Finally, even fewer statistical tests involve the mode than the median; once we've specified the most frequently used category, there is little else we can do with it.

Variations on a Theme: Geometric and Harmonic Means

It is so ingrained to think of the AM when the term "average" is used that many people find it difficult to believe that there are, in fact, several different means and that, in some situations, these alternatives are preferable. One of these, *the geometric mean* (GM), is defined as

$$\text{Geometric Mean} = \sqrt[n]{\Gamma X_i}, \qquad [2]$$

where Γ (the Greek capital gamma) means the product of all the Xs (that is, $X_1 \times X_2 \times \ldots \times X_n$) and n before the radical indicates the nth root. For example, the geometric mean of 3, 4, and 5 is

$$\text{GM} = \sqrt[3]{3 \times 4 \times 5} = 3.91, \qquad [3]$$

which is smaller than the AM of 4.0.

The GM finds the most use when we look at data that increase exponentially over time. For example, Figure 1.1 shows the per capita expenditure for outpatient hospital services in the US in 1980, 1985, and 1990.

Fig. 1.1 Relationship between the arithmetic, geometric, and harmonic means

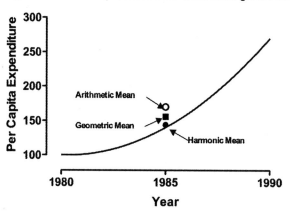

If we had data only for the years 1980 and 1990 and used the AM to esti-mate the 1985 expenditure, the result would be the value indicated by the open circle. When we use the GM, however, the result would be the filled square, which is much closer to the actual amount, represented by the line. The AM assumes that the change between 1980 and 1990 is best approximated by a straight line (the equal interval assumption of interval and ratio data), whereas in reality it follows an exponential growth curve. Because the GM is always smaller than the AM (except when all the values are the same, in which case the AM and the GM are identical), it gives a more accurate estimate with data of this sort, which we often encounter in looking at changes in populations over time (remember Malthus?). Be aware, though, that if any of the num-bers is 0, your computer will have an infarction because the root of 0 is indeterminate; and if any number is negative, the results won't make sense (if an odd number of values is negative, an even more massive infarction will occur).

The *harmonic mean* (M_H) is defined as

$$\text{Harmonic Mean} = \frac{n}{\sum \frac{1}{X_i}}.$$ [4]

Using the same numbers as before, the M_H of 3, 4, and 5 is

$$M_H = \frac{3}{\dfrac{1}{3} + \dfrac{1}{4} + \dfrac{1}{5}} = 3.83, \qquad\qquad [5]$$

which is smaller than both the AM of 4.00 and the GM of 3.91. This is always the case: unless all the numbers are identical (in which case the three means are identical), the AM yields the largest number, the M_H yields the smallest, and the GM is somewhere in between (Figure 1.1). It is used primarily in figuring out the mean sample size across groups, where each group has a different number of subjects.

Robust Estimators of the Mean

Let's take a closer look at some of the implicit assumptions of the various means and the median. With the mean, each number contributes equally to the final result. In other words, it is as if we multiplied each number by 1. As we saw, though, this can be a disadvantage when the data are skewed; very extreme values can pull the mean away from where the bulk of the data are. To get around this problem, we use the median, or the one central value that divides the number of data values into equal halves. In this case, it is tantamount to multiplying that single value of the median by 1 and all of the other numbers by 0. The disadvantage here is that we are disregarding almost all of the data. Even if we were to add 1000 to each of the values above the median or multiply the most extreme values by 1,000,000, the median itself would not shift: 50% of the values would still be above and 50% below it. This definitely seems to be an overreaction to the problem of the mean.

Over the years, several variants of the mean have emerged, called *robust estimators* because extreme values influence them much less than they influence the AM; that is, they are "robust" against the effects of long tails on one or both sides of the distribution. They fall intermediately between the mean and the median: not all numbers are given a weight of 1, as is the case with the mean. By the same token, however, they make use of all or most of the data, which the median does not.

The simplest robust estimator is the *trimmed mean*. "Trimmed" refers to the fact that the extreme 5% or 10% of the data are discarded. One form of this statistic is symmetric: both ends of the distribution are trimmed equally. If the distribution itself is roughly symmetrical, then the trimmed mean and the AM will yield equivalent estimates. However, the standard deviation (SD) of the trimmed mean will be smaller (sometimes quite a bit smaller) than that of the AM. Consequently, because the SD is part of the error term in most statistical tests, you may find significance with the trimmed mean when you don't with the more traditional mean. Another form of the trimmed mean deletes data from only one end of the distribution, which is useful if the data are highly skewed. We often find this to be true when there is a "barrier" at one end, where numbers cannot be smaller or larger than some value, but there is no barrier at the other end. For example, there is a natural lower limit on the number of days in hospital or in jail (that is, 0) but no upper limit. It is quite common to find that most people in a study cluster around a relatively low number of days, but a few people have been in hospital or behind bars for extended periods of time, highly skewing the data to the right (that is, towards longer times). It makes sense not to trim the lower end of the distribution, but only the upper end. In this case, the trimmed mean and the AM would differ , and again the SD of the former is lower than that of the latter.

With the trimmed mean, we give 90% or 95% of the data a weight of 1 and assign a weight of 0 to the trimmed values. There is no reason for the weights to be either 0 or 1; they can take any value between these extremes. This is the rationale behind a large class of robust estimators, of which the best known is the *bisquare weight mean*, also referred to as the *biweight mean* (Mosteller & Tukey, 1977). The name comes from the way it is calculated. First, we determine how much each value deviates from the AM, and then we square the result. If the squared deviation is less than some criterion (that is, it is near the mean), then the results are squared again (hence "bisquare"), and this becomes the weight for that value; the nearer to the mean, the closer the weight is to 1.

If the deviation exceeds the criterion, then the weight is 0. The mean is then recalculated using the original values multiplied by their weights. The procedure is repeated using this new estimate of the mean until further iterations have a minimal effect on the mean. In essence, this (and other robust estimators) gives higher weight to numbers that are near the mean and lower (or no) weight to numbers that deviate considerably from it.

There are two limitations of the biweight mean. First, the need to iterate makes it quite labour intensive; it must therefore be done on a computer or programmable calculator. Second, the user must supply the values for two constants used in the formula and also determine when the change in the mean from one iteration to the next is small enough to stop. Mosteller and Tukey (1977) provide guidelines for these decisions, but others have criticized the subjectivity involved (e.g., Glickman & Noether, 1997). In most situations, though, different values for the constants do not affect the final results very much.

Summary

Measures of central tendency should not be used blindly, nor should we necessarily trust the one printed out by a computer program. The choice depends on the type of data (nominal, ordinal, or interval and ratio); the distribution of the data (symmetrical or skewed); the presence or absence of outliers; and whether the trend is linear, exponential, or some other shape. Nothing takes the place of looking at the data, knowing what they represent, and using good judgment.

REFERENCES

Barber, K. (Ed.). (1998). *The Canadian Oxford dictionary*. (2nd ed.). Toronto: Oxford University Press.

Beck, A.T., Steer, R.A., & Brown, G.K. (1996). *Manual for the Beck Depression Inventory – II*. San Antonio, TX: Psychological Corporation.

Glickman, M.E., & Noether, M. (1997, Aug). An examination of cross-specialty linkage applied to the resource-based relative value scale. *Medical Care*, 35(8), 843–866. http://dx.doi.org/10.1097/00005650-199708000-00009 Medline:9268256

Mosteller, F., & Tukey, J. (1977). *Data analysis and regression: A second course in statistics*. Reading, MA: Addison-Wesley.

Spielberger, C.D., Gorsuch, R.L., Lushene, R.E., Vagg, P.R., & Jacobs, G.A. (1983). *Manual for the State-Trait Anxiety Inventory*. Palo Alto, CA: Consulting Psychologists Press.

TO READ FURTHER

Norman, G.R., & Streiner, D.L. (2008). *Biostatistics: The bare essentials*. (3rd ed.). Shelton, CT: PMPH USA. Chapter 3

2 Maintaining Standards: Differences between the Standard Deviation and Standard Error and When to Use Each

DAVID L. STREINER, PH.D.

Canadian Journal of Psychiatry, 1996, *41*, 498–502

Imagine that you've just discovered a new brain protein that causes otherwise rational people to continually mutter words like "re-engineer," "operational visioning," and "mission statements." You suspect that this new chemical, which you call LDE for Language Destroying Enzyme, would be found in higher concentrations in the cerebrospinal fluid (CSF) of administrators than in that of other people. Difficult as it is to find volunteers, you eventually get samples from 25 administrators and an equal number of controls and find the results shown in Table 2.1. Because you feel that these data would be more compelling if you showed them visually, you prepare your paper using a bar graph. Just before you mail it off, though, you vaguely remember something about error bars, but can't quite recall what they are; you check with a few of your colleagues. The first one tells you to draw a line above and below the top of each bar so that each part is equal to the standard deviation. The second person disagrees, saying that the lines should reflect the standard errors, while the third person has yet another opinion: the lines should be plus and minus two standard errors, that is, two standard errors above and two below the mean. As you can see in Figure 2.1, these methods result in very different pictures of what's going on. So, now you have two problems: first, what is the difference between the standard error and the standard deviation; second, which should you draw?

Table 2.1 Levels of LDE in the CSF of administrators
and controls

Group	Number	Mean	SD
Administrators	25	25.83	5.72
Controls	25	17.25	4.36

Fig. 2.1 Data from Table 2.1, plotted with different types of error bars

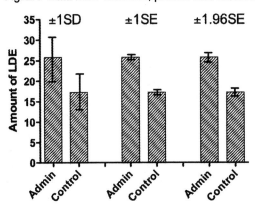

The Standard Deviation

The standard deviation, which is abbreviated variously as S.D., SD, or s (just to confuse people), is an index of how closely the individual data points cluster around the mean. If we call each point X_i, so that X_1 indicates the first value, X_2 the second value, and so on, and call the mean M, then it may seem that an index of the dispersion of the points would be simply $\Sigma(X_i - M)$, which means to sum (that's what Σ indicates) how much each value of X deviates from M; in other words, an index of dispersion would be the *Sum of (Individual Data Points – Mean of the Data Points)*. Logical as this approach may seem, it has two drawbacks. The first difficulty is that the answer will be zero – not just in this situation, but in every case. By definition, the sum of the values above the mean is always equal to the sum of the values below it, and thus they'll cancel each other out. We can get around this problem by taking the absolute value of each difference (that is, we can ignore the sign whenever it's negative), but for a number of arcane reasons, statisticians don't like to use absolute numbers. Another way to eliminate negative values is to square them, since the square of any number – negative or positive – is always positive. So, what we now have is $\Sigma(X_i - M)^2$.

The second problem is that the result of this equation will increase as we add more subjects. Let's imagine that we have a sample of 25 values, with an SD of 10. If we now add another 25 subjects who look exactly the same, it makes intuitive sense that the dispersion of these 50 points should stay the same. Yet the formula as it now reads can result only in a larger sum as we add more data points. We can compensate by dividing by the number of subjects, N, so that the equation now reads $\Sigma(X_i - M)^2/N$. In the true spirit of Murphy's Law, what we've done in solving these two difficulties is to create two new ones. The first (or should we say third, so we can keep track of our problems) is that now we are expressing the deviation in squared units; for instance, if we were measuring IQs in children with autism, we might find that their mean IQ is 75 and their dispersion is 100 squared IQ points. But what in heaven's name is a squared IQ point? At least this problem is easy to cure: we simply take the square root of the answer, and we'll end up with a number that is in the original units of measurement. So in this example the dispersion would be 10 IQ points, which is much easier to understand.

The last problem (yes, it really is the last one) is that the results of the formula as it exists so far produce a biased estimate, that is, one that is consistently either higher or (as in this case) lower than the "true" value. The explanation is a bit more complicated and requires somewhat of a detour. Most of the time when we do research, we are not interested so much in the samples we study as in the populations they come from. That is, if we look at the level of expressed emotion (EE) in the families of young schizophrenic males, our interest is in the families of all people who meet the criteria (the population), not just those in our study. What we do is estimate the population mean and SD from our sample. Because all we are studying is a sample, however, these estimates will deviate by some unknown amount from the population values. In calculating the SD, we would ideally see how much each person's score deviates from the population mean, but all we have available to us is the sample mean. By definition, scores deviate less from their own mean than from any other number. So, when we do the calculation and subtract each score from the sample mean, the result will be smaller than if we subtracted each score from the population mean (which we don't know); hence, the result is biased downwards. To correct for this bias, we divide by $N - 1$ instead of N. Putting all of this together, we finally arrive at the formula for the standard deviation:

$$SD = \sqrt{\frac{\Sigma(X_i - M)^2}{N-1}}. \qquad [1]$$

(By the way, don't use this equation if, for whatever bizarre reason, you want to calculate the SD by hand, because it leads to too much rounding error. There is another formula, mathematically equivalent and found in any statistics book, which yields a more precise value.) Now that we've gone through all this work, what does it mean? If we assume that the data are normally distributed, then knowing the mean and the SD tells us everything we need to know about the distribution of scores. In any normal distribution, roughly two-thirds (actually, 68.2%) of the scores fall between −1 and +1 SD, and 95.4% fall between −2 and +2 SD. For example, most of the tests used for admission to graduate or professional schools (the GRE, MCAT, LSAT, and other instruments of torture) were originally designed to have a mean of 500 and an SD of 100. That means that 68% of people score between 400 and 600 and just over 95% score between 300 and 700. Using a table of the normal curve (found in most statistics books), we can figure out exactly what proportion of people get scores above or below any given value. Conversely, if we want to fail the lowest 5% of test-takers (as was done with the LMCCs), then knowing the mean and SD of this year's class and armed with the table, we can work out what the cut-off point should be. So, to summarize, the SD tells us the distribution of individual scores around the mean. Now, let's turn our attention to the standard error.

The Standard Error

I mentioned previously that the purpose of most studies is to estimate some population parameter, such as the mean, the SD, a correlation, or a proportion. Once we have that estimate, another question then arises: How accurate is our estimate? This may seem an unanswerable question; if we don't know what the population value is, how can we evaluate how close we are to it? Mere logic, however, has never stopped statisticians in the past, and it won't stop us now. What we can do is resort to probabilities: what is the probability (Pr) that the true (population) mean falls within a certain range of values? (To cite one of our mottos, "Statistics means you never have to say you're certain.")

One way to answer the question is to repeat the study a few hundred times, which will give us many estimates of the mean. We can then take the mean of these means, as well as figure out what the distribution of means is; that is, we can get the standard deviation of the mean values. Then, using the same table of the normal curve that we used previously, we can estimate what range of values would encompass 95% or 99% of the means. If each sample had been drawn from the population at random, we would be fairly safe in concluding that the true mean also falls within this range 90% or 95% of the time. We assign a new name to the standard deviation of the means: we call it the *standard error of the mean* (abbreviated as SEM or, if there is no ambiguity that we're talking about the mean, SE).

But first, let's deal with one slight problem: replicating the study a few hundred times. Nowadays, it's hard enough to get money to do a study once, much less replicate it this many times (even assuming you would actually want to spend the rest of your life doing the same study over and over). Ever helpful, statisticians have figured out a way to determine the SE based on the results of a single study. Let's approach this first from an intuitive standpoint: what would make us more or less confident that our estimate of the population mean, based on our study, is accurate? One obvious factor would be the size of the study: the larger the sample size, N, the less chance there is that one or two aberrant values are distorting the results and the more likely it is that our estimate is close to the true value. So, some index of N should be in the denominator of SE, since the larger N is, the smaller SE would become. Second, and for similar reasons, the smaller the variability in the data, the more confident we are that one value (the mean) accurately reflects them. Thus, the SD should be in the numerator: the larger it is, the larger SE will be, and we end up with the equation:

$$SE = \frac{SD}{\sqrt{N}}. \qquad [2]$$

(Why does the denominator read $\sqrt{N}$ instead of just N? Because we are really dividing the variance, which is SD^2, by N, but we end up again with squared units, so we take the square root of everything. Aren't you sorry you asked?)

So, the SD reflects the variability of individual data points, and the SE is the variability of means.

Confidence Intervals

In the previous section on the SE we spoke of a range of values in which we were 95% or 99% confident that the true value of the mean fell. Not surprisingly, this range is called the *confidence interval*, or CI. Let's see how it's calculated. If we turn again to our table of the normal curve, we'll find that 95% of the area falls between −1.96 and +1.96 SDs. When we go back to our example of GREs and MCATs, which had a mean of 500 and an SD of 100, 95% of scores fall between 304 and 696. How did we get those figures? First, we multiplied the SD by 1.96, subtracted it from the mean to find the lower bound, and added it to the mean for the upper bound. The CI is calculated in the same way, except that we use the SE instead of the SD. So, the 95% CI is

$$95\% \ CI = M \pm (1.96 \times SE). \qquad [3]$$

For the 90% CI, we would use the value 1.65 instead of 1.96, and for the 99% CI, 2.58. Using the data from Table 2.1, we see that the SE for administrators is $5.72 / \sqrt{25}$, or 1.14, and thus the 95% CI would be 25.83 ± (1.96 × 1.14), or 23.59 to 28.07. We would interpret this to mean that we are 95% confident that the value of LDE in the population of administrators is somewhere within this interval. If we wanted to be more confident, we would multiply 1.14 by 2.58; the penalty we pay for our increased confidence is a wider CI, so that we are less sure of the exact value.

The Choice of Units

Now we have the SD, the SE, and any one of a number of CIs, and the question becomes: which do we use, and when? Obviously, when we are describing the results of any study we've done, it is imperative that we report the SD. Just as obviously, armed with this and the sample size, it is a simple matter for the reader to figure out the SE and any CI. Do we gain anything by adding them? The answer, as usual, is yes and no.

Essentially, we want to convey to the reader that there will always be sample-to-sample variation and that the answers we get from one study wouldn't be exactly the same if the study were replicated. What we would like to show is how much of a difference in findings we can expect: just a few points either way, but not enough to substantially alter our conclusions, or so much that the next study is as likely to show results going in the opposite direction as to replicate the findings. To some degree, this is what significance testing does – the lower the p level, the less likely the results are due simply to chance and the greater the probability that they will be repeated the next time around. Significance tests, however, are usually interpreted in an all-or-nothing manner: either the result was statistically significant or it wasn't, and a difference between group means that just barely squeaked under the $p < 0.05$ wire is often given as much credence as a result that is highly unlikely to be due to chance.

If we used CIs, either in a table or in a graph, it would be much easier for the reader to determine how much variation in results to expect from sample to sample. But which CI should we use? We could draw the error bars on a graph or report them in a table to show a CI that is equal to exactly one SE. These methods have the advantages that we don't have to choose between the SE or the CI (they're identical) and that not much calculation is involved. Unfortunately, this choice of an interval conveys very little useful information. An error bar of plus and minus one SE is the same as the 68% CI; we would be 68% sure that the true mean (or difference between two means) fell within this range. The problem is that we're more used to being 95% or 99% sure, not 68%. So, to begin with, let's forget about showing the SE; it tells us little that is useful, and its sole purpose is in calculating CIs.

What about the advice to use plus and minus two SEs in the graph? This makes more sense: two is a good approximation of 1.96, at least to the degree that graphics programs can display the value and our eyes discern it. The advantages are twofold. First, this method shows the 95% CI, which is more meaningful than 68%. Second, it allows us to do an "eyeball" test of significance, at least in the two-group situation. If the top of the lower bar (the controls in Figure 2.1) and the bottom of the higher bar (the administrators) don't overlap by more than about half their length, then the difference between the groups is significant at the 5% level or better (Cumming & Finch, 2005). (If they don't overlap at all, the difference is significant at the 1% level.) Thus, we would say that, in this example, the two groups were significantly different from one another. If we actually did a t-test, we would find this to be true: $t(48) = 2.668, p < 0.05$. A t-test doesn't work too accurately if there are more than two groups, since we have the issue of multiple tests to deal with (for example, Group 1 versus Group 2, Group 2 versus 3, and Group 1 versus 3), but it gives a rough indication of where the differences lie. Never do this eyeball test when the data reflect repeated measurements (for example, pretest and posttest); it will give the wrong answer. Needless to say, when presenting the CI in a table, you should give the exact values (multiply by 1.96, not 2).

Wrapping Up

The SD indicates the dispersion of individual data values around their mean and should be given any time we report data. The SE is an index of the variability of the means that would be expected if the study were exactly replicated a large number of times. By itself, this measure doesn't convey much useful information. Its main function is to help construct 95% and 99% CIs, which can supplement statistical significance testing and indicate the range within which the true mean or difference between means may be found. Some journals have dropped significance testing entirely and replaced it with the reporting of CIs; this is probably going too far, since both have advantages and both can be misused to equal degrees. For example, a study using a small sample size may report that the difference between the control and experimental group is significant at the 0.05 level. Had the study indicated the CIs, however, it would be more apparent to the reader that the CI is very wide and the estimate of the difference is crude, at best. By contrast, the much-touted figure of the number of people affected by second-hand smoke is actually not the estimate of the mean. The best estimate of the mean is zero, and it has a very broad CI; what is reported is the upper end of that CI.

To sum up, SDs, significance testing, and 95% or 99% CIs should be reported to help the reader; all are informative and complement, rather than replace, each other. Conversely, "naked" SEs alone don't tell us much and more or less just take up space in a report. Conducting our studies with these guidelines in mind may help us to maintain the standards in research.

REFERENCE

Cumming, G., & Finch, S. (2005, Feb-Mar). Inference by eye: Confidence intervals and how to read pictures of data. *American Psychologist, 60*(2), 170–180. http://dx.doi.org/10.1037/0003-066X.60.2.170 Medline:15740449

TO READ FURTHER

Altman, D.G., Machin, D., Bryant, T.N., & Gardner, M.J. (2000). *Statistics with confidence: Confidence intervals and statistical guidelines.* (2nd ed.). London: British Medical Journal.

Cumming, G., & Finch, S. (2005, Feb-Mar). Inference by eye: Confidence intervals and how to read pictures of data. *American Psychologist, 60*(2), 170–180. http://dx.doi.org/10.1037/0003-066X.60.2.170 Medline:15740449

Norman, G.R., & Streiner, D.L. (2008). *Biostatistics: The bare essentials.* (3rd ed.). Shelton, CT: PMPH USA. Chapter.

3 Breaking Up Is Hard to Do: The Heartbreak of Dichotomizing Continuous Data

DAVID L. STREINER, PH.D.

Canadian Journal of Psychiatry, 2002, 47, 262–266

Those of you who are old enough may remember Neil Sedaka singing "Breaking Up Is Hard to Do." If only that were true when it comes to the variables we use in research! Many times (I would say far too many), a researcher uses a continuous measure, such as a depression inventory, as an outcome variable and then dichotomizes it – above or below some cut-point, for example, or the number of people who did and did not show a 50% reduction in their scores from baseline to follow-up (e.g., Keller et al., 2000). Less often, but again far too frequently, researchers may assign patients to different groups by dichotomizing or trichotomizing scores from a continuous scale.

Over the years, several arguments have tried to justify this practice. Perhaps the most common one runs something like this: "Clinicians have to make dichotomous decisions to treat or not to treat, so it makes sense to have a binary outcome." Another rationale that is offered is "Physicians find it easier to understand the results when they're expressed as proportions or odds ratios. They have difficulty grasping the meaning of beta weights and other indices that emerge when we use continuous variables." In this chapter, I'll try to show that you pay a very stiff penalty in terms of power or sample size when continuous variables are broken up, with the consequent risk of a Type II error (that is, failing to detect real differences). But before we begin, let me assume the role of a marriage counsellor and see whether the arguments in favour of splitting up are really viable.

The rationale for dichotomizing outcomes because clinical decisions are binary fails on three grounds. The primary reason is that it confuses measurement with decision making. The purpose of most research is to discover relations – relations between or among variables or between treatment interventions and outcomes. The more accurate the findings, the better the decisions that we can make; that is, the findings come first and the decision making follows. As we will see, findings come more readily and more accurately when we retain the scaling of continuous variables. The second reason is that all the research using the old dichotomy becomes useless if the cut-point changes. For example, the definition of hypertension used to be 160/95 (World Health Organization, 1978). If we defined the outcome of intervention trials dichotomously – above 160/95 being hypertensive and below 160/95 being normotensive – then those findings would become useless after the definition changed to 140/90 (Zanchetti, 1995). If we expressed the outcome as a continuum, however, the values of beta coefficients and similar indices showing the effects of various risk and protective factors would not change at all; if we wanted to use statistics such as odds ratios (ORs) or the percentage of patients who improved, it would be a trivial matter to recalculate the results. We have a similar situation in psychiatry. The diagnosis of antisocial personality disorder (ASP), for example, is a binary one: the person either does or does not satisfy the diagnostic criteria (that is, a certain number of symptoms are present). However, Livesley and others maintain that ASP and many other disorders should actually be seen as a continuum: the more symptoms that are checked off, the more of the trait the person has (Livesley, Schroeder, Jackson, & Jang, 1994). If the number of symptoms necessary to meet the criteria were to change, as occurred when DSM-IV replaced DSM-III-R, then much previous research using a dichotomous diagnosis would have to be discarded. If the diagnosis were expressed as the number of symptoms present, though, it would be relatively easy to reinterpret the findings using the new criteria. Finally, whether to hospitalize a patient with suicidal ideation or to discharge a patient with symptoms of schizophrenia may be binary decisions, but many treatments – perhaps most – fall along a continuum involving the dosage or strength of a medication and the number and frequency of therapy sessions.

As for the argument that physicians are more comfortable with statistics based on categorical measures, we are likely dealing with both a base canard that they, like old dogs, cannot learn new tricks and a vicious circle. As long as the belief persists, studies will be designed, analysed, and reported using proportions and ORs, meaning that physicians will not have the opportunity to become more comfortable with other approaches.

Table 3.1 Data on an outcome measure for two groups

Group 1	Group 2
9	16
14	12
13	25
12	14
5	16
5	9
12	10
22	23
13	22
12	21

Table 3.2 The number of people in each group above and below a cut-point of 15/16

	Group 1	Group 2
15 and below	9	4
16 and above	1	6

First, I'll give some examples of how dichotomizing can lead us astray, and then I'll use these examples to discuss why this is the case.

Example 1

Let's look at the data in Table 3.1, which shows scores on a scale for two groups, each with 10 subjects. Let's assume that, if we were to dichotomize the scale, we would use a criterion for "caseness" of 15/16: people with scores from 1 to 15 would be considered normal, and those with scores of 16 and over would be defined as cases. The mean for Group 1 is 11.70, and the mean for Group 2 is 16.80. There is slightly more than a 5-point difference between the groups, and the average of the first group is well below the cut-off of 15/16, while the average of the second group is above the cut-point. If we used a t-test to compare the groups, we'd find that $t(18) = 2.16$, $p = 0.045$. That is, there is a statistically significant difference between the means. Now, let's dichotomize the results and count the number of people above and below the cut-point in each group. What we'd find is shown in Table 3.2. Because two of the cells have frequencies below 5, we'd use a Fisher's exact test, rather than a

Table 3.3 Correlations among four variables[a]

	A	B	C	D
A		0.59[b]	0.56[b]	0.70[b]
B	0.30		0.28	0.84[b]
C	0.16	0.25		0.39
D	0.45[b]	0.55[b]	0.20	

[a] Correlations above the diagonal are for the variables
treated as continua; below the diagonal as dichotomized.
[b] $p < 0.05$

chi-square test, and we'd find that the p level is 0.057. In other words, the difference is not statistically significant.

Example 2

In the second example, we have 40 subjects, measured on four variables, A through D. If we were to correlate these variables, we'd find the results shown in the upper triangle of Table 3.3. Of the six correlations, five are significant at the $p < 0.01$ level. Now, we'll do a median split on each of these variables, so that roughly one-half of the subjects fall above and one-half below the cut-point. If we reran the correlations, we would find the results in the lower triangle of the same table. In every case, the correlations are lower – sometimes substantively so – and only two of the six correlations are significant at the $p < 0.01$ level.

Taking this example a bit further, we can run a regression equation, with A as the dependent variable (DV) and B through D as the predictors. Keeping the variables as continua, we'd find the multiple R is 0.767 and $R^2 = 0.588$, which would lead to thoughts of publication and promotion for most people. If we dichotomized the variables, however, we'd find that the multiple R is 0.460, with an associated R^2 of 0.211, which might jeopardize that promotion by at least a year. (Purists might say that we should really use a logistic regression with a dichotomous DV. If we did, we'd find the Cox and Snell pseudo-R^2 to be an even more disappointing 0.20.)

Why This Occurs

These examples illustrate two points. First, the magnitude of the effects (for example, the differences between groups, the correlations between variables, and the amount of variance explained by the regression) were lower – sometimes dramatically lower – when we took continuous variables and treated them as dichotomies. Second, findings that were significant using continuous variables were sometime not significant when we dichotomized those variables. Let's examine each of these issues separately.

Dichotomizing variables results in a tremendous loss of information. If the values in Example 1 were scores on a Beck Depression Inventory (BDI), the possible range would be between 0 and 69. When we dichotomize this scale, we are saying, in essence, that there is no difference between a score of 0 and one of 15 (both would be coded as 1) or between scores of 16 and 69 (both coded as 2). At the same time, we are making a qualitative difference between scores of 15 and 16. This doesn't seem conceptually logical and ignores the problem of measurement error. As we discuss in other places [Streiner, 1993 (see Chapter 22); Streiner & Norman, 2008], every observed score (for example, a numerical value on a questionnaire, a blood level, or the number of diagnostic criteria that are satisfied) is made up of two parts: a "true" score, which is never seen, plus some error. The more reliable the scale, the smaller the error and the closer the observed score is to the true score. But, since no measurement has a reliability of 1.00 (including lab as well as paper-and-pencil tests), every score has some degree of error associated with it. We also assume that the errors are random and have a mean of 0; that is, over a large number of people or over many observations of the same person (or both), the errors will tend to cancel each other out. This means that, if we treat the scores as numbers along a continuum, we may misplace a person to some degree, which will be reflected in, for example, a lower correlation between the scale score and some other variable. However, because the errors are random with a mean of 0, there will not be any bias in the relation.

But the situation is different when we dichotomize the scale. Now, for people near the cut-point, the measurement error may result not just in a score that's slightly off but in their being misclassified into the wrong group. A person suffering from depression, with a true score of 16 and a relatively small error of −1 point, would end up in the group without depression. Thus, we can see that using a scale as a continuum will present us with some degree of random error (which is inevitable), but dichotomization can easily result in misclassification error.

Another reason dichotomizing variables puts us behind the eight ball is a function of the statistical tests themselves. All statistical procedures can be seen as a ratio between a signal and noise (Norman & Streiner, 2008). The "signal" is the information that we've captured in the measurement – the difference between group means, the relation between two variables, and so forth. The "noise" is the error, usually captured by the differences among the subjects within the same group (when we're comparing means), deviations from a linear relation (in correlational tests), or misclassifications (in procedures such as chi-square, ORs, and relative risks). As we mentioned, dichotomization results in a loss of information, so that the "signal" is weaker than when we use continua. Not surprisingly, tests based on dichotomous variables are generally less powerful than those based on continuous variables. Suissa (1991) determined that a dichotomized outcome is at best only 67% as efficient as a continuous one; that is, if you need 50 subjects in each group to demonstrate statistical significance with a continuous scale, you would need 75 subjects per group to show the same effect after dichotomizing. In fact, though, most clinical scales are split at a clinically important point that doesn't usually correspond to the best place from a statistical point of view, with the result that the efficiency rarely approaches even 67% and may drop to as low at 10% (that is, the required sample size is 10 times as large). Similarly, if the dichotomy is statistically ideal, resulting in one-half of the people being in one group and one-half in the other, the correlation of that variable with another one is reduced by about 20%. The more the split deviates from 50:50, the more the correlation is reduced. By the time the division is 90:10, the correlation is reduced by 41% (Hunter & Schmidt, 1990).

It's Not All Bad

Up to now, we've treated categorization of a continuum as an unmitigated disaster with no redeeming features. At the risk of appearing to be a Pollyanna, who can find positive things to say about the worst situations, I can see a few situations wherein we actually could divide a continuous variable into a trichotomy or an ordinal variable. These situations, though, are based on statistical considerations; they are not based on clinical considerations or on what is convenient.

Most parametric statistical tests assume that the variables are normally distributed. While we can often get away with variables that deviate from normality to some degree – and, as Micceri (1989) has shown, almost all do – there are limits. One of these is found when a variable resembles a J-shaped distribution; that is, most of the subjects clump at one end, and the rest trail off in the opposite direction. This occurs most frequently if there is a "wall," or limit, at one end but not at the other. For example, a population survey may find that most people have had no psychiatric admissions, and a small proportion have had a single admission. Then the numbers trickle off, with a few people having a large number of admissions. There's a lower limit, in that you can't have fewer than 0 admissions, but no upper limit. We can try to transform the variable, but if it's very highly skewed, even this change won't help. The only solution is to trichotomize it (for example, none, 1 or 2, 3 or more), and treat it as an ordinal variable.

Similarly, we may feel that the relation between two variables is not linear. For example, we may suspect that, within the range of low income (say up to $10,000 a year), the actual dollar amount is unimportant, insofar as it buffers against stress, while above a certain amount ($60,000, for example), more money doesn't provide more protection. Within the middle range, however, we may suspect that there is a linear relation. In other words, the relation between income and buffering looks like an elongated S. We can try to model this with a complicated, higher-order equation, but it's often easier to divide income into three categories and, again, treat it as if it were an ordinal variable.

However, even in these two cases, there must be a minimum of three categories for there to be any improvement by categorizing a continuous variable. Since we can always draw a straight line between two points, dichotomizing a variable never yields better results than keeping the variable continuous, no matter how non-linear it is (DeCoster, Iselin, & Gallucci, 2009).

Conclusions

Except when the variable deviates considerably from normal, splitting a variable into categories results in lost information, the requirement to use less powerful non-parametric tests, and increased probability of a Type II error. We are most often much further ahead to retain the continuous nature of the variable and analyse the data using the appropriate statistics.

This discussion has focused primarily on taking data that were gathered as continua and then splitting them into categories. The other implication of this is that we should gather the data as continua whenever possible. For example, an item on a questionnaire might look like the following:

How old were you on your last birthday?

❑ 15–19
❑ 20–29
❑ 30–39
❑ 40–49
❑ 50–59
❑ 60–65
❑ Over 65

It would be better, however, to ask the question

"How old were you on your last birthday?": _____ years.

If you use the first format, you lose fine-grained information, and you're forced to use those categories in all subsequent analyses. By using the second format, you can later split age any way you want (although I don't know why you would want to, after all that's been said), and you'll have all the advantages of a continuous variable. The only possible exception may be income: people may feel more comfortable reporting it within a range, rather than reporting the exact amount, but the jury is still out on this.

So, in conclusion, the one word of advice about turning continuous variables into dichotomies is – don't!

REFERENCES

DeCoster, J., Iselin, A.-M.R., & Gallucci, M. (2009, Dec). A conceptual and empirical examination of justifications for dichotomization. *Psychological Methods*, 14(4), 349–366. http://dx.doi.org/10.1037/a0016956 Medline: 19968397

Hunter, J.E., & Schmidt, F.L. (1990). Dichotomization of continuous variables: The implications for meta-analysis. *Journal of Applied Psychology*, 75(3), 334–349. http://dx.doi.org/10.1037/0021-9010.75.3.334

Keller, M.B., McCullough, J.P., Klein, D.N., Arnow, B., Dunner, D.L., Gelenberg, A.J., ..., & Zajecka, J. (2000, May 18). A comparison of nefazodone, the cognitive behavioral-analysis system of psychotherapy, and their combination for the treatment of chronic depression. *New England Journal of Medicine*, 342(20), 1462–1470. http://dx.doi.org/10.1056/NEJM200005183422001 Medline:10816183

Livesley, W.J., Schroeder, M.L., Jackson, D.N., & Jang, K.L. (1994, Feb). Categorical distinctions in the study of personality disorder: Implications for classification. *Journal of Abnormal Psychology, 103*(1), 6–17. http://dx.doi.org/10.1037/0021-843X.103.1.6 Medline:8040482

Micceri, T. (1989). The unicorn, the normal curve, and other improbable creatures. *Psychological Bulletin, 105*(1), 156–166. http://dx.doi.org/10.1037/0033-2909.105.1.156

Norman, G.R., & Streiner, D.L. (2008). *Biostatistics: The bare essentials.* (3rd ed.). Shelton, CT: PMPH USA.

Streiner, D.L. (1993, Mar). A checklist for evaluating the usefulness of rating scales. *Canadian Journal of Psychiatry, 38*(2), 140–148. Medline:8467441

Streiner, D.L., & Norman, G.R. (2008). *Health measurement scales: A practical guide to their development and use.* (4th ed.). Oxford: Oxford University Press.

Suissa, S. (1991). Binary methods for continuous outcomes: A parametric alternative. *Journal of Clinical Epidemiology, 44*(3), 241–248. http://dx.doi.org/10.1016/0895-4356(91)90035-8 Medline:1999683

World Health Organization. (1978). *Arterial hypertension. Report of WHO expert committee.* Technical Report Series, No. 628. Geneva: WHO.

Zanchetti, A., & World Health Organization. International Society of Hypertension. (1995, Aug). Guidelines for the management of hypertension: The World Health Organization/International Society of Hypertension view. *Journal of Hypertension, 13*(2 Suppl), S119–S122. http://dx.doi.org/10.1097/00004872-199508001-00020 Medline:8576782

TO READ FURTHER

DeCoster, J., Iselin, A.-M.R., & Gallucci, M. (2009, Dec). A conceptual and empirical examination of justifications for dichotomization. *Psychological Methods, 14*(4), 349–366. http://dx.doi.org/10.1037/a0016956 Medline: 19968397

4 Pick a Number: Sample Size and Power in Psychiatric Research

DAVID L. STREINER, PH.D.

Canadian Journal of Psychiatry, 1990, 35, 616–620

We usually do a study to determine whether or not some intervention is effective, or whether there is a relationship among a set of variables. Each investigation is an attempt to determine the true state of affairs (for example, whether or not treatment A is better than treatment B, or whether or not there is a genetic component to a certain disorder). However, it's often infeasible or impossible to test every person in the population of interest, so the study consists of a sample of individuals that ideally is representative of the population. Since each sample is somewhat different from every other one, we can never be absolutely sure whether the results of a specific study are an accurate reflection of reality or are due to sampling error (that is, that the result was due simply to chance differences between the groups). We can only hope that if the different aspects of the sampling, design, and analysis are sufficiently rigorous, the correct conclusion will be drawn most of the time.

Most clinicians are familiar with the notion that we can at times wrongly conclude that the results of a specific study are statistically significant when, in fact, they are really due to chance or random sampling error – a Type I or an α-type error. If we adopt an α level of 0.05, which is traditional in most fields, we will make this false positive error about 5% of the time.

However, there is another type of error that can be made, which is less familiar to clinical researchers. This is called the Type II or β-type error. It is the converse of a Type I error and is made if we conclude from our study that in reality there is no difference between groups or any association between variables when, in fact, there is a difference or

Table 4.1 The four types of conclusions which can be drawn by a study

		True state of affairs	
		Difference	No difference
Results of the study	Difference	Correct conclusion (A)	Type I (α) error (B)
	No difference	Type II (β) error (C)	Correct conclusion (D)

a correlation. These different outcomes are illustrated in Table 4.1. If the true state of affairs (which we can never know) is that there is a difference, and our results show a statistically significant difference, then we have drawn the correct conclusion from our data (cell A in Table 4.1). Similarly, if our results correctly indicate that there is no difference (cell D), we have again made an accurate conclusion. Cells B and C show the Types I and II errors, respectively.

It is just as important to minimize the probability of a Type II error as that of a Type I error, although it is only relatively recently that studies have been designed with this in mind. A study should maximize the *power* of the statistical test, where power is the probability of correctly concluding that there is a difference. That is, power is defined as the complement of β, or $1 - \beta$, and is the probability of correctly rejecting the null hypothesis (cell A). The determination of the power of a statistical test (a "power analysis") can be used in two ways: prospectively, when a study is designed; and retrospectively, in an attempt to determine whether or not negative findings were a true or a false failure to reject the null hypothesis.

The power of a statistical test is a function of three factors: (1) the magnitude of the effect; (2) the α level; and (3) the sample size (N). When power analysis is used prospectively, we select the desired power beforehand and then calculate the sample size needed in order to achieve that power. When used retrospectively, we base our calculations on the actual sample size and calculate the power the study had.

Magnitude of Effect

The magnitude of the effect is the difference between, for example, the mean score of the treated group and that of the control group. However, simply saying that the two groups differed by four points doesn't tell us too much, since the various outcomes used in research differ in terms of their range of possible scores, means, and standard deviations. For example, in examining the effectiveness of a new anxiolytic agent, two studies could use different outcome measures; one, the Hamilton Anxiety Scale (HAS; Hamilton, 1959), and the other, the State-Trait Anxiety Inventory (STAI; Spielberger, Gorsuch, & Lushene, 1970). The scores on the HAS range from 0 to 52 based on 13 items, while the scores on the STAI range from 20 to 80 and are derived from 20 questions. It would be highly unlikely that a 4-point difference on one instrument is equivalent to a 4-point difference on the other.

To make sense of these differences among scales, we transform the study outcomes into an *effect size* (ES), expressed in standard deviation (SD) units. In general, the effect size is calculated by the formula:

$$\text{Effect Size} = \frac{\bar{X}_T - \bar{X}_C}{SD_C}, \tag{1}$$

where $\bar{X}_T$ is the mean of the treatment group, $\bar{X}_C$ is the mean of the control group, and SD_C is the standard deviation of the outcome measure for the control group. Since the standard deviation of the STAI is approximately 8 points (Knight, Waal-Manning, & Spears, 1983), then a 4-point difference between the groups is equivalent to one-half of a standard deviation, or 0.5.

When a power analysis is done retrospectively, these numbers are (or should be) provided in the report. If a sample size calculation is being done prospectively, though, the researcher must determine a priori what the minimum effect size should be. This minimum-effect size is the smallest difference between the groups that would still be seen as being clinically important. Given a large enough sample size, any difference, no matter how small, may be statistically significant. However, the magnitude of that difference may be so small as to be clinically meaningless. A multi-centre study involving 400 patients may have shown, for example, that five group therapy sessions a week led to a reduction of 0.2 standard deviations in the patients' depression scores, compared with conventional treatment. Most clinicians would likely feel, though, that in order to justify the large expenditure of time and personnel needed to undertake such a clinical program, it would have to demonstrate a much larger effect.

It should be emphasized that the decision regarding the magnitude of the minimum effect size is a clinical one, not a statistical one. It is usually the point at which the clinician is willing to sit up, take notice, and change his or her clinical practice if the results prove to be true. This point may vary from one study to the next, depending on the cost of the intervention and the outcome itself. An effect size of 0.2 may be clinically meaningless when the intervention is expensive and the outcome is a score on a depression inventory. The same effect size may be very important if the intervention consisted of choosing between two otherwise equivalent medications and the outcome is a reduction in the proportion of patients who develop agranulocytosis.

There are no firm rules regarding what is an acceptable effect size. Cohen (1988), who is credited with introducing the notion of power analysis to the social sciences, stated that a small value of effect size would be 0.2; a value of 0.5 would be medium; and 0.8 would be large. However, it is not uncommon to see sample size calculations based on effect sizes of 0.75 or even 1.0, as in the study by Elkin, Parloff, Hadley, and Autry (1985). This reduces the required sample size, but the danger is that if a smaller effect is found, it won't be statistically significant.

The α or Type I Error

As mentioned earlier, the α level sets the probability of falsely rejecting the null hypothesis that is, the proportion of times we erroneously conclude that there is an effect, when, in fact, it was due to chance. By convention, it is set at 1 in 20, or 5%. Although this figure is somewhat arbitrary, it does seem to coincide with our intuitive sense of chance and probability, as we can see with a simple "mind experiment." Assume we are playing a betting game; I'll flip a coin and pay you $1 if the coin comes up tails, and you'll pay me $1 if it comes up heads. The first toss comes up heads, as does the second, the third, and so on. At what point do you begin to get suspicious that this run of heads is more than you would expect by chance, and that perhaps I am using a biased coin or lying about the results? For most people, this point is somewhere between the fourth and fifth flips. The probability of four heads in a row is 0.5^4 (that is, $0.5 \times 0.5 \times 0.5 \times 0.5$), or 0.0625; the probability of five in a row is 0.5^5, or 0.03125; a probability of 0.05 fits neatly between 0.03 and 0.06.

We can reduce the probability of a Type I error by adopting a more stringent α level, such as 0.01 or even 0.001. This is often done when we're running a large number of statistical tests and want to reduce the chances of reporting a false-positive result. A commonly used technique is called the Bonferroni correction (Pocock, Geller, & Tsiatis, 1987), which divides the α level by the number of tests conducted; if 20 tests are done, then a result will be taken as statistically significant only if the p level is less than 0.05/20, or 0.0025. Nowadays, Bonferroni is being replaced by "sequential" procedures, which adjust the p level with each test (e.g., Holm, 1979). They are not as conservative as the Bonferroni correction and not as liberal as using 0.05 for everything; like Goldilocks's porridge, they're just right. The penalty we pay for adjusting α, however, is that decreasing the probability of a Type I error increases the probability of committing a Type II error.

The β or Type II Error

By convention, the β level is usually set at three or four times the α level, at 0.15 or 0.20, which gives a power of between 80% and 85% (power = $1 - \beta$). This implies that it is more important to avoid a Type I than a Type II error. Cohen (1988), who proposed this level, defended it on two grounds. First, increasing the power requires relatively large increases in the required sample size. For instance, setting α at 0.05 and with a β of 0.20, a researcher would need 63 subjects in each of two groups to detect an effect size of 0.50; keeping the same ES but decreasing the β level to 0.10 (that is, raising the power from 80% to 90%) would necessitate a sample size of 84 per group, a 33% increase. As one perhaps extreme example, the GISSI study of streptokinase in acute myocardial infarction (MI) (GISSI, 1986), used a β of 0.05; their sample size was 11,806!

The second reason for setting β higher than α is that, while a power of 0.80 (80%) may seem low, it represents a significant improvement over current practice. For example, Peto (1987) reported that, of the 24 trials testing the effectiveness of long-term beta blockade with post-MI patients, 21 (87.5%) did not have sufficient power to have demonstrated a clinically important effect. Not surprisingly, only 2 of these 21 trials showed statistical significance. Within the field of psychiatry, King (1985) reviewed six articles investigating the purported link between wheat gluten consumption and schizophrenia. The three articles that reported an association had powers over 70%, while the three articles with negative findings had powers at or below 54%.

Sample Size

The sample size of a study, usually abbreviated as N, can be thought of as equivalent to the power of a microscope: the larger N is, the more easily the study can detect differences between groups. Put another way, the smaller the value of ES we wish to detect, the larger the sample size we need. As one example, the ISIS study of atenolol in acute MI

(ISIS-1, 1986) needed well over 20,000 subjects, and the researchers considered themselves lucky to have been able to enrol 16,027. While this figure may be a bit extreme compared with most studies, since the initial infarction rate was low and the change that was deemed clinically important was small, it does demonstrate the need for large samples in order to pick up small differences.

Determining the sample size required for a study is the major reason for doing power analyses. Indeed, granting agencies increasingly are requiring applicants to justify the number of subjects to be included in a trial. The reasons are twofold. On the one hand, a study with an insufficient sample size stands a large chance of committing a Type II error. Hence, the money would have been spent arriving at results that at best are inconclusive and that at worst may delay further investigation of a potentially fruitful field. On the other hand, it is equally wasteful and unethical to study many more subjects than are needed to show a clinically important effect.

Calculating Sample Size and Power

Determining Sample Size Prospectively

Over the past two decades, a number of books and articles have appeared that provide sample size tables or equations covering various types of research designs (there's a list of resources at the end of the chapter). Of these, the most comprehensive are the books by Cohen (1988) and by Kraemer and Thiemann (1987).

Although this chapter cannot present all of the equations for computing sample sizes for different research designs. the majority of cases fall into one of two categories: studies that try to show differences between the means of two groups on some variable and those that compare the proportions of people in the two groups. The first situation is more common in psychiatry, where the outcome usually is measured on some scale or consists of other numbers that can be assumed to be normally distributed, such as the degree of depression, a serum level, or the number of psychotic symptoms. The equation for the sample size in this case is

$$N = 2 \left[\frac{\left(z_{a/2} + z_b \right) s}{d} \right]^2 \qquad [2]$$

Table 4.2 Some commonly used values for z_α and z_β

α level	$z_{\alpha/2}$	β level	z_β
0.001	3.29	0.05	1.64
0.005	2.81	0.10	1.28
0.010	2.58	0.15	1.04
0.050	1.96	0.20	0.84
0.100	1.64	0.25	0.67

where d is the difference between the two groups; s is the standard deviation of the measure; and $z_{\alpha/2}$ and z_β are taken from a table of the normal curve in order to set the Type I and Type II error rates, respectively. Some of the more commonly used values for these two parameters are given in Table 4.2 for a two-tailed test; more complete tables can be found in most introductory statistics texts. It should be noted that it is not necessary to know the exact values of d and s to use this formula. Since s/d is the reciprocal of the ES (that is, ES = d/s), any two numbers that yield the desired ratio can be used. For example, for an ES of 0.5, it is easiest to set s at 2 and d at 1, simplifying the calculations. Thus, the equation can be used if either s and d or ES is specified.

Let's work through one calculation, the sample size needed for a study comparing two groups, using the example mentioned previously about the effectiveness of an anxiolytic, with an α of 0.05 and a β of 0.2. Remember that we were interested in a 4-point difference ($d = 4$) when the standard deviation was 8 points ($s = 8$). From Table 4.2 we see that $z_{\alpha/2} = 1.96$ and $z_\beta = 0.84$. The equation would now read

$$N = 2\left[\frac{(1.96+0.84)\times 8}{4}\right]^2 = 63 \text{ subjects per group.} \qquad [3]$$

(If N is not a whole number, it's always rounded up to the next integer; to be conservative, we do not round down if the decimal part is less than 0.5.) Note that if we set s at 2 and d at 1 to get an ES of 0.5, we would come up with exactly the same result.

Now that you've bent your mind around that formula, let me simplify your life. If we use $\alpha = 0.05$ and $\beta = 0.20$, then we get a very good approximation of the sample size with

$$N = 16s^2/d^2, \qquad [4]$$

which gives us 64 instead of 63. Just remember it doesn't work for other values of α and β.

The second case we'll consider consists of comparing the proportions of subjects in two groups who have some outcome, such as showing an improvement, developing side effects, returning to work, or committing suicide. There are a number of equations to determine the required sample size, all of which yield somewhat different results. The easiest computational formula is

$$N = \frac{2\bar{p}\left(1-\bar{p}\right)\left(z_{a/2}+z_\beta\right)^2}{\left(p_T - p_C\right)^2},$$ [5]

where p_T is the proportion of subjects in the treatment or experimental group who are expected to show the outcome; p_C is the proportion in the control groups; $\bar{p}$ is the average of the two (that is, $\bar{p} = (p_T + p_c)/2$); and $z_a/2$ and z_β have the same meaning as before.

To work through an example, assume that 20% of patients develop uncomfortable side effects on drug A. The new drug promises to reduce this to 10%. How many subjects would be necessary to demonstrate that this is true? In this example, $p_C = 0.20$ and $p_T = 0.10$ ($\bar{p}$ is therefore 0.15), and again we'll set α at 0.05 and β at 0.20. Putting these numbers into Equation [5], we have

$$N = \frac{2\times(0.15)\times(0.85)\times(1.96+0.84)^2}{(.20-.10)^2} = 199.92,$$ [6]

or 200 subjects per group.

Determining Power Retrospectively

Power is calculated after a study has been completed when the results were negative (for example, concluding that the intervention had no effect or there was no association between two variables), and you want to determine the probability that this was a Type II error. It can also be done to check the author's claim that the two groups were equivalent at baseline in terms of demographic or clinical characteristics. Often, the "equivalence" is a result of insufficient power to detect clinically meaningful differences (Streiner, 2003; see Chapter 18). Before we proceed further, it should be pointed out that it's not necessary to do a power analysis when a difference or an association has been shown; by definition, there was sufficient power to have demonstrated that effect. Whether or not the magnitude of the effect is of clinical importance is another issue, which is best left to the judgment of the reader.

It's possible to do this in one of two ways: calculating the actual power of the study or determining the sample size that would have been necessary to show a difference. In the latter case, you can use Equation [2] or [6] to see how far the study was from having the necessary number of subjects.

The more direct method is to calculate the power directly, by solving the previous equations for z_β. For the case of comparing the means of two groups we get

$$z_\beta = \frac{|d|\sqrt{N}}{2s} - z_{\alpha/2}, \qquad [7]$$

where N is the total number of subjects in both groups. The values of d and s are the actual values of the mean difference and the standard deviation that should have been reported in the paper, and the vertical bars around d indicate the absolute value (disregard the sign). You would then look up z_β in Table 4.1 and read the corresponding value of β.

As an example of a power calculation comparing means, we can use a study by Peet et al. (1981). They reported that propranolol was no better than placebo in relieving schizophrenic symptoms, and that "the effects of chlorpromazine (CPZ) were small and inconsistent" (p. 105), as measured by a standard rating scale, the Brief Psychiatric Rating Scale (BPRS) (Overall & Gorham, 1962). However, since there were only 18 patients in the placebo group and 16 in the CPZ group, this surprising negative result could have been a Type II error. From their data, the value of s was 8.91. Setting $\alpha = 0.05$ gives $z_\alpha = 1.96$. To detect an effect size of 0.5, d would have to be a 4.45 point difference on the BPRS. Putting these numbers into the equation, we get

$$\frac{4.45\sqrt{34}}{2 \times 8.91} - 1.96 = -0.50. \qquad [8]$$

If we look this up in a table of the normal curve, we'd find that the area to the left of −0.50 is about 0.31, so the power of the Peet et al. (1981) study to detect an effect size of 0.50 was 31%; it's not surprising that they didn't find a difference.

If the goal is to calculate the power of two proportions, the appropriate formula is

$$z_\beta = \frac{\sqrt{N}\,|p_T - p_C|}{2\,\sqrt{[\bar{p}\,(1-\bar{p})]}} - z_{\alpha/2}. \tag{9}$$

In the same study, Peet et al. concluded that there were no major differences among the groups in terms of the number of side effects. We can calculate the power of detecting a decrease from 50% ($p_T = 0.50$) in the CPZ group to 25% ($p_C = 0.25$) in the propranolol group. Because of dropouts and missing data, there were only 11 patients in the former group and 13 in the latter for this comparison, so that N is 24. Putting these values into Equation [9] we get

$$z_\beta = \frac{\sqrt{24} \times |0.50 - 0.25|}{2 \times \sqrt{(0.375)\,(0.625)}} - 1.96 = -0.695. \tag{10}$$

This result is checked in a table of the normal curve, yielding a value of β of approximately 0.24 – again, woefully inadequate. In actuality, there would have to have been 77 subjects per group for the study to have had a power of 80% (Streiner, 1982).

Summary

It is important (if not mandatory) to calculate the sample size necessary to show a clinically important result before a study is designed. Too small a sample size leads to an increased risk of committing a Type II error, while too large a sample size leads to unnecessary expenditures of time, effort, and money. Similarly, negative results may be a reflection of a Type II error, so the reader should determine whether what appears to be a clinically important but statistically non-significant finding was a true one or not. The calculation of sample size and power is not an arcane art, but one that can be easily mastered. It should be part of the repertoire of every reader of research and every researcher.

Further Thoughts

Since this chapter was written in 1990, computers have changed how we do things. Now it's no longer necessary to haul out paper, pencil, and calculators. There are many programs that are free or can be bought that do sample size and power calculations. Even better, there are now a multitude of websites that provide online assistance. Just use your browser and enter terms such as "sample size" or "power" plus "calculator," and follow the links.

REFERENCES

Cohen, J. (1988). *Statistical power analysis for the social sciences*. (2nd ed.). Hillsdale, NJ: Lawrence Earlbaum.

Elkin, I., Parloff, M.B., Hadley, S.W., & Autry, J.H. (1985, Mar). NIMH treatment of depression collaborative research program: Background and research plan. *Archives of General Psychiatry, 42*(3), 305–316. http://dx.doi.org/10.1001/archpsyc.1985.01790260103013 Medline:2983631

GISSI (Gruppo Italiano Per Lo Studio Della Streptochinasi Nell'infarto Miocardio) (1986, Feb 22). Effectiveness of intravenous thrombolytic treatment in acute myocardial infarction. *Lancet, 1*(8478), 397–402. Medline:2868337

Hamilton, M. (1959). The assessment of anxiety states by rating. *British Journal of Psychiatry, 32*(1), 50–55. http://dx.doi.org/10.1111/j.2044-8341.1959.tb00467.x Medline:13638508

Holm, S. (1979). A simple sequential rejective multiple test procedure. *Scandinavian Journal of Statistics, 6*, 65–70.

ISIS-1 (First International Study of Infarct Survival) Collaborative Group (1986). Randomised trial of intravenous atenolol among 16,027 cases of suspected acute myocardial infarction: ISIS-I. *Lancet, ii*, 57–66.

King, D.S. (1985, Jul). Statistical power of the controlled research on wheat gluten and schizophrenia. *Biological Psychiatry, 20*(7), 785–787. http://dx.doi.org/10.1016/0006-3223(85)90157-X Medline:3839143

Knight, R.G., Waal-Manning, H.J., & Spears, G.F. (1983, Nov). Some norms and reliability data for the State-Trait Anxiety Inventory and the Zung Self-Rating Depression scale. *British Journal of Clinical Psychology, 22*(Pt 4), 245–249. http://dx.doi.org/10.1111/j.2044-8260.1983.tb00610.x Medline:6640176

Overall, J.E., & Gorham, D.R. (1962). The Brief Psychiatric Rating Scale. *Psychological Reports, 10*, 799–812.

Peet, M., Bethell, M.S., Coates, A., Khamnee, A.K., Hall, P., Cooper, S.J., ..., & Yates, R.A. (1981, Aug). Propranolol in schizophrenia. I. Comparison of propranolol, chlorpromazine and placebo. *British Journal of Psychiatry, 139*(2), 105–111. http://dx.doi.org/10.1192/bjp.139.2.105 Medline:7030442

Peto, R. (1987, Apr-May). Why do we need systematic overviews of randomized trials? *Statistics in Medicine, 6*(3), 233–244. http://dx.doi.org/10.1002/sim.4780060306 Medline:3616281

Pocock, S.J., Geller, N.L., & Tsiatis, A.A. (1987, Sep). The analysis of multiple endpoints in clinical trials. *Biometrics, 43*(3), 487–498. http://dx.doi.org/10.2307/2531989 Medline:3663814

Spielberger, C.D., Gorsuch, R.L., & Lushene, R. (1970). *Manual for the State Trait Anxiety Inventory.* Palo Alto, CA: Consulting Psychologists Press.

Streiner, D.L. (1982, Aug). Propranolol in schizophrenia. [Letter to the editor]. *British Journal of Psychiatry, 141,* 212–213. Medline:7116066

Streiner, D.L. (2003, Dec). Unicorns *do* exist: A tutorial on "proving" the null hypothesis. *Canadian Journal of Psychiatry, 48*(11), 756–761. Medline:14733457

TO READ FURTHER

Bird, K.D., & Hall, W. (1986, Jun). Statistical power in psychiatric research. *Australian and New Zealand Journal of Psychiatry, 20*(2), 189–200. http://dx.doi.org/10.3109/00048678609161331 Medline:3533036

Cohen, J. (1988). *Statistical power analysis for the social sciences.* (2nd ed.). Hillsdale, NJ: Lawrence Earlbaum.

Donner, A., & Eliasziw, M. (1987, Jun). Sample size requirements for reliability studies. *Statistics in Medicine, 6*(4), 441–448. http://dx.doi.org/10.1002/sim.4780060404 Medline:3629046

Friedman, H. (1982). Simplified determinations of statistical power, magnitude of effect and research sample sizes. *Educational and Psychological Measurement, 42*(2), 521–526. http://dx.doi.org/10.1177/001316448204200214

Kraemer, H.C., & Thiemann, S. (1987). *How many subjects?* Beverly Hills, CA: Sage.

Lachin, J.M. (1981, Jun). Introduction to sample size determination and power analysis for clinical trials. *Controlled Clinical Trials, 2*(2), 93–113. http://dx.doi.org/10.1016/0197-2456(81)90001-5 Medline:7273794

Medler, J.F., Schneider, P.R., & Schneider, A.L. (1981). Statistical power analysis and experimental field research: Some examples from the National Juvenile Restitution Evaluation. *Evaluation Review, 5*(6), 834–850. http://dx.doi.org/10.1177/0193841X8100500607

Overall, J.E., & Dalal, S.N. (1968, Oct). Empirical formulae for estimating appropriate sample sizes for analysis of variance designs. *Perceptual and Motor Skills, 27*(2), 263–267. http://dx.doi.org/10.2466/pms.1968.27.2.363 Medline:5701398

Pasternack, B.S., & Shore, R.E. (1982, May). Sample sizes for individually matched case-control studies: A group sequential approach. *American Journal of Epidemiology, 115*(5), 778–784. Medline:7081206

Runyon, R. (1969). Minimum sample size required to achieve power $1 - \beta$ in testing for the significance of a difference in independent proportions. *Perceptual and Motor Skills, 28*(1), 247–250. http://dx.doi.org/10.2466/pms.1969.28.1.247

5 Speaking Graphically: An Introduction to Some Newer Graphing Techniques

DAVID L. STREINER, PH.D.

Canadian Journal of Psychiatry, 1997, 42, 388–394

In the 1630s René Descartes developed a radically new way of displaying data, a technique that we now eponymously call Cartesian coordinates. As it is currently used, an independent variable (IV), such as time of day, is plotted along a horizontal axis (the X-axis, or abscissa), and a point is placed corresponding to the value of the dependent variable (DV), such as melatonin level, on the vertical axis (the Y-axis, or ordinate). If we now connect the points, the result is a *line graph*, which shows how changes in one variable relate to changes in the other, for example, how melatonin level varies as a function of time of day. Another version of the graph, used mainly but not exclusively when the IV consists of categories, has a vertical bar, extending upwards from the X-axis, to indicate the value of the DV. This is called a *bar chart* if the IV is a non-continuous, categorical variable, such as diagnosis, treatment group, or sex, and the bars have spaces between them; it is referred to as a *histogram* if the IV is continuous (for example, age) and the bars abut one another. (For more details about drawing these graphs, see Norman and Streiner, 2008.)

This new way of looking at the world was so revolutionary that not much happened for the next 300 years or so. If Descartes were still around, he would have no difficulty recognizing the vast majority of graphs that appear in psychiatric journals. Over the past three decades, however, a number of new techniques have been developed and are beginning to appear in the literature and in the output of many statistical computer programs. Some of these methods, such as stem-and-leaf plots and box plots (described below) are "simply" attempts to convey more aspects of the data than do conventional graphs or to present them in more understandable ways (Tukey, 1977); other methods, such as horizontal bar charts, are based on empirical studies of human perception and try to minimize errors that people make in reading line and bar charts (Cleveland, 1994). The purpose of this chapter is to introduce some of these newer methods, as well as to rail against some common but erroneous "improvements" in the traditional techniques, alterations attributable mainly to the wide availability of computerized graphing packages that are poorly designed for scientific work.

Variations on a Bar Chart

Bar charts seem so simple, elegant, and straightforward that there doesn't seem to be much room left for improvement. What could be easier than a graph where the heights of the bars are proportional to some value? Actually, there are a number of ways to improve the picture. First, as we discussed in a previous essay (Streiner, 1996; see Chapter 2), adding error bars showing the width of the 95% confidence interval gives some indication of the precision of our estimate and allows us to do "eyeball" tests of the data. Another change turns the world not quite on its head, but only on its side. Drawing the graph so that the bars project horizontally from the left side accomplishes two things. First, a traditional, vertical bar chart can get very messy below the axis if there are many groups; the legends under each bar can run into each other, unless they are turned 45 or 90 degrees, which then makes reading them difficult. Placing the legends on the left side of the chart eliminates this problem, although at the expense of leaving less room on the page for the bars themselves. The second advantage of *horizontal bar charts* is based on research about perception. People can more accurately gauge the magnitude of the differences among the bars if the numerical axis is on the bottom than if it is on the side (Cleveland, 1994).

Another variation of the horizontal bar chart is the *horizontal dot chart*, devised by Cleveland (1994). Instead of drawing the entire bar, a large dot is placed at the end, often with smaller dots leading up to it, as in Figure 5.1, which shows the relative use of different psychological tests. If there aren't many data points (a number determined more by aesthetics than by counting), the smaller dots can be omitted. When the graph has a meaningful zero point on the left, then the smaller dots should start at the axis and end at the large dot. If the left axis does not begin at zero, however, the visual impression could be mis-

Fig. 5.1 A horizontal dot chart

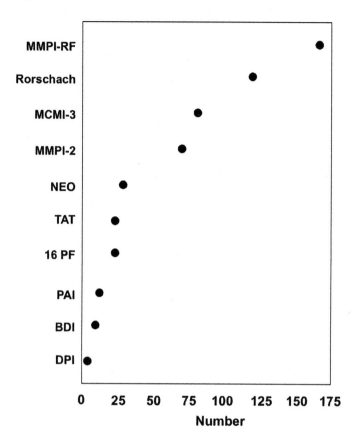

leading, since the relative lengths of the lines do not reflect true ratios. For example, if all the values in the graph fall between 310 and 350, you would not want to start the graph at zero, since most of the graph would be empty and all the end points would cluster near each other, making it difficult to detect differences among them. It would make more sense to start the axis at 300, but a line from the base of 300 to a score of 330 would appear on the graph to be three times as long as the line from 300 to 310, even though the difference between 310 and 330 is less than 7%. To minimize this misleading visual effect, the small dots should start at the arbitrary base, go through the large dot, and end at the right-hand side of the graph.

Table 5.1 A stem-and-leaf plot of the ages of 69 people

0	1	1	2	3	3	7	8						
1	0	0	1	2	4	4	4	5	8	9			
2	0	2	2	3	3	4	5	7	7	8	9		
3	1	3	4	5	5	6	7	8	9	9	9	9	9	9
4	2	3	3	5	6	6	7	8					
5	0	1	1	2	4	5	5	7	9				
6	0	0	2	3	3	5	6						
7													
8	4												
9	8												
10	4												

Histograms, which are used primarily to display continuous data, usually have between 5 and 15 bars, mainly for aesthetic reasons (Norman & Streiner, 2008). This means that if the variable we are plotting (for example, age) has more than this many values, we have to combine categories, such as plotting the number of people who fall within each decade rather than each year. But this involves a trade-off: what we gain in appearance we lose in information. The graph may tell us that there are, for instance, 47 people in the sample between the ages of 30 and 39, but we cannot tell how many were exactly 30, how many were 31, and so on. (Of course, a very large peak at 39 may alert us to the fact that some people are incapable of counting above this number, especially when it's their years on this planet that they're reporting.)

To eliminate this problem, Tukey (1977) devised a form of a horizontal histogram called a *stem-and-leaf plot*. Continuing with our example of age, let's take a look at Table 5.1. The left-hand column, which is the *stem*, indicates the decade (that is, the most significant digit, both mathematically and, for age, psychologically), so that the row that has 0 in this column reflects the number of people between birth and 9 years of age, the row with a 1 in the left column counts the number of people between 10 and 19, and so on. Then, the numbers to the right, the *leaves*, are the least significant digits of all people in that decade. Reading across the first row, we see 0 1123378, which means that there are two children who are 1 year old, one 2-year-old child, two 3-year-olds, and one child each of ages 7 and 8. If each digit takes up the same amount of space (you should not do this with a "smart" word processor, which uses proportional spacing and assigns more room to an 8 than to a 1), then the result is both a horizontal histogram, as well as a table preserving the original data. If the sample is very large, resulting in very long strings of numbers, you can divide each stem in half; that is, you can have two rows of 1s, for instance, where the top row is reserved for ages 10 to 14 and the bottom for ages 15 through 19.

Over the years, there have been a number of refinements to the stem-and-leaf plot that have appeared in various computer programs. For example, to the left of the stem, you can indicate the cumulative percentage of people: for the first row, it would be the percentage of people who fall in that range; for the second row, it would be the percentage of people who fall in the first and second rows; and so on. This makes it easy to determine where the 50th percentile is or where the 5th and 95th percentiles are. To make life even easier, some programs put an asterisk next to the stem that contains the 50th percentile; how much more can a person ask for?

Stem-and-leaf plots haven't shown up often in articles, possibly because they aren't as pretty as histograms. However, you will encounter them in almost every major statistical program, such as Minitab, SPSS, SAS, and Stata.

Before we leave the area of histograms, bar charts, and their variants, let me inveigh against three "modifications" that should be avoided: 3-D graphs, stacked graphs, and pie charts. Computerized graphics programs have become extremely popular, rivalling computerized poker or solitaire as ways of keeping jaded academics amused. Unfortunately, they're designed for people (who shall remain unidentified, but who usually have MBA following their names) for whom style takes precedence over substance.

It's easy to see the allure of 3-D graphs: you can fool around with the depth and colour of the shading and pretty them up in other ways. Unfortunately, they are as misleading as they are "sexy." Take a look at Figure 5.2; what is the value of the middle bar? The answer is 60, but your eye is drawn to the uppermost edge, which is closer to 70. The greater the 3-D effect, the more your eye will be deceived. Even worse, two graphing packages made by the same company, PowerPoint and Excel, use different conventions for plotting 3-D graphs, making a murky situation even more confusing. So, use 2-dimensional graphs in articles and talks and save those 3-D graphs for making a budget presentation to administration (oops, we let slip who the nameless ones are).

Another variant of bar charts regrettably made possible by graphics programs and popularized by newspapers and magazines is the *stacked bar chart*, which is shown in Figure 5.3. At first glance, this appears to be a useful graph, since we can present, in this case, five different values for

Fig. 5.2 A 3-D bar chart

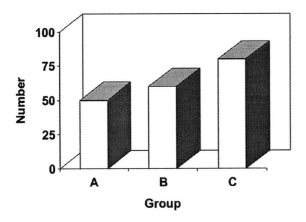

Fig. 5.3 A stacked bar chart

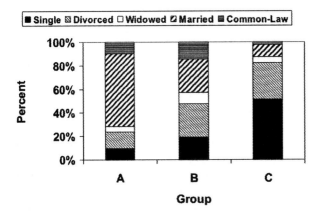

each of the three groups; quite a lot of information in one figure. The difficulty arises when we try to compare categories across groups. There is no problem with the bottom category (single), since the base is the same for all groups and we can easily tell for which group that segment of the graph is highest. But are the numbers of widowed people the same in all three groups and, if not, in which group are they highest? Now the comparison is more difficult. Because the lower two categories have different numbers in each group, the bottom of the widowed segments start

Fig. 5.4 A 3-D pie chart

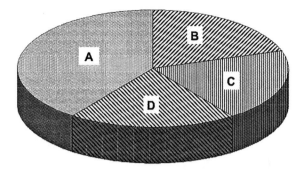

at different places for each group. We have to mentally move them to a common baseline and then compare the heights. This becomes progressively more difficult to do as the number of groups and the number of categories increase. Again, it looks sexy, but it can be quite misleading.

A similar problem exists with pie charts. A single pie chart, showing the proportion of people in different categories, is fine and can be quite informative. The problem begins as soon as we try to compare two pie charts. If comparable segments in each pie start with one edge of the wedge exactly at the 12 o'clock position and extend in the same direction (that is, clockwise or counterclockwise), then, like the bottom segment of a stacked bar chart, we can compare them without too much difficulty. If they begin at different places in their respective pies, however, as in the segment labelled "Widowed," then it becomes almost impossible to see if their areas are equal or not. Some people try to get around this problem by also printing out the actual number or percentage of cases inside the wedges. This simply turns the graph into two funny-looking round tables, which is redundant; just present the table and make the journal editor happy, since it costs less money to print a table than a graph. The bottom line is, if you need numbers in order to make the graph tell its story, then either you don't need a graph or you're using the wrong kind of graph (such as stacked bar charts or pie charts). As the old saying goes, "The only time a pie chart is appropriate is at a baker's convention."

If we combine the worst attributes of 3-D charts and pie charts, we end up with a 3-D pie chart, one of the worst abominations foisted on viewers. Take a look at Figure 5.4. Can you rank order the four slices from largest to smallest? You probably can – A is the largest, followed by D, then C, and then B. The only problem is that B, C, and D are the same. They look different, because tilting the graph distorts the angles between the slices. It looks sexy as all get-out, but it's terrible for presenting data. Just remember the admonition of Howard Wainer: "Although I shudder to consider it, perhaps there is something to be learned from the success enjoyed by the multi-colored, three-dimensional pie charts that clutter the pages of *USA Today, Time,* and *Newsweek.* I sure hope not much" (1990, p. 345).

Box Plots and Notched Box Plots

If we use a bar chart to display the mean age of people in a treatment condition and a control condition, for example, we are showing only one piece of data per group – the mean (or median if the data are ordinal or highly skewed). We can go a step further and add bars indicating the confidence intervals, but we are still showing only a small amount of the data. Can we convey more information about the groups and still keep the graph readable? Obviously, the answer is yes, or we wouldn't have bothered to ask the question. Let's return to the data in Table 5.1, which lists the ages of 69 people. To begin with, instead of starting the bar at the bottom of the graph and extending it upward to the mean, let's draw a short horizontal line at the median of the group (for those who have forgotten, the median is the value that divides the group, so that half the people have higher values and half have lower ones). In this case, the median age is 37; 34 people are younger and 34 are older. Next, let's look at those 34 more mature (the euphemism for "older") people and find the median for them. This is at age 51, so we draw another short, horizontal line (which we call the *upper quartile,* or Q_U) at this level. Finally, we'll do the same thing for the younger 50% of the people, drawing a line for the *lower quartile* (Q_L) at their median, which is at age 19.5. We have thus divided the group into fourths, with roughly an equal number of people in each quarter: 25% above Q_U; 25% between the median and Q_U; 25% between the median and Q_L; and the remaining 25% below Q_L. If we now draw vertical lines joining the upper and lower quartiles, we'll end up with a rectangle, which is labelled "Box" in Figure 5.5. What we've accomplished so far is to display the median of the group (37 years); where the upper quartile falls (age 51); where the lower quartile is (age 19.5); and what the interquartile range (IQR) is, namely, the difference between the upper and lower quartiles (that is, 51 minus 19.5, or 31.5). By definition, the IQR includes the middle 50% of the subjects. (The IQR, by the way, is the

Fig. 5.5 The functional anatomy of a box plot

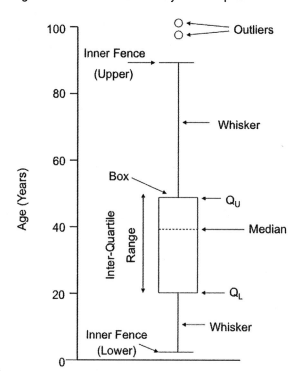

measure of variability used with the median, in the same way that the standard deviation is used with the mean.)

This has increased the informational value of the chart quite a bit, but we can go even further by drawing "whiskers" above and below the rectangle. Based on some arcane math which we won't bother to elaborate on here but which is explained in more detail elsewhere (Tukey, 1977), 95% of the sample falls within the range of scores of the median ± 1.5 × IQR (in our example, that is 37 ± 47.25). By convention (and for the sake of confusion), we don't actually draw the lines at these levels; the upper line is drawn to correspond to the largest actual value in our data that is below this higher limit, and the lower line is at the smallest actual value above the lower limit. The upper limit is 37 + 47.25, or 84.25 years. If we go back to Table 5.1, we find that the highest age in our data below 84.25 is 84, so that's where the line is drawn. The lower limit is 37 − 47.25, or −10.25 (obviously a very young person), and the first real value above this is 1, so that's where we draw the lower line. In the somewhat convoluted language of box plots, those horizontal lines at the ends of the whiskers are called the *inner fences*. Next, we define (but don't draw) the *outer fences*, which are 3.0 times the IQR, and put some symbol, such as a circle, for each subject whose score falls between the inner and outer fences. These cases (there were two in our example) are called *outliers* and have scores that are below the 5th or above the 95th percentile for that group. *Extreme outliers*, whose scores fall below the 1st or exceed the 99th percentile and lie outside the outer fence, are identified with a different symbol, such as an asterisk; we didn't have any in our data set. (Just to confuse you even more, every computer program uses a different set of symbols or even letters, but they are usually labelled.) Some computer programs even print the case numbers of the outliers and extreme outliers. This makes it extremely easy to identify subjects with very deviant scores, so that the researcher can determine if the data are real or reflect a coding or data entry error.

If more than one group is shown on a graph, we can display even more information: the sample size. This is useful for a number of reasons: estimates of the mean and standard deviation are usually more accurate when based on larger samples, and if groups do not differ, it may be due to a lack of power caused by too few subjects (Streiner, 1990; see Chapter 4). Seeing the differences in sample size across the groups helps us to make these determinations. The sample size is reflected by making the width of the box proportional to the square root of the number of subjects. The square root is used more for perceptual than for mathematical reasons; if one group is twice the size of another, drawing the box twice as wide would actually make it look three or four times larger, since we are representing a one-dimensional number (sample size) with a two-dimensional figure (the box).

Even with all the information we have displayed so far, two important pieces are still missing: the mean and the 95% confidence interval (CI) around the mean. We can easily accommodate them with a variant of the box plot called the *notched box plot*, which is shown in Figure 5.6. The point of the notch falls at the mean, and the height of the V corresponds to the 95% confidence interval, which is defined as

$$95\% \ CI = \overline{X} \pm 1.96 \ \frac{SD}{\sqrt{N}}, \qquad [1]$$

Fig. 5.6 A notched box plot

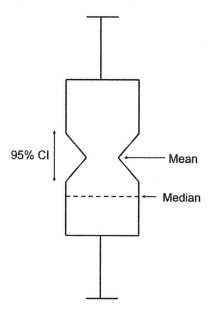

where $\bar{X}$ is the mean, SD is the standard deviation, and N is the sample size.

As you can see, box plots and notched box plots can display a large amount of data in a small space: (1) the mean; (2) the 95% confidence interval around the mean; (3) the median; (4) the skewness of the data, by how much the mean is displaced from the middle of the box; (5) the upper quartile; (6) the lower quartile; (7) the inter-quartile range, within which 50% of the subjects fall; (8) the distance between the fences, which spans 95% of the subjects; and (9) the number and values of outlying data points. These graphs are becoming more common in statistical and psychological journal, and hopefully will soon find their place in psychiatry.

Getting Rid of Those Ugly Bumps

No, we haven't changed the focus of this chapter to look at weight-loss procedures. The topic is much more mundane and prosaic (and also much easier to accomplish): how to smooth out graphs in order to uncover trends more easily. This technique is used most often with measures taken repeatedly over time, such as a person's melatonin levels over a course of 24 hours or the diurnal variation in subjective mood. The problem is that any trend in the data may be obscured by errors in measurement, errors attributable to limitations of the measuring tool, normal biological variation, inaccurate recording, and so forth. To illustrate the effectiveness of this technique, we'll use some data whose probable content we know ahead of time: the 11-year sunspot activity cycle (Andrews & Herzberg, 1985).

The top part of Figure 5.7 shows the number of sunspots per month, averaged over a three-month span (that is, the first dot is the average of January, February, and March 1981; the second dot is the average of the next three months, and so on). The data do tend to follow a sinusoidal path, but it's hard to discern the pattern among all the point-to-point variability. We'll try to reduce some of that clutter with a technique called *moving averages*. The raw data, which are plotted in the top part of Figure 5.7, are in the "Number of sunspots" column of Table 5.2. The next column, "Moving average 3," is where the smoothing begins. The first number in this column (411.8) is the average of the first three numbers of the previous column (390.8, 374.8, and 469.8); the second value (431.5) is the average of the second (374.8), third (469.8), and fourth (450.0) raw data points; and so on down the table. The results of this averaging are shown in the middle part of Figure 5.7.

As you can see, the sinusoidal shape is more evident, because the large fluctuations have been reduced considerably. The reason is that if one data point is discrepant, its effect is lessened by averaging it with two other (hopefully more typical) values. This is readily apparent in the case of the 12th data point (the 3rd quarter of 1983 in Table 5.2): it is 122.5, while those on either side of it are 204.3 and 225.9. In the top graph of Figure 5.7, it is responsible for the sharp downward spike at the left, which has been virtually eliminated in the middle graph. If we feel that the data are still too "lumpy," we can smooth them further by averaging over five values, which is done in the "Moving average 5" column of Table 5.2 and shown in the bottom part of Figure 5.7. Now the pattern appears very clearly.

Should we then average over six or seven numbers? Obviously, there is a trade-off. We can reach a point where we are smoothing out "lumps" that represent useful data rather than error. In fact, if we averaged over 15 numbers in this data set, even the 11-year cycle would disappear. So, we have to rely on our eyeball and clinical judgment to tell us when enough is enough and when any further smoothing would

Fig. 5.7 The effect of moving averages

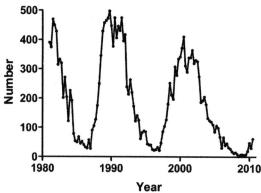

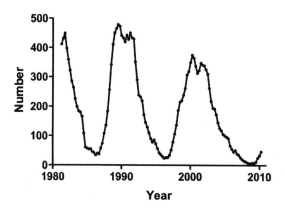

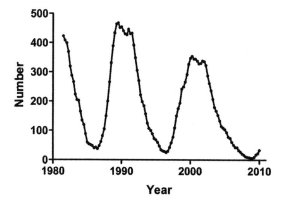

Table 5.2 Average monthly sunspot activity in three-month blocks

Year	Quarter	Number of sunspots	Moving average 3	Moving average 5
1981	1	390.8		
	2	374.8	411.8	
	3	469.8	431.5	422.8
	4	450.0	449.5	407.6
1982	1	428.6	397.7	399.1
	2	314.6	358.6	369.1
	3	332.5	322.2	319.5
	4	319.8	284.7	287.9
1983	1	201.8	264.2	265.9
	2	271.0	225.7	223.9
	3	204.3	199.3	205.1
	4	122.5	184.2	203.2

result in the loss of meaningful information. The second negative feature is that we lose some data points. When we average three numbers, we lose two data points; in general, if we are averaging k values, we lose $k - 1$ points. (We don't see the lost data points at the bottom of Table 5.2 because we have used the actual values for 1984; if we didn't use them, we would lose one extra value in the "Moving average 3" column, and two in the "Moving average 5" set.) If the data set is large, this may not matter too much, but if we start off with only 15 points and average over four values, we would lose 20% of the data.

Summary

In the past, we were fairly limited in the number of ways in which we could present our findings. Newer techniques allow us to show the data so that they are less prone to misinterpretation (the horizontal and dot charts); to minimize the amount of data lost through graphing (stem-and-leaf plots); to present a more complete description of the data (box plots and notched box plots); and to reduce the visual clutter due to variation (smoothing). Especially since many statistical programs can output these graphs directly into drawing programs, researchers should learn to use them and, in many cases, replace the more traditional but less informative bar and line charts.

REFERENCES

Andrews, D.F., & Herzberg, A.M. (1985). *Data: A collection of problems from many fields for the student and research worker.* New York: Springer-Verlag.

Cleveland, W.S. (1994). *The elements of graphing data.* (2nd ed.). Summit, NJ: Hobart Press.

Norman, G.R., & Streiner, D.L. (2008). *Biostatistics: The bare essentials.* (3rd ed.). Shelton, CT: PMPH USA.

Streiner, D.L. (1990, Oct). Sample size and power in psychiatric research. *Canadian Journal of Psychiatry, 35*(7), 616–620. Medline:2268843

Streiner, D.L. (1996, Oct). Maintaining standards: Differences between the standard deviation and standard error, and when to use each. *Canadian Journal of Psychiatry, 41*(8), 498–502. Medline:8899234

Tukey, J.W. (1977). *Exploratory data analysis.* Reading, MA: Addison-Wesley.

Wainer, H. (1990). Graphical visions from William Playfair to John Tukey. *Statistical Science, 5*(3), 340–346. http://dx.doi.org/10.1214/ss/1177012102

TO READ FURTHER

Tufte, E.R. (2001). *The visual display of quantitative information.* (2nd ed.). Cheshire, CT: Graphics Press.

Tufte, E.R. (2006). *The cognitive style of PowerPoint: Pitching out corrupts within.* (2nd ed.). Cheshire, CT: Graphics Press.

Tukey, J.W. (1977). *Exploratory data analysis.* Reading, MA: Addison-Wesley.

6 Let Me Count the Ways: Measuring Incidence, Prevalence, and Impact in Epidemiological Studies

DAVID L. STREINER, PH.D.

Canadian Journal of Psychiatry, 1998, 43, 173–179

According to Dohrenwend and Dohrenwend (1982), there have been three generations of psychiatric epidemiology. The first generation, which dates back to the mid-1800s, grew out of the recognition that simply counting people in mental institutions would underestimate the number of individuals who had serious emotional problems because not all mentally ill people were hospitalized. These early researchers supplemented agency records with reports from key informants, such as general practitioners and clergymen, to estimate the amount and distribution of psychiatric disorders in the community. The second generation of studies, which Weissman (1995) called the "golden age of social epidemiology," began after the Second World War. Rather than accepting the judgments of others regarding who was ill, this research relied on direct interviews with members of the public. Small groups of interviewers, who were often clinicians, randomly assessed selected individuals within a circumscribed location. In most cases, either the clinical interviewers themselves determined the diagnoses, or the subjects filled out forms that yielded global ratings of psychopathology but not a diagnosis. Perhaps the two most famous studies from the second generation were the Midtown Manhattan study in the United States (Srole, Langner, Michael, Opler, & Rennie, 1962) and the Stirling County study in Canada (Leighton, Harding, Macklin, Hughes, & Leighton, 1963). In the third generation, there was greater acknowledgment of the possibility of interviewer variability and error, and a consequent increase was seen in the reliance on structured interviews, such as the Diagnostic Interview Schedule (DIS), which was used in the Epidemiologic Catchment

Area (ECA) study (Regier et al., 1984). Weissman (1995) has added two more generations to this lineage. The fourth generation studies, which are underway now, rely on probability sampling of large populations, such as the National Comorbidity Study (NCS) in the United States (Kessler et al., 1994), the Mental Health Supplement study in Ontario, Canada (Goering, Lin, Campbell, Boyle, & Offord, 1996), and the Canadian Community Health Survey Cycle 1.2 – Mental Health and Wellbeing (Gravel & Béland, 2005). The last generation, appropriately enough, focuses on children (e.g., Boyle et al., 1987). (For a fuller history of psychiatric epidemiology, see Streiner & Cairney, 2010.)

One unintentional side effect of these studies is their introduction of new terms, such as incidence, point prevalence, and etiologic fraction, into psychiatrists' vocabularies. These are terms with which Freud, Horney, Sullivan, and our other forebears never had to contend. In this chapter, we discuss what these and other terms mean and why it is important for researchers, clinicians, and administrators to know them. Before discussing incidence and prevalence, however, let us start off by defining some other terms we encounter that are used incorrectly, even by researchers, as often as they are used properly.

Basic Definitions

A *proportion* is a fraction in which the people in the numerator also appear in the denominator. For example, Stewart and Streiner (1995) reported that of the 545 pregnant women in one study, 89 smoked regularly during the second half of their pregnancy. The proportion of smokers is therefore 89/545 or 16.3%; that is, the 89 smokers appear in the numerator, and they are also counted in the denominator as part of the total sample size of 545. A proportion is always a positive number and can never exceed 1.00 (or 100%). The people in the numerator, however, are not part of the denominator when we form a *ratio*. Using the same figures, we can say that the ratio of non-smokers to smokers is roughly 5 to 1 (actually, 456 to 89). Technically, this is called a *dimensionless* ratio because the value 5:1 applies whether we are talking about 100 people or 1,000,000 people. A *dimensional* ratio usually has a fixed denominator, such as the number of psychiatric beds per 1000 people. Finally, a *rate* always has a unit of time in the denominator; for example, the number of new cases per 1000 person years (that is, 1000 people followed for one year or 500 people followed for two years). With that as background, we are ready to look at measures of incidence, prevalence, and impact.

Measures of Frequency Incidence

To set the scene and to keep the numbers manageable, imagine that we are living in a very small country whose entire population is 1000 people. A study is undertaken to determine the number of people who have photonumerophobia (PNP). This severe, non-fatal condition, which was first described by Norman and Streiner (2008), characterizes patients' fear that their fear of numbers would come to light. The initial survey asked people if they currently had symptoms of PNP, if they had ever had symptoms in the past but had got over them, and, as best as they could determine, when the symptoms began and ended. People were re-interviewed annually for the next four years to determine how many new cases had developed and how many people who had symptoms at the previous interview had recovered. The time course for the 20 people who had symptoms at any time during the five-year study is shown in Figure 6.1. In addition, another 25 people who said they had been photonumerophobic in the past but who were fully recovered by the time the study began were included in the study.

Let us first look at the *incidence* of PNP, which, roughly speaking, is the number of new cases of a disorder in a given period. I say "roughly speaking" because incidence can be measured in two ways. The first way, called *cumulative incidence* (abbreviated as CI, which in other contexts is the abbreviation for confidence interval), is defined as

$$CI = \frac{\text{Number of new cases in a given period}}{\text{Total number of people at risk}}. \qquad [1]$$

Using Figure 6.1, we see that the number of new cases in 2006 is four (cases D, J, L, and Q). The denominator is a bit trickier. The total population is 1000, but if we look again at Figure 6.1, it is apparent that seven people (cases E, F, G, I, K, O, and P) had PNP when the year began, so they cannot be considered "at risk" for developing it during that year. Therefore, the CI for 2006 is

$$CI = \frac{4}{993} = 0.004 = 0.4\%. \qquad [2]$$

Although the CI is sometimes called the incidence rate, it is actually a proportion, not a rate. The number that emerges at the end is the proportion of people who developed the disorder within the given period (in this case, one year).

Fig. 6.1 Time course of photonumerophobia for 20 people who had the disorder at some time during the study

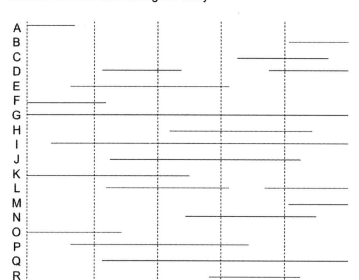

Because it is a proportion, the CI can never exceed 1.0 (or 100%), but the magnitude of the CI does depend on the length of the period: obviously, if we were to count only those cases that came to light between 12:00 a.m. and 12:01 a.m. on January 1, the numerator would be extremely small (if for no other reason than few of us can remember anything from New Year's Eve). The longer the time span, the greater the opportunity for new cases to appear. Thus, the incidence across studies can appear to be very different, simply because each one used a different period. One solution is to choose an arbitrary time span, such as one month or one year. In many cases, the one-year incidence rate is simply 12 times the one-month rate; however, this is not true when seasonal variation is involved. As an extreme example, an estimate of the yearly incidence of the flu would be grossly inflated if we multiplied by 12 the one-month incidence based on February's cases, and it would be seriously underestimated if the incidence were estimated in

June. Since seasonality has been postulated for a number of psychiatric disorders (Boyd, Pulver, & Stewart, 1986; Torrey, Rawlings, Ennis, Merrill, & Flores, 1996), such an extrapolation may be problematic. For this reason, and by convention, the CI usually uses a period of one year.

The second measure of incidence is the *incidence density* (ID), which has the same numerator but a different denominator:

$$ID = \frac{\text{Number of new cases in a given period}}{\text{Total person-time of observation of people at risk}}. \qquad [3]$$

"Person-time of observation" means that if a person is followed for two years before developing the disorder, he or she contributes two person-years to the denominator. Someone followed for 18 months would add 1.5 person-years, and so on, with the proviso that all people are followed for at least the given period, which in this case is one year. Statistically, it does not matter whether 20 people are followed for five years or 50 people are followed for two years because both would result in 100 person-years of observation. In very large studies, in which there are wide distributions of ages and other risk factors, the results would likely be similar with both sampling strategies. In studies that enrol people within a narrow age range, however, we may obtain very different results. For example, if we followed even a large sample of 20-year-olds for two years, we might find a very low ID for depression because they would not have entered the period of highest risk by the time the follow-up ended. Thus, the sampling strategy for studies of incidence must take into account not only the total number of person-years in the denominator, but also the composition of the sample, specifically whether or not it includes a sufficient number of people followed through the period of highest risk.

Before we actually plug numbers into the equation, we have to make another decision common to both measures of incidence: who to include in the denominator. As an obvious case, men would be excluded from a study of the incidence of cervical cancer because they are not at risk. In psychiatry, having had certain diagnoses in the past disqualifies people from other diagnoses. For example, DSM-IV states that a diagnosis of major depressive disorder, single episode (MDDSE), cannot be made if there has ever been a manic, mixed, or hypomanic episode in the person's life (American Psychiatric Association, 1994). Thus, such people would not be considered to be at risk in determining the incidence of MDDSE.

We are still not quite ready to do any calculations; we have to make one more decision about whom to count. Needless to say, we would exclude the 20 people who have PNP at the time the study began because they cannot be "at risk" for developing it during the follow-up time. What should we do with the 25 people who had PNP in the past but recovered before the survey began? Would we consider them to be at risk or not? Part of the difficulty in answering these questions is historical: many of the first epidemiological studies looked at fatal disorders, such as cancer and heart disease, in which people were not expected to recover. In psychiatry, the decision is somewhat arbitrary and dictated by our knowledge (or theory) of the disorder and by the aim of the study. For example, if we believe that schizophrenia, bipolar disorders, or obsessive-compulsive disorders are the result of chemical imbalances that can only be ameliorated by therapy but not cured, then, obviously, these people can enter into the equation only once because, once they develop the disorder, they can no longer be considered at risk. Conversely, if we feel that people can be cured of a phobia, only to develop it again, then we should include the 25 people who had PNP in the past. It becomes a bit trickier if we believe that a person can recover from a disorder but that he or she is then more susceptible to it in the future. Including these people in the denominator means that we are treating them in the same way as those who have never had the problem and, therefore, we would overestimate the ID. There is no easy solution except to calculate two IDs: one for first-timers and one for repeaters. In the current example, we are making two assumptions: one can have PNP any number of times and the risk does not change if the person had a previous episode of PNP. Consequently, we will include all of these 25 people.

Finally, we are ready to calculate the ID. Using Figure 6.1 and calculating the rate over the five-year interval starting in 1990, we would have 980 people (the total population minus the 20 who had PNP at some time during the period) followed for five years, so they would contribute 4900 person years to the denominator. Subject A would not be counted because he had PNP at the start of the study, whereas Subject B would add 4.2 person-years until she was stricken with PNP. Adding in the times of the remaining eligible subjects, we find a total of 4932 person-years and 15 new cases. Therefore, the average ID is

$$ID = \frac{15}{4932} = 0.003/\text{person-year}. \hspace{2cm} [4]$$

The result of this calculation is a rate: the number of cases per person-year (Essex-Sorlie, 1995).

You would think that with all the decisions we had to make about whom to count, there would be little left to discuss about the ID; this would seriously underestimate the ability of statisticians to say, "Yes, but ..." In this case, the "but" is an assumption we are making when we calculate the average rate over a five- or ten-year period: that the rate is the same each year, except for fluctuations due to sampling error. For most psychiatric problems, this is a fairly safe assumption because the rates for various disorders are fairly stable over time (Hagnell, 1989; Murphy, Sobol, Neff, Olivier, & Leighton, 1984).

There are exceptions, however, such as when a new edition of DSM or ICD results in a change of criteria or when there is an increase in cases following the introduction of a new disorder (for example, post-traumatic stress disorder). When the ID changes by more than approximately 10% from one year to the next, it is probably better to calculate it separately for each year (Thompson & Weissman, 1981). In fact, we can make the same argument regarding any variable that may affect the ID, such as age or gender: if the estimates differ at various levels of the variable, it is best to figure out the stratum-specific incidence and then add over all the strata.

Prevalence

Prevalence refers to the proportion of people who have the disorder at a given point:

$$\text{Prevalence} = \frac{\text{Number of cases at time } t}{\text{Population at time } t}. \qquad [5]$$

Like the CI, prevalence is often referred to as a rate, but it is actually a proportion. Also, it is usually expressed as the number of cases in relation to some "base," such as per 1000, 10,000, or even 1,000,000 people. The smaller the prevalence, the larger the base that is used in order to make the number comprehendible to the reader. Also, as in the case of incidence, there are a few variations on the theme. *Point prevalence* is the proportion of people who are a case at time t and would include both people who have the disorder for the first time and people who may have had it in the past, recovered, and have it again. If we choose the point to be January 1, 2010, then the numerator will consist of seven cases (E, F, G, I, K, O, and P), which yields a point prevalence of

$$\text{Point prevalence} = \frac{7}{1000} = 0.007 = 7 \text{ per } 1000. \qquad [6]$$

Note that because prevalence is a proportion, the denominator is the total population; it includes both the affected and the unaffected people.

Point prevalence is most useful in conditions with well-defined onsets and a clear distinction between illness and health. In psychiatry, however, many disorders develop insidiously, and improvement is equally gradual. Consequently, estimates of point prevalence may be subject to error because of the problem of dating the beginning and end of the disorder. As a result, surveys like the ECA study place a greater reliance on *period prevalence* (Regier et al., 1984). This refers to the proportion of people who had the disorder at any time during a fixed period, which is usually six or twelve months. Figure 6.1 shows that 11 people in 2010 had PNP. Some had it for the entire year (subjects E, G, I, K, and P), some had it and later recovered (subjects F and O), and some developed it after the year began (D, J, L, and Q). All of these people are included in the numerator. Thus, the one-year prevalence in 2010 is

$$\text{Prevalence}_{1\text{Year}} = \frac{11}{1000} = 0.011 = 11 \text{ per } 1000. \qquad [7]$$

One problem with this index, however, is that it counts cases whose onset preceded the start of the interval as well as cases that developed during the interval. Consequently, the final number is a mix of both prevalent and incident cases (Kleinbaum, Kupper, & Morgenstern, 1982).

Another variant of point prevalence is *lifetime prevalence,* which is the proportion of people who have had the disorder at some time during their lives. Thus, cases would include people who currently carry the diagnosis, people who have recovered, and people who are in remission (Kleinbaum et al., 1982). In our example, the numerator would consist of the 20 people who had or developed PNP during the course of the study, plus the 25 people whose episodes ended before the study began, which leads to a lifetime prevalence of 0.045. Lifetime prevalence is not used very often in more traditional medical areas, but it is quite common in psychiatry. One reason for its popularity, which we mentioned within the context of period prevalence, is the difficulty in determining exactly when a disorder started or ended. Another reason, mentioned when we were discussing ID, is that it avoids having to deal with the issue of whether one is ever "cured" of a specific disorder. If a person is diagnosed twice as having schizophrenia, the lifetime prevalence is the same whether we regard this as two separate, independent "attacks" of the disorder or one episode with a period of remission between exacerbations.

Despite its popularity, though, lifetime prevalence may be a fatally flawed index. A number of studies have found that the lifetime prevalence of various psychiatric disorders decreases with age (e.g., Streiner, Cairney, & Veldhuizen, 2006), which is obviously impossible, unless people with the disorder die at a much higher rate than the general population. After looking at various alternative explanations for the decline, we have concluded that it is likely artefactual and due to problems with recall (Streiner, Patten, Anthony, & Cairney, 2009).

These prevalence indices are, as their names and definitions indicate, *proportions* of people who develop a specific disorder. Closely related is a series of indicators that reflect the *risk* of the onset of a disorder up to a certain age. That last qualifier, "up to a certain age," reflects the fact that while some diagnoses have age spans of increased risk, there does not seem to be an age after which the chances of developing the disorder are zero. Since everyone may succumb to the disorder if they live long enough, the total lifetime risk is usually unknowable (Thompson & Weissman, 1981). Moreover, the risk varies with the age of the individual. For example, since the median age for a first psychotic episode of schizophrenia occurs in the 20s, 15-year-olds have a greater risk for schizophrenia than people who are in their 40s and have passed through the period of highest risk without incident (American Psychiatric Association, 1994). Given these considerations, we define the *lifetime risk* (LR or LTR) as

$$\mathrm{LR}_x = \frac{\text{Probability of a disorder between age } x \text{ and age } (x + \Delta x)}{\Delta x}, \quad [8]$$

in which Δx means some span of time (for example, one year) and given that the person does not have the disorder at age x. The technical term for this type of expression is a *hazard function*. We saw a hazard function in another paper on survival analysis in this series, and the concept is the same: it describes the probability that a disease-free individual will develop the disorder within a specified interval (Streiner, 1995; see Chapter 13).

One problem with LR is that it assumes that if we measure the risk up to some age x, no one – affected or unaffected with the disorder – has died up to that point. There is no easy way around this problem. One index that does not assume this is the *proportion of survivors affected* (PSA$_x$), where the subscript x means "at a given age." If the age-specific mortality rates in the affected and unaffected groups are the same, then PSA$_x$ and LR are the same. If the disorder is associated with a high mortality rate, however, as is the case with depression, PSA$_x$ can be considerably lower than LR (Thompson & Weissman, 1981). At the extreme, if the mortality rate is 100%, the PSA$_x$ will be 0. Another way around the problem is to look at the *proportion of the cohort affected* (PCA$_x$), which is based on all members of the cohort, whether or not they are still alive at age x. Although it does not depend on the mortality rate in the affected group, it is affected by the death rate in the unaffected group. That is, if a sizeable proportion of people without the disorder die before they reach age x, then PCA$_x$ will be smaller than LR, because it does not include people who may have developed the disorder sometime between the age at which they died and age x.

One solution is to build in a correction factor that takes into account the age-adjusted mortality rate among unaffected people. This is called the *morbidity risk ratio* (MRR$_x$), which is defined as

$$MRR_x = \frac{PCA_x}{PCA_x + q(1 - PCA_x)},$$ [9]

in which q is the correction factor. This is probably the most widely used index in psychiatry for estimating the risk of developing a disorder as of a specific age, x. More details on how q is calculated are available in Thompson and Weissman (1981).

Factors That Influence Prevalence

Many factors can make the observed prevalence of a disorder increase or decrease (Beaglehole, Bonita, & Kjellström, 1993). The first factor is the movement of people into or out of the area. For example, if a hospital admits patients from a wide catchment area but discharges them to nearby nursing homes, then the prevalence would increase in the region near the hospital and decrease in the surrounding areas. Another factor is improved diagnosis and reporting. For example, a partial explanation for the recent increase in breast cancer is that the newer mammograms are more sensitive than the older ones, which allows radiographers to detect lesions that previously would have been missed (Harris, Lippman, Veronesi, & Willett, 1992; Miller, Feuer, & Hankey, 1991). Similarly, new diagnostic interview schedules may be more sensitive in detecting subtler forms of the disorder. Furthermore, a change in criteria may increase or decrease the prevalence, depending on whether they make it easier or harder for a patient to satisfy the criteria. For example, slight differences in the format of the DIS may be responsible for the fact that, in the ECA study, the lifetime and six-month prevalence rates of phobias in Baltimore are two to three times higher than those in other sites (Myers et al., 1984; Robins et al., 1984). Finally, treatment may influence the prevalence of a disorder. If the newer antidepressants, for instance, are more effective in preventing suicides than the older ones, but they do not cure the underlying problem, then the incidence of suicide would decrease, but the prevalence of severe affective disorders would increase because the patients are now living longer with the depression.

The Relationship between Prevalence and Incidence

There is a direct relationship between incidence and prevalence:

$$\text{Prevalence} = \text{Incidence} \times \text{Duration.} \qquad [10]$$

By simple arithmetic, then,

$$\text{Incidence} = \frac{\text{Prevalence}}{\text{Duration}}. \qquad [11]$$

And

$$\text{Duration} = \frac{\text{Prevalence}}{\text{Incidence}}. \qquad [12]$$

Thus, if improved treatment of PNP leads to a shorter duration of the disorder, then its prevalence will decrease. Similarly, an observed decrease in prevalence could also be caused by a decrease in the incidence. Furthermore, a constant prevalence rate over time or similar prevalences in different locales could reflect very different patterns in the disorder: a high incidence combined with a short duration in one place and a low incidence and a long duration in the other.

Finally, we estimated the one-year prevalence to be 0.011 and the average incidence density to be 0.003 annually. Thus, we can estimate the duration of PNP to be, on average, 3.67 years.

When to Use Each Measure

As we discussed, there are many variables that could increase the prevalence of a disorder: migration of cases into the area, improvements in diagnosis, and an increase in the duration of the disorder caused by changes in treatment or other factors. For these reasons, indices of prevalence are not very useful when we are trying to determine the causes of a disorder, whereas measures of incidence provide much better clues. Conversely, people who are trying to anticipate demand for service would be more interested in prevalence than incidence. In planning for how many hospital beds or therapists are needed, it rarely makes much difference if the patient is seeking help for the first time or the fifth time; the important factor is how many people are in need of the service at any one time.

The choice between cumulative incidence or incidence density depends on the quality of the available data. If the exact dates of onset and remission are known, then ID provides a more accurate estimate than CI. As we have mentioned, however, these dates are rarely known with any precision for psychiatric disorders, and we may have to resort to using the CI.

Measures of Impact

Primary prevention programs are predicated on the belief that reducing the risk factor for a disorder will result in a corresponding decrease in its prevalence. For example, it has been hypothesized that some cases of schizophrenia are the result of perinatal trauma (Mednick & Schulsinger, 1971). Not all cases of schizophrenia are due to birth-related injuries, however, so even if we were 100% successful in eliminating such damage, people would still develop schizophrenia because of other causes. The *etiologic fraction* (EF; also referred to as the "attributable risk" or "attributable fraction," among other terms) is the proportion of all new cases within a given period that is attributable to the risk factor (Kleinbaum et al., 1982):

$$EF = \frac{\text{Number of new cases during the period attributable to the risk factor}}{\text{Total number of new cases during the period}}. \quad [13]$$

This requires that we know two values: the incidence density of schizophrenia in the total population (ID_T) and the ID of schizophrenia in the exposed population that had perinatal trauma (ID_E). From this we can calculate

$$EF = \frac{ID_E - ID_T}{ID_E}. \qquad [14]$$

For example, if the ID of schizophrenia is 0.0002 annually, and the ID of schizophrenia among those who had birth problems is twice as high (0.0004 annually), then the EF is

$$EF = \frac{0.0004 - 0.0002}{0.0004} = 0.50. \qquad [15]$$

If these (fictitious) figures were correct and we could totally eliminate head traumas at birth, the incidence of schizophrenia would drop by 50%. In another chapter in this book, we'll discuss other indices of risk in greater depth (Streiner, 1998; see Chapter 7).

Summary

Epidemiology has introduced a new vocabulary into the language of psychiatry. Unlike other phrases that have recently crept in, such as "inner child," "silos," or "front loading," however, these terms have agreed-upon meanings and provide information that can be used to understand the distribution of disorders in the community and the potential effectiveness of intervention programs. Indices of incidence relate to the number of new cases in a given time; prevalence relates to the total number of people with the disorder; risk refers to the probability of developing the disorder by a certain age; and the etiologic fraction estimates the maximum impact a prevention program can have if one cause of the disorder were eliminated.

REFERENCES

American Psychiatric Association. (1994). *Diagnostic and statistical manual of mental disorders*. (4th ed.). Washington, DC: American Psychiatric Association.

Beaglehole, R., Bonita, R., & Kjellström, T. (1993). *Basic epidemiology*. Geneva: World Health Organization.

Boyd, J.H., Pulver, A.E., & Stewart, W. (1986). Season of birth: Schizophrenia and bipolar disorder. *Schizophrenia Bulletin, 12*(2), 173–186. Medline:3520803

Boyle, M.H., Offord, D.R., Hofmann, H.G., Catlin, G.P., Byles, J.A., Cadman, D.T., ..., & Szatmari, P. (1987, Sep). Ontario child health survey: Part 1. Methodology. *Archives of General Psychiatry, 44*(9), 826–831. http://dx.doi. org/10.1001/archpsyc.1987.01800210078012 Medline:3632257

Dohrenwend, B.P., & Dohrenwend, B.S. (1982, Nov). Perspectives on the past and future of psychiatric epidemiology. The 1981 Rema Lapouse Lecture. *American Journal of Public Health, 72*(11), 1271–1279. http://dx.doi. org/10.2105/AJPH.72.11.1271 Medline:7125030

Essex-Sorlie, D. (1995). *Medical biostatistics and epidemiology*. Norwalk, CT: Appleton and Lange.

Goering, P.N., Lin, E., Campbell, D., Boyle, M.H., & Offord, D.R. (1996, Nov). Psychiatric disability in Ontario. *Canadian Journal of Psychiatry, 41*(9), 564–571. Medline:8946079

Gravel, R., & Béland, Y. (2005). The Canadian Community Health Survey: Mental health and wellbeing. *Canadian Journal of Psychiatry, 50*, 573–579.

Hagnell, O. (1989). Repeated incidence and prevalence studies of mental disorders in a total population followed during 25 years: The Lundby study, Sweden. *Acta Psychiatrica Scandinavica, 79*(348 Suppl), 61S–78S. http:// dx.doi.org/10.1111/j.1600-0447.1989.tb05216.x

Harris, J.R., Lippman, M.E., Veronesi, U., & Willett, W. (1992, Jul 30). Breast cancer. *New England Journal of Medicine, 327*(5), 319–328. http://dx.doi. org/10.1056/NEJM199207303270505 Medline:1620171

Kessler, R.C., McGonagle, K.A., Zhao, S., Nelson, C.B., Hughes, M., Eshleman, S., . . ., & Kendler, K.S. (1994, Jan). Lifetime and 12-month prevalence of DSM-III-R psychiatric disorders in the United States. Results from the National Comorbidity Survey. *Archives of General Psychiatry, 51*(1), 8–19. http://dx.doi.org/10.1001/archpsyc.1994.03950010008002 Medline:8279933

Kleinbaum, D.G., Kupper, L.L., & Morgenstern, H. (1982). *Epidemiologic research: Principles and quantitative methods*. Belmont, CA: Lifetime Learning Publications.

Leighton, D.C., Harding, J.S., MacKlin, D.B., Hughes, C.C., & Leighton, A.H. (1963, May). Psychiatric findings of the Stirling County Study. *American Journal of Psychiatry, 119*, 1021–1026. Medline:13929431

Mednick, S., & Schulsinger, F. (1971). Breakdown in individuals at high risk for schizophrenia: Possible predispositional perinatal factors. *Mental Hygiene, 54*, 50–63.

Miller, B.A., Feuer, E.J., & Hankey, B.F. (1991, Mar). The increasing incidence of breast cancer since 1982: Relevance of early detection. *Cancer Causes & Control, 2*(2), 67–74. http://dx.doi.org/10.1007/BF00053123 Medline:1873438

Murphy, J.M., Sobol, A.M., Neff, R.K., Olivier, D.C., & Leighton, A.H. (1984, Oct). Stability of prevalence. Depression and anxiety disorders. *Archives of General Psychiatry, 41*(10), 990–997. http://dx.doi.org/10.1001/archpsyc.1984.01790210072009 Medline:6332592

Myers, J.K., Weissman, M.M., Tischler, G.L., Holzer, C.E., III, Leaf, P.J., Orvaschel, H., …, & Stoltzman, R. (1984, Oct). Six-month prevalence of psychiatric disorders in three communities 1980 to 1982. *Archives of General Psychiatry, 41*(10), 959–967. http://dx.doi.org/10.1001/archpsyc.1984.01790210041006 Medline:6332591

Norman, G.R., & Streiner, D.L. (2008). *Biostatistics: The bare essentials.* (3rd ed.). Shelton, CT: PMPH USA.

Regier, D.A., Myers, J.K., Kramer, M., Robins, L.N., Blazer, D.G., Hough, R.L., …, & Locke, B.Z. (1984, Oct). The NIMH Epidemiologic Catchment Area program. Historical context, major objectives, and study population characteristics. *Archives of General Psychiatry, 41*(10), 934–941. http://dx.doi.org/10.1001/archpsyc.1984.01790210016003 Medline:6089692

Robins, L.N., Helzer, J.E., Weissman, M.M., Orvaschel, H., Gruenberg, E., Burke, J.D., Jr., & Regier, D.A. (1984, Oct). Lifetime prevalence of specific psychiatric disorders in three sites. *Archives of General Psychiatry, 41*(10), 949–958. http://dx.doi.org/10.1001/archpsyc.1984.01790210031005 Medline:6332590

Srole, L., Langner, T.S., Michael, S.T., Opler, M.K., & Rennie, T.A.C. (1962). *Mental health in the metropolis.* New York: McGraw-Hill. http://dx.doi.org/10.1037/10638-000

Stewart, D.E., & Streiner, D.L. (1995, Dec). Cigarette smoking during pregnancy. *Canadian Journal of Psychiatry, 40*(10), 603–607. Medline:8681257

Streiner, D.L. (1995, Oct). Stayin' alive: An introduction to survival analysis. *Canadian Journal of Psychiatry, 40*(8), 439–444. Medline:8681267

Streiner, D.L. (1998, May). Risky business: Making sense of estimates of risk. *Canadian Journal of Psychiatry, 43*(4), 411–415. Medline:9598280

Streiner, D.L., & Cairney, J. (2010). The social science contribution to psychiatric epidemiology. In J. Cairney & D.L. Streiner (Eds.), *Mental disorder in Canada: An epidemiological perspective* (pp. 11–28). Toronto: University of Toronto Press.

Streiner, D.L., Cairney, J., & Veldhuizen, S. (2006, Mar). The epidemiology of psychological problems in the elderly. *Canadian Journal of Psychiatry, 51*(3), 185–191. Medline:16618010

Streiner, D.L., Patten, S.B., Anthony, J.C., & Cairney, J. (2009, Dec). Has 'lifetime prevalence' reached the end of its life? An examination of the concept. *International Journal of Methods in Psychiatric Research, 18*(4), 221–228. http://dx.doi.org/10.1002/mpr.296 Medline:20052690

Thompson, W.D., & Weissman, M.M. (1981). Quantifying lifetime risk of psychiatric disorder. *Journal of Psychiatric Research, 16*(2), 113–126. http://dx.doi.org/10.1016/0022-3956(81)90026-1 Medline:7265008

Torrey, E.F., Rawlings, R.R., Ennis, J.M., Merrill, D.D., & Flores, D.S. (1996, Sep 18). Birth seasonality in bipolar disorder, schizophrenia, schizoaffective disorder and stillbirths. *Schizophrenia Research, 21*(3), 141–149. http://dx.doi.org/10.1016/0920-9964(96)00022-9 Medline:8885042

Weissman, M.M. (1995). The epidemiology of psychiatric disorders: Past, present, and future generations. *International Journal of Methods in Psychiatric Research, 5*, 69–78.

TO READ FURTHER

Kleinbaum, D.G., Kupper, L.L., & Morgenstern, H. (1982). *Epidemiologic research: Principles and quantitative methods.* Belmont, CA: Lifetime Learning Publications.

Streiner, D.L., & Norman, G.R. (2009). *PDQ epidemiology.* (3rd ed.). Shelton, CT: PMPH USA.

7 Risky Business: Making Sense of Estimates of Risk

DAVID L. STREINER, PH.D.

Canadian Journal of Psychiatry, 1998, 43, 411–415

Imagine that you were offered a pill that would improve your quality of life, but, as is the case with most treatments, there are side effects. In this case, the major adverse reaction is that it increases the chances that you will be appointed the next associate dean of education (ADE). Needless to say, there are a number of questions you would want answered before taking the first pill: How much will the intervention improve my quality of life? How long must I remain the ADE? Is there life after an associate deanship? But perhaps the most important question ("most important" because it is the one we will be discussing here) is "what do we mean by 'increases the chances'?" Although this specific example might be fanciful, the general situation is a common one. For instance, there has been research showing that women who use the birth control pill are at an increased risk for a thromboembolic event (Inman & Vessey, 1969). Some of the reports indicated that the risk is doubled, which resulted in a 20% decline in the number of prescriptions for oral contraceptives for women in the 20- to 45-year age bracket.

On the other hand, different people have looked at the same data and said that, while it is true that there is an increased risk, the absolute level of risk for thromboembolism in this age group is so low to begin with (roughly 3 per 100,000 women annually) that doubling a very small risk results in a risk that is still very small and one that can be ignored. Conversely, some new and very expensive drugs (such as ticlopidine) have been heralded as able to reduce the risk of reinfarction by half compared with acetylsalicylic acid, and this has been the basis for aggressively advertising them (Gent et al., 1989). The counter-

Table 7.1 Abbreviations used in this chapter

AR	Absolute risk (also see CI)
AR%	Attributable risk percent
ARR	Absolute risk reduction (also see RD)
CI	Cumulative incidence (also see AR)
NNT	Number needed to treat
OR	Odds ratio (also called relative odds)
RD	Risk difference (also see ARR)
RR	Relative risk or risk ratio

argument again is that, with a relatively small initial risk, the medication may be doing more for the financial health of the drug company than for the cardiac well-being of the patient.

There are at least two issues raised by these examples. First, and perhaps the easier one to deal with, is what exactly do we mean by the term "risk"? The second issue involves the best way to present estimates of risk and, more particularly, the ideal way to compare risk estimates – as a difference in the absolute levels between conditions, as relative changes in risk, or in some other way.

Originally, risk was used in a fairly restricted sense to mean the chance that a healthy individual will develop some outcome. For example, the lifetime risk of developing schizophrenia is slightly below 1% (Slater & Cowie, 1971). Those who have read (and still remember) a previous chapter in this series on indices of incidence and prevalence (Streiner, 1998; see Chapter 6) will recognize that this definition of risk is identical to what is called the *cumulative incidence* (CI):

$$CI = \frac{\text{Number of new cases in a given period}}{\text{Total number of people at risk}}. \qquad [1]$$

(To help keep you – and me – sane, a list of abbreviations used in this chapter is provided in Table 7.1.)

We can go further and define the risk for people who have been exposed to certain factors or who have various clinical, genetic, or demographic characteristics (Fletcher & Fletcher, 2005). For example, people who have two schizophrenic parents have a *conditional risk* (that is, the risk, given this condition of family history) of 37% (Slater & Cowie, 1971). When we have two groups that we want to compare, we would create a 2 × 2 table in which we cross-classify people who (1) do or do not have the exposure or factor and (2) do or do not have the

Table 7.2 Cross-tabulation of taking a new drug and becoming
associate dean of education (ADE)

		Became dean		
		Yes	No	Total
	Yes	30 (A)	120 (B)	150 (A + B)
Took pill	No	50 (C)	550 (D)	600 (C + D)
	Total	80 (A + C)	670 (B + D)	750

diagnosis. Let's go back to our original example and classify people as to whether or not they were ADEs and whether or not they had ever been exposed to the drug in question. We would get something that looks like Table 7.2. Even though there are only four numbers in the body of the table, we are able to generate dozens of different indices; fortunately, we will not be concerned with the majority of them here, but let us look at a few that are of interest to us.

The *absolute risk* (AR) for people who took the pill is A/(A + B), or 30/150 = 0.200. Similarly, for those who did not take it, the AR is C/(C + D), or 50/600 = 0.083. That is, your chances of becoming the ADE are 20% if you abuse the pill. Not abusing it does not protect one completely, because 8.3% of abstainers still end up as an ADE, but, obviously, the risk is lessened. How much it is lessened can be expressed by the *risk difference* (RD), which is also called the *attributable risk reduction* (ARR) and is simply the difference between the two:

$$RD = ARR = CI_{\text{With factor}} - CI_{\text{Without factor}} \qquad [2]$$

$$= AR_{\text{With factor}} - AR_{\text{Without factor}} \qquad [3]$$

$$= \frac{A}{A + B} - \frac{C}{C + D}, \qquad [4]$$

which in this case is 0.200 − 0.083 = 0.117. This means that people who use this medication have an increased risk for terminal associate deanship of 11.7%. We can also estimate the proportion of cases of deanism among drug users that can be attributed to using the pill. Not surprisingly, this is called the *attributable risk percent* (AR%) and is defined as

$$AR\% = \frac{RD}{AR_{\text{With factor}}} \times 100. \qquad [5]$$

If we use the same data, this works out to be

$$\frac{0.117}{0.200} \times 100 = 58.5. \qquad [6]$$

If becoming an ADE were a preventable condition, we could say that eliminating the exposure factor (use of this drug) would reduce these people's chances of becoming an ADE by 58.5%; the other 41.5% is due to factors other than exposure to the pill. (Unfortunately, because deans have an uncontrollable urge to have underlings, the prevalence of ADEs would stay the same; simply the risk factors would change.)

To repeat ourselves a bit, the AR% is the reduction in the chances of experiencing the outcome among people who are exposed to the risk factor (that is, using the pill).. However, not everyone on the faculty uses it (the other people use alcohol or other methods to improve their happiness); let us say that 5% do use it. To determine how much of a reduction there would be in becoming an ADE in the general population of university professors, we would have to multiply the AR% by the prevalence of drug use; that is, 58.5% × 5% = 2.93%. This is called the *population attributable risk percent*, or PAR%. So, once becoming an ADE is finally classified in the *Diagnostic and Statistical Manual of Mental Disorders* (DSM-V or DSM-VI) as a health hazard to be eliminated, we would say that stopping people from using the pill would (1) reduce the prevalence of ADE among pill abusers by 58.5% (AR%) and (2) reduce the prevalence of ADE in the general population by 2.93% (PAR%).

We can also ask the question "how many times more likely is it for a drug user to become an ADE than for a non-drug user?" Unfortunately, how we go about answering this question depends on how we gathered the sample. Because ethical considerations prevent us from conducting a randomized controlled trial, since we would be deliberately exposing people to serious adverse events, we are left with two possibilities. First, we could use a cohort design in which we gather a group of pill users and another group of non-users when they are still lowly faculty. We would follow them over a period of years and note which ones became ADEs and which ones did not. The other approach, called a case-control study, would take a group of ADEs and another group of non-ADEs and ask them about prior use of this drug (ignoring the possibility that one of these groups – we won't say which – may be somewhat cavalier with the truth). In other words, using a cohort study, we sample people on the basis of exposure and follow them forward in time, whereas when we use a case-control study, we sample on the basis of the outcome and look backwards to see how many in each group were exposed. We will soon see why this distinction is important.

Assuming that we used a cohort design (or an RCT), the way to answer the question is with a statistic called the *relative risk*, or risk ratio (RR). Basically, what it does is look at the ratio of the risks (or CIs) for the exposed and unexposed groups; hence its name.

$$RR = \frac{A/(A+B)}{C/(C+D)}. \qquad [7]$$

In our example, this works out to be

$$RR = \frac{30/150}{50/600} = 2.4, \qquad [8]$$

which means that pill users are 2.4 times more likely to develop ADE-itis than non-users. Risk ratios of 1.0 show no difference in risk between the groups; by convention, RRs over 2.0 (or below 0.5) are viewed as clinically important. When we are dealing with a disorder that affects many people, however, even smaller RRs may be important, as long as they are first statistically significant.

Why can't we do the same thing with a case-control study? The reason has to do with how we sampled. In a cohort study, by sampling people on the basis of exposure, we can answer the questions "what proportion of people who used the pill became ADEs?" (A/A + B), and "what proportion of people who did not use the pill ended up in this sorry state?" (C/C + D). That is, the two proportions are dependent on the effects of the exposure (or the intervention, in an RCT). In a case-control study, though, because we sample people based on the outcome, we can elect to have any number of people in cells B and D – we can have one control for each case, two controls per case, or whatever number we want. Thus, the two ratios are a function of our sampling scheme, not the effects of the exposure. So, we have to address somewhat different questions: "what proportion of people who became ADEs used the pill?" (A/A + C) and similarly, "what proportion of people who did not become ADEs used the pill?" (B/B + D).

For some arcane reasons that need not concern us here, rather than using proportions, we use something very similar called *odds*. The odds of pill use among people who became an ADE is A/C, and the odds of having used the pill among the lumpen proletariat (dean talk for non-deans) is B/D. The ratio of these two, not surprisingly, is called the *odds ratio* (OR), or *relative odds*:

$$OR = \frac{A/C}{B/D} = \frac{AD}{BC}. \qquad [9]$$

The OR is interpreted a bit differently from the RR. The OR tells us how many times more likely it was that a person with the outcome (a case) was exposed to the risk factor than was a control subject. If the prevalence of the disorder is actually low in the population, then the OR is a good estimator of what we really want to know, which is the RR. Based on the data in Table 7.1, the OR is 2.75, compared with the RR of 2.40. The measures are this close because the "prevalence" of being an ADE in our example is 80/750, or just under 11%.

Up to this point, we have defined RD, RR, OR, and the other expressions in terms of the increased risk of contracting some disorder because of exposure to a harmful agent or a background variable such as genetic loading. The same formulae, however, can be used in discussing the (hopefully) positive results from some therapeutic intervention. The only difference is in the interpretation. An OR or RR of 2.0 would show a twofold probability of improving among people receiving the new treatment, that is, twice the "risk" of improving.

So, returning to the question with which we opened this paper, is it better to use an absolute difference in risks when comparing groups (for example, the RD) or to use some relative measure, such as the OR or RR? As is true for much of statistics, the answer is "yes." Relative indices have the property that they are related to the level of the baseline, incident level of risk. That is, equal RDs translate into very different ORs or RRs, depending on the level of risk in the non-exposed group. For example, the left side of Table 7.3 shows an AR for the exposed group of 0.20 and of 0.10 for the non-exposed group, which leads to an ARR of 0.10. The OR for this table is 2.25, which would be regarded as clinically important because it is above the (somewhat arbitrary) cutoff of 2.0. On the right side of the table, the AR for the exposed group is 0.60 and is 0.50 for the

Table 7.3 Tables with the same risk difference and different odds ratios (ORs)

| | Outcome | | | Outcome | | |
	+	−		+	−	
Exposed	20	80	100	60	40	100
Not exposed	10	90	100	50	50	100
Total	30	170	200	110	90	200

non-exposed group: again an ARR of 0.10. The OR in this case is only 1.50, however, which falls below the level of 2.0 deemed to be exciting. Thus, what may be a meaningful intervention in some circumstances (for example, the OR or RR is over 2.0) may be unimportant in others.

Conversely, blind reliance on relative indices can also lead to bad decisions. Reducing the risk of a disease from 2 in 1,000,000 to 1 in 1,000,000 has very different policy implications than reducing it from 2 in 100 to 1 in 100, even though the risk has been halved in both cases. In such situations, it may be better to use an index of the absolute difference in risks: in the first case it is 0.000001, and in the second case it is 0.01. The bottom line is that it is usually preferable to report both absolute and relative change if there is any chance of misinterpretation (and 999 times out of 1000 there is such a chance).

When we are dealing with treatments, there is another measure we can use that is extremely informative: the *number needed to treat* (NNT) (Laupacis, Sackett, & Roberts, 1988). The NNT is simply the reciprocal of the RD; that is,

$$\text{NNT} = \frac{1}{\text{RD}} = \frac{1}{\text{ARR}}. \quad [10]$$

As the name implies, it shows the number of patients who must be treated in order for one additional patient to derive any benefit. This can be a very humbling way of viewing the results of a study. For example, an RD of 0.10 means that 10 patients must receive the treatment for one additional patient to benefit; the other nine either will not improve (if they were in the treatment group), or, more often, would have improved even without our intervention (if they were in the control group). That is, not everyone benefits from treatment and, despite the ads on TV, not everyone who forgoes therapy does badly. At the same time, those taking the drugs have been exposed to all of the side effects of the treatment, which range from dry mouth to neutropenia and seizures (Kumra et al., 1996). In fact, though, psychiatric interventions compare quite favourably with medical ones in terms of NNT. For example, only two patients with chronic fatigue syndrome need to be treated with cognitive-behavioural therapy in order for one patient to show improved functioning (Sharpe et al., 1996). Conversely, 850 patients need to be treated with benzoflurazide in order to prevent one person from having a stroke over a one-year period (Medical Research Council, 1985), and 641 hypercholesterolemic men must take privastatin in order for one person to benefit (Shepherd et al., 1995). Number needed to treat is a number that is much easier to comprehend than RD, RR, or OR. Within the last decade, several journals have appeared that summarize the results of well-designed studies (*ACP Journal Club, Evidence Based Medicine, Evidence Based Mental Health*), and the findings for therapeutic trials include an estimate of the NNT. I imagine that this trend will increase and will include the primary journals as clinicians become more familiar with the term.

Summary

Over 50 years ago, a delightful book was published titled *How to Lie with Statistics* (Huff, 1954). It consists of many examples of how one can present data in such a way that the results are somewhat misleading (at best) or deceptive (at worst). Indices of risk, while not designed to be either deceptive or misleading, can very easily be misinterpreted. Indices of relative risk or risk reduction (the RR and OR) reflect how many times better or worse one condition is in comparison with another, which is a very useful property when we want to assign blame (for example, to our parents for making us the way we are) or credit (for example, for an effective treatment). The problem is that relative indices do not tell us the magnitude of the problem – "twice as much" means going from 0.1% to 0.2% and from 10% to 20%. Absolute risks do reflect the baseline, but they are more difficult for the non-statistically minded to understand. To avoid confusion (deliberate or unintentional), it is best to include both numbers in presentations of results and, when treatments are involved, to include the NNT, which reflects the number of people who must be treated to help one of them.

REFERENCES

Fletcher, R.W., & Fletcher, S.W. (2005). *Clinical epidemiology: The essentials.* (4th ed.). Baltimore, MD: Williams and Wilkins.

Gent, M., Blakely, J.A., Easton, J.D., Ellis, D.J., Hachinski, V.C., Harbison, J.W., ..., & Turpie, A.G. (1989, Jun 3). The Canadian American ticlopidine study (CATS) in thromboembolic stroke. *Lancet, 333*(8649), 1215–1220. http://dx.doi.org/10.1016/S0140-6736(89)92327-1 Medline:2566778

Huff, D. (1954). *How to lie with statistics.* New York: Norton.

Inman, W., & Vessey, M.P. (1969). Investigation of deaths from pulmonary, coronary, and cerebral thrombosis and embolism in women of child-bearing age. *British Medical Journal, 2,* 651–657. Medline:5783122

Kumra, S., Frazier, J.A., Jacobsen, L.K., McKenna, K., Gordon, C.T., Lenane, M.C., ..., & Rapoport, J.L. (1996, Dec). Childhood-onset schizophrenia. A double-blind clozapine-haloperidol comparison. *Archives of General Psychiatry, 53*(12), 1090–1097. http://dx.doi.org/10.1001/archpsyc.1996. 01830120020005 Medline:8956674

Laupacis, A., Sackett, D.L., & Roberts, R.S. (1988, Jun 30). An assessment of clinically useful measures of the consequences of treatment. *New England Journal of Medicine, 318*(26), 1728–1733. http://dx.doi.org/10.1056/ NEJM198806303182605 Medline:3374545

Medical Research Council Working Party (1985, Jul 13). MRC trial of treatment of mild hypertension: Principal results. *BMJ, 291*(6488), 97–104. http://dx.doi.org/10.1136/bmj.291.6488.97 Medline:2861880

Sharpe, M., Hawton, K., Simkin, S., Surawy, C., Hackmann, A., Klimes, I., ..., & Seagroatt, V. (1996, Jan 6). Cognitive behaviour therapy for the chronic fatigue syndrome: A randomized controlled trial. *BMJ (Clinical Research Ed.), 312*(7022), 22–26. http://dx.doi.org/10.1136/bmj.312.7022.22 Medline:8555852

Shepherd, J., Cobbe, S.M., Ford, I., Isles, C.G., Lorimer, A.R., MacFarlane, P.W., ..., Packard, C.J., & West of Scotland Coronary Prevention Study Group. (1995, Nov 16). Prevention of coronary heart disease with pravastatin in men with hypercholesterolemia. *New England Journal of Medicine, 333*(20), 1301–1307. http://dx.doi.org/10.1056/NEJM199511163332001 Medline:7566020

Slater, E., & Cowie, V. (1971). *The genetics of mental disorder.* Oxford: Oxford University Press.

Streiner, D.L. (1998, Mar). Let me count the ways: Measuring incidence, prevalence, and impact in epidemiological studies. *Canadian Journal of Psychiatry, 43*(2), 173–179. Medline:9533971

TO READ FURTHER

Kleinbaum, D.G., Kupper, L.L., & Morgenstern, H. (1982). *Epidemiologic research: Principles and quantitative methods.* Belmont, CA: Lifetime Learning Publications.

Streiner, D.L., MacPherson, D.W., & Gushulak, B.D. (2010). *PDQ public health.* Shelton, CT: PMPH USA.

PART TWO

More Advanced Statistics

8 The Case of the Missing Data: Methods of Dealing with Dropouts and Other Research Vagaries

DAVID L. STREINER, PH.D.

Canadian Journal of Psychiatry, 2002, 47, 68–75

Imagine this situation: you've just completed a study that involved two groups, one of which received a new drug while the other received standard therapy. They were followed for three months, during which time each patient completed a weekly self-report scale and had blood drawn once monthly. At the end of the trial, you have complete data on all the subjects who were initially enrolled. I said "imagine this situation," because you will have to imagine it – it rarely occurs in real life. There are very few large studies with realistic follow-up times and real patients that come even close to the 100% follow-up of the NASCET trial (North American Symptomatic, 1991). The more usual situation is that subjects miss appointments or drop out of the study entirely, questionnaires get misplaced, blood samples get lost or the equipment breaks down, and data are entered incorrectly into the computer (and, needless to say, the original forms cannot be found after the errors are detected). In other words, missing data are a fact of life in most treatment studies. This raises two issues: why is it important, and what can we do about it?

Why Missing Data Is an Important Issue

Effect on Sample Size

When data are missing, the validity of a study can be compromised in several ways. The first we will discuss is the effects on sample size. Well-planned studies begin by calculating the number of subjects needed to

Table 8.1 Example of missing data points for ten subjects and five variables

Subject	Variable				
---	A	B	C	D	E
1	✓	✓	✓		✓
2		✓	✓	✓	✓
3	✓	✓	✓	✓	✓
4	✓	✓	✓	✓	✓
5	✓		✓	✓	✓
6	✓	✓	✓	✓	✓
7	✓	✓		✓	✓
8	✓	✓	✓	✓	✓
9	✓	✓	✓	✓	
10	✓	✓	✓	✓	✓

demonstrate statistical significance, based on some assumptions (realistic, we hope) made about the magnitude of the effect we expect to see (Streiner, 1990; see Chapter 4). Because enrolling, following, and assessing subjects is an expensive proposition, we try to keep the sample size as close to this number as possible. If we lose data points along the way, the effective sample size at the end may not be sufficient to show significance. At first glance, the solution to this problem seems simple: assume ahead of time that some subjects will drop out and increase the initial sample size to accommodate the attrition. So, if we estimate that we'll need 60 subjects, but that 15% may not complete the study, we will actually enrol 71 people. How did we get 71? By the following equation:

$$\text{Number to enrol} = \frac{\text{Desired sample size}}{\text{Estimated completion rate}} = \frac{60}{0.85} = 70.6. \quad [1]$$

This formula partly gets around the problem of subjects dropping out (we'll see later why it's only a partial solution), but it leaves a more insidious problem: subjects who remain in the study, but perhaps with some of their data missing. If we look at Table 8.1, we can see why the difficulty is insidious. It shows which data are present for five variables (A through E) and 10 subjects. One-half of the subjects are missing only one value, no one is missing more than one number, and no variable has more than one subject with a missing data point. This situation looks relatively innocuous, because we can easily live with a variable that has 10% of its values missing. But, let's say we want to factor analyse these data or do a multiple regression, with variable A, for example, as the dependent variable and B through E as the predictors. Here is where we run into trouble. Statistics that use two or more variables at once use what is called a *listwise* or a *casewise* deletion; that is, if any subject is missing a value for any variable in the analysis, then that person is eliminated, along with all of his or her valid data. So, even though only 10% of the data points are missing, the analyses will eliminate 50% of the subjects and their data in this example. One simulation found that when only 2% of the data were missing at random, over 18% of the total data set was lost using listwise deletion; over 59% of cases were lost with a 10% missing data rate (Kim & Curry, 1977). (Do not be tempted by this result to use an option present in some statistical software packages called *pairwise* deletion, which deletes only the pairs of variables for which one value is missing. This means that each correlation may be based on different combinations of subjects, which leads to far more problems than it solves, such as negative variances and correlations greater than 1.0.) So, even a few missing values, if spread across several subjects and variables, can result in a large decrease in the sample size for many analyses.

Effect on Validity of the Study

The second way in which missing data compromise the validity of the results cannot be solved by the simple expedient of enrolling more subjects than we need or by replacing the missing subjects with new ones. This is because data are rarely missing for trivial reasons. That is, people often drop out of a study because they aren't getting any better and look for a different form of treatment, they find the side effects of the treatment too onerous to deal with, or they have gotten better and don't see any purpose in wasting their time coming into the clinic just to fill out some questionnaires and have blood drawn – or half a dozen other reasons, all of which are related to the intervention itself. This is a particular problem if subjects drop out of the groups at different rates or for different reasons. Let's work through a few examples.

It is often the case that patients in one condition do less well than those in the other arm of the study. If patients drop out of the trial because they do not feel that they are getting better, there will be more unsuccessful cases who will leave the first group than the second. This will decrease the magnitude of the treatment effect. We can illustrate this with the data in Table 8.2. To keep the example easy, assume that

Table 8.2 Change scores for two groups

Treatment A		Treatment B	
Subject	Change	Subject	Change
1	10	1	10
2	10	2	10
3	10	3	0
4	10	4	0
5	10	5	0
6	0	6	0
7	0	7	10
8	10	8	0
9	10	9	10
10	10	10	0

either patients improve, in which case their change score is 10.0, or they don't improve, in which case their score is 0.0. If we take the average improvement score for all subjects in both groups, it is 8.0 for Treatment A and 4.0 for Treatment B. But, if one-half of those who do not improve drop out of the study, the mean change score for the remaining subjects will be 8.9 for Treatment A (based on nine subjects, of whom eight improve) and 5.7 in Treatment B (based on seven subjects, of whom four improve). So, the original difference of 4.0 points is reduced to 3.2 points, and the estimates of the intervention's effectiveness in both groups are biased upwards. Although this is an extreme example, the effect is the same if not all the change scores are identical; only the magnitude of the effect will be somewhat less.

Conversely, if one-half of the people who improve drop out, there will be four people with scores of 10.0 and two people with scores of 0.0 in Group A, for a mean of 6.7, and there will be two people with scores of 10, and six with scores of 0 in Group B, yielding a mean of 2.5. Again, the magnitude of the difference is reduced (3.5 instead of 4.0), and the estimates of the treatment's true effects are erroneous (in this case, biased downward). Replacing lost subjects with new ones doesn't help in either situation, because the same factors that influence dropping out will affect them too; we'll simply end up with more people providing a biased and untrustworthy estimate of the treatment means.

The situation becomes even worse if people drop out of each group for different reasons. That is, if those who improve drop out of the group with the more effective treatment because they've gotten better, while those who do not improve quit the other group because they are not improving, the estimate of the treatment effect in the experimental group will be biased downward and that of the control group biased upward. Again, the groups will appear to be more similar than is actually the case.

Types of Missing Data

Before discussing the cures, we should consider a little more about etiology. Medicine is replete with terms that seem designed to confuse. (For example, who has ever seen a red rash that looks like a wolf, even in patients with systemic lupus erythematosus?) Not to be outdone, statistics, too, has its fair share of confusing terminology. Three such terms are important here: data can be *missing completely at random* (MCAR), *missing at random* (MAR), or *missing not at random* (MNAR) (Little & Rubin, 1987). The first two terms are not synonymous. For a change, the first term, MCAR, means exactly what it says: the probability of the "missingness" (an ugly statistical jargon term) of a variable is not related either to the value of that variable or to any other variable (such as group membership, sex, or duration of the disorder). This may occur if, for example, a piece of lab equipment broke down, spoiling some of the samples; if a water leak ruined a batch of questionnaires; if a subject was out of the country on a follow-up day for a reason unrelated to the disorder; or if people didn't show up for an appointment because of bad weather (a particular problem in Canada). Because the data are MCAR, their loss doesn't bias the results in favour of one group or the other. This is a fairly stringent criterion for missingness. We often act as if missing data are MCAR, but they rarely are.

More commonly, missingness is related to some variable that we've measured, but not to the outcome (the situation called MAR). For example, older people may miss more appointments than younger people do because of difficulty in getting to the session in bad weather. As long as age is not related to depression, the data are MAR. Data that are MCAR or MAR are *ignorable* (another ugly statistical term) because, as we'll see, we're able to fill in the blanks using the other variables in the data set.

Even more often, though, the probability of missingness is related to values that themselves are missing. This is the case when, for example, people drop out of a study because they are not getting better or, conversely, they have gotten better. That is, the probability of having missing values on a depression scale is related to the degree of depression. In this situation, the missing data are MNAR; these missing data are also called *non-ignorable*. The distinctions among MCAR, MAR, and MNAR data are important, because the different techniques for dealing with the problem make various assumptions about why they are missing.

What to Do about It

Testing for Differences

Actually, this section should have the more unwieldy, but also more descriptive, heading, "What's Always Done, but Why Bother, Because It Doesn't Tell Us Anything in Any Case, Although It Keeps the Editors Happy." In almost every trial that has dropouts (that is, in almost every trial), the "Results" section begins by comparing those who completed the study with those who did not. And, in almost every case, the conclusion is that there are no significant differences between these two groups of people. Why shouldn't we bother to do this? Mainly, because the conclusion is most often wrong. If we assume that people do not drop out for trivial reasons (other than moving out of the region or dying for causes unrelated to the disorder or the treatment), then, by definition, those who dropped out are different; we simply haven't found those differences. There are at least two reasons for this. The first is, again, sample size. If we based the sample size on a calculation of how many subjects are necessary to show a clinically important difference, then sample sizes that are smaller than this figure are, by definition, less likely to detect important differences. Unless the dropouts form a large proportion of the total sample size (which would call into question the validity of the study as a whole), there will not be a sufficient number of people in that group to see statistical significance for even large and clinically important differences with any degree of certainty.

The second reason for the almost universal failure to find differences between dropouts and completers is like the proverbial drunk looking for his keys under the lamp post – not because he lost them there, but rather because the light is better than where he actually dropped them. Similarly, we're often looking in the wrong place to find differences between those who do and those who do not remain in a study. We perform tests on variables for which we have data, such as age, duration of illness, or number of previous hospitalizations, not because we expect that these are the crucial variables that affect retention in the study but because they are available. We rarely measure the factors that may be important, such as the person's intention to comply or what he or she expects to gain from participating.

The bottom line is that testing for differences between completers and non-completers is often a ritual we feel obligated to perform (or are made to feel obligated to perform by the editors), but it is one that rarely yields any useful information.

Filling in the Blanks

Missing data can occur in one of two ways: subjects start the study, but drop out before the trial is done, or they do stay in the study to the end, but some of their data may be missing. This may occur for several reasons, such as failure to appear for an appointment, equipment failure, loss of data sheets, or the omission of some items in a questionnaire. Until recently, such a loss would have resulted either in relatively crude attempts at *imputing* the data (a fancy term for "inventing numbers") or in dropping them entirely from some of the analyses. Let's begin with the easier situation – the subject remains in the study, but with some missing values.

Perhaps the easiest way of filling in the blanks is to replace the missing values with the mean of the group. For example, if a Beck Depression Inventory (BDI) score were missing for a few people (under, say, 10%), then the mean BDI score of the remaining subjects would be assigned to them. We can even be somewhat more sophisticated and try to get more accurate estimates based on group characteristics. For example, because women tend to have slightly higher depression scores than men, we can use the mean of the female subjects to replace women's missing values and do the same for men. This method has several attractive features. First, it is easy to understand and to implement with most statistical packages. Second, it does not bias the estimate of the mean, since the replaced value is the mean itself. When things seem this easy and straightforward in statistics, it is usually a sign that there are major problems waiting in the wings, so we should not be surprised to find some. The first is that replacing with the mean assumes that the data are MCAR, which is very rarely the case. Second, and more important, is that it reduces the estimate of the standard deviation (SD) of the variable, because the imputed values do not differ at all from the mean. Since all parametric statistical tests use the standard error of the mean (the SD divided by the square root of the sample size [Streiner, 1996; see Chapter 2]) in their calculations, this results in inflation of the test's value, in confidence intervals (CIs) that are too narrow, and in an increased probability of a Type I error (that is, concluding that there is a difference, when in fact there isn't one).

A step up in sophistication, called hot-deck imputation, involves finding a similar person among the subjects and using that person's score. For example, let's say Subject A is missing her third BDI score. We would look for a woman who has similar scores to Subject A's on the first two BDIs and use this person's third testing as the value for Subject A. If there are several such people (as we hope there are), one is selected at random. This results in a more accurate estimate of the score, because the value is realistic and includes some degree of measurement error. The downside of this approach is again that it reduces the estimate of the SD and also requires a large sample size to find people with similar scores.

Taking this method to its logical end, we can use multiple regression to predict the missing values, based on several other variables in the data set. This means that we don't have to find subjects with similar scores, which is both easier and more practical, especially with a limited number of people in the study. In fact, this is the approach used by many statistical software packages. It also has the advantage of requiring data that are only MAR, which is more reasonable than the more stringent MCAR requirement. It assumes, though, that we are able to predict the missing value from other scores in the data and, again, has the drawback that it is biased towards the mean. This results in a reduced estimate of the SD and in CIs that are too narrow. An improvement is to use the value predicted by the regression equation and then add a "fudge factor," which is some degree of error based on the SD of the predicted values. For example, if the predicted value of the BDI is 10 for a subject, we would add or subtract something to this value, where how much is added or subtracted is consistent with the amount of error in the regression equation; the more accurate the prediction (that is, the higher the value of the R^2), the smaller the fudge factor. This means that if two people have predicted scores of 10, each would get somewhat different imputed scores and we would better preserve the SD of the variable. It requires a bit more work, but we are repaid in that the resulting statistical tests aren't quite as biased (Norman & Streiner, 2008).

Within the past few years, even more sophisticated and accurate methods, called *multiple imputation*, have been developed (Little & Rubin, 1987; Rubin, 1987). These approaches use maximum likelihood and Markov Chain Monte Carlo procedures (about which the less said the better). Basically, they estimate the missing values based on regression-like statistics, but they do it many times, with different starting values each time. The final imputed value is the mean of these guesses. Multiple imputation's power derives from the fact that not only does it estimate the mean, but, based on how much the guesses differ from each other, it can build in the variability that is present in the data. The end result is that the final data set, with the imputed values, gives unbiased estimates of means, variances, and other parameters.

It is often said that you don't get something for nothing. In the case of computer programs that do multiple imputation, however, you actually do get something for nothing. There is a commercially available program, called SOLAS (Statistical Software Solutions, n.d.), that costs over $1000, but some programs that are free and can be downloaded from the Web actually work better (Allison, 2000). The most powerful one is called Amelia II (Honaker, King, & Blackwell, n.d.), in honour of that famous missing person who could not be brought back, even with a computer program. Another, called NORM (Schafer, n.d.), is much easier to use but is limited to data that are normally distributed. CAT (Schafer, n.d.), written by the same group, deals with categorical data.

Trying It Out

Until now, we've been talking in general about how some imputation methods result in smaller values for the SD than do others. Let's take a look at how much the methods vary. I began with some real data for 10 variables from 174 subjects. For one of those variables, I randomly deleted 20% of the values (creating the most optimal situation, in that the data are MCAR). Then, the missing values were imputed four ways: (1) they were replaced by the mean; (2) they were estimated with a regression equation, where the other variables were predictors; (3) they were estimated with a regression, where the imputed values were varied based on the SD of the predicted value; and (4) they were estimated using the multiple imputation package NORM. As we can see in Table 8.3, all the methods gave very good estimates of the mean. Where they differed, though, was in estimating the SD. As expected, replacement with the mean resulted in the lowest value; it underestimated the SD by nearly 13% and produced the narrowest CI. Multiple regression did marginally better, followed by multiple regression plus error. The multiple imputation approach, though, yielded an estimate of the SD that differed from the original by less than 0.3% and resulted in a CI nearly identical to that of the original data.

Table 8.3 Means, SDs, and 95% CIs of data imputed various ways

	Mean	SD	95% CI
Original data	575.93	85.32	563.25 – 588.61
Replaced with the mean	575.68	74.47	564.61 – 586.75
Replaced with regression estimate	575.05	76.33	563.71 – 586.39
Replaced with regression plus error	573.07	79.31	561.29 – 584.85
Multiple imputation	575.93	85.07	563.29 – 588.57

The bottom line is that replacement with the mean is the poorest option (other than listwise deletion). If you do not have access to a multiple imputation program, replace the missing values with a regression estimate after modifying that estimate with some error based on the regression equation itself.

Saving Those Who Are Lost

This sounds like an invitation to a revival meeting, and in a way it is. The techniques we have just described are useful for filling in the blanks when the subjects remain in the study but some of their data are missing. They are much less useful when there are repeated measurements over time, and the subjects either miss some follow-up visits or entirely drop out of the study. In this situation, there are also several options, ranging from abysmal to quite acceptable.

The worst option is to drop the subject entirely, for the reasons that we discussed earlier. However, if most statistical procedures are done without thinking (something none of us would ever do, but we're not too sure about some of our colleagues), this is exactly what happens. Repeated-measures analyses of variance (and all of their variants, such as multivariate analysis of variance) require that all the subjects have complete data: if even one value is missing, the programs eliminate that person and all of his or her data.

Within recent years, many researchers have adopted the strategy of "the last observation carried forward" (LOCF). This means that if, for example, there were six follow-up visits, but the subject dropped out after the third visit, the value at Time 3 is "carried forward" and presumed to be the score at Times 4, 5, and 6. In Figure 8.1, the dotted line shows what we would expect to see if the subject remained in the study, while the solid line shows the score that is actually recorded for that person. The rationale behind this approach is that it is conservative;

Fig. 8.1 Assumed and recorded values for the last observation carried forward method

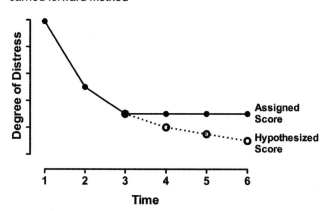

that is, it operates against the hypothesis that people will improve over time, and so we are underestimating the degree of improvement.

The advantages of this approach are obvious. It is easy to do, and we do not lose subjects from the analyses. Unfortunately, the disadvantages aren't as obvious. First, let us take a closer look at the assumption of no change outside the study. While it may be conservative insofar as the experimental group is concerned, it is actually quite liberal when applied to subjects in the control or comparison group. It ignores the fact that the natural history for many disorders, such as depression, is improvement over time, even in the absence of medication. This is especially true if the person is on a comparator drug. The selective serotonin reuptake inhibitors (SSRIs), for example, are no more effective than the older tricyclic antidepressants (TCAs); their advantage is in their side-effect profile. Consequently, patients may drop out of the TCA arm, not because they aren't improving but because they have problems with dry mouth or drowsiness. Assuming they will not continue to improve may underestimate the efficacy of these drugs. So, when applied to the control group, LOCF may artificially inflate the difference between the groups in favour of the experimental one. Second, when LOCF is used with negative outcomes, such as adverse drug reactions, it underestimates their consequences by assuming that they will not get worse over time. The third limitation, which is related to the first two, is that it does not make optimal use of all of the data points before the last one; that is, it ignores the "trajectory" of how the subject was improving or getting worse. Bad as these limitations are, the pale in comparison to one other – LOCF should *never* be used when the goal of therapy is to slow a decline in function. For example, the so-called memory-enhancing drugs are meant to slow the cognitive decline in Alzheimer's disease. If a patient drops out of the study early, the worst possible thing to do is to carry forward his or her values, because that assumes no further decline will occur, which is nonsensical. This drawback, though, hasn't stopped people from using LOCF or the Food and Drug Administration from approving it (e.g., Rogers et al., 1998). From the drug manufacturer's perspective, the ideal trial would be one where all of the patients drop out early and the researchers used LOCF.

A more optimal way of dealing with dropouts in longitudinal studies is a class of statistics with many names: growth curve analysis, random effects modelling, structured covariance matrix analysis, hierarchical regression modelling, and the like (Norman & Streiner, 2008). However, the first two terms – growth curve analysis and random effects modelling – are perhaps the most descriptive when used for analysing data from dropouts. "Growth curve" analysis is so called because it fits a line through the existing data points for each subject individually. If there are three follow-up visits (the minimum number for this type of analysis), we can derive the parameters for a straight line; with four data points, we can fit a quadratic line; and with five points, we can fit a cubic one. An added advantage is that these points do not have to be consecutive. If a patient misses one or two appointments in the middle, it will simply limit the complexity of the curve that can be fitted, and we do not have to use the imputation methods we discussed earlier. The term "random effects" derives from the fact that, when we usually fit a regression line to some data, we assume that the parameters (the intercept and slopes) are "fixed," that is, the same for all of the subjects. In a random effects model, we allow them to differ for each person. This means that we do not expect that the curves for people who drop out will be the same as for people who complete the study. We already suspect that they may differ, and this allows us to model those differences and account for them in the analysis.

The major disadvantage at this time is that random effects requires specialized software and more than just a passing knowledge of statistics (although statisticians see this as a definite plus, ensuring their continued employment for at least a few more years). It also cannot deal with situations where people drop out of a study because of a dramatic worsening of their condition or a sudden increase in side effects after their last visit (nor, for that matter, can any other procedure, other than asking the person). For longitudinal data, however, it makes fewer unrealistic assumptions than the LOCF and better use of the existing data.

Summary

As long as researchers use real people as subjects, there will be problems with missing data. We cannot ignore them; even replacing subjects or eliminating them from the analysis means that we have made a decision about how they should be treated, and these are probably the worst of all the alternatives. When we have cross-sectional data (for example, demographic and background variables or only one outcome measurement time), replacement of missing values with the group mean preserves the estimate of the mean, but results in an underestimate of the SD, a CI that is too narrow, and an increased probability of a Type I error. A regression equation that estimates the missing values is slightly better and can be improved further if some error is artificially added to the imputed value. The best alternative is to use multiple imputation, which gives more accurate estimates of the mean and SD, even when 20% to 30% or more of the data are missing. For longitudinal follow-up measures, LOCF is better than eliminating the subject from the analysis, but some of the assumptions it makes about the missing data are unwarranted. This can bias the results, either in favour of or against the hypothesis, depending on the nature of the outcome and the group membership of the subjects with missing values. It should never be used if the aim of the intervention is to slow a decline rather than to improve functioning. A preferred strategy is to use growth curve analysis, which makes optimal use of the existing data, can handle data points that are missing in the middle, and assumes that the best predictor of future behaviour is past behaviour.

Let me end on a note of caution, though. The wider availability of these new and powerful imputation techniques should not blind us to the fact that the best way of dealing with missing data is not to have them in the first place. Good research methodology includes doing everything possible to ensure that we have as complete follow-up as possible. These imputation methods should be used only when everything else has failed and should not be seen as an excuse to let subjects slip through our fingers.

REFERENCES

Allison, P.D. (2000). Multiple imputation for missing data: A cautionary tale. *Sociological Methods & Research, 28*(3), 301–309. http://dx.doi.org/10.1177/0049124100028003003

Honaker, J., King, G., & Blackwell, M. (n.d.). *Amelia II: A program for missing data.* Available at: http://GKing.Harvard.edu/amelia/

Kim, J.O., & Curry, J. (1977). The treatment of missing data in multivariate analysis. *Sociological Methods & Research, 6*(2), 215–240. http://dx.doi.org/10.1177/004912417700600206

Little, R.J., & Rubin, D.B. (1987). *Statistical analysis with missing data.* New York: Wiley.

Norman, G.R., & Streiner, D.L. (2008). *Biostatistics: The bare essentials.* (3rd ed.). Shelton, CT: PMPH USA.

North American Symptomatic Carotid Endarterectomy Trial Collaborators (1991, Aug 15). Beneficial effect of carotid endarterectomy in symptomatic patients with high-grade carotid stenosis. *New England Journal of Medicine, 325*(7), 445–453. http://dx.doi.org/10.1056/NEJM199108153250701 Medline:1852179

Rogers, S.L., Farlow, M.R., Doody, R.S., Mohs, R., Friedhoff, L.T., & Donepezil Study Group. (1998, Jan). A 24-week, double-blind, placebo-controlled trial of donepezil in patients with Alzheimer's disease. *Neurology, 50*(1), 136–145. Medline:9443470

Rubin, D. (1987). *Multiple imputation for nonresponse in surveys.* New York: Wiley.

Schafer, J.L. (n.d.). *NORM: Multiple imputation of incomplete multivariate data under normal model, Version 2.* Available at: http://stat.psu.edu/~jls/misoftwa.html

Statistical Software Solutions (n.d.). *SOLAS for missing data analysis. Version 1.1.* Available at: http://www.statistical-solutions-software.com/products-page/solas-for-missing-data-analysis/

Streiner, D.L. (1990, Oct). Sample size and power in psychiatric research. *Canadian Journal of Psychiatry, 35*(7), 616–620. Medline:2268843

Streiner, D.L. (1996, Oct). Maintaining standards: Differences between the standard deviation and standard error, and when to use each. *Canadian Journal of Psychiatry, 41*(8), 498–502. Medline:8899234

TO READ FURTHER

Little, R.J., & Rubin, D.B. (1987). *Statistical analysis with missing data.* New York: Wiley.

McKnight, P.E., McKnight, K.M., Sidani, S., & Figueredo, A.J. (2007). *Missing data: A gentle introduction*. New York: Guilford Press.

Rubin, D. (1987). *Multiple imputation for nonresponse in surveys*. New York: Wiley.

Schafer, J.L., & Graham, J.W. (2002, Jun). Missing data: Our view of the state of the art. *Psychological Methods, 7*(2), 147–177. http://dx.doi.org/10.1037/1082-989X.7.2.147 Medline:12090408

Sinharay, S., Stern, H.S., & Russell, D. (2001, Dec). The use of multiple imputation for the analysis of missing data. *Psychological Methods, 6*(4), 317–329. http://dx.doi.org/10.1037/1082-989X.6.4.317 Medline:11778675

9 An Introduction to Multivariate Statistics

DAVID L. STREINER, PH.D.

Canadian Journal of Psychiatry, 1993, *38*, 9–13

As research becomes more sophisticated, so do the statistical techniques that are used to analyse the results. Until recently, it was sufficient for researchers and those interested in research to be aware of procedures such as the *t*-test, analysis of variance (ANOVA), Pearson's chi-square test, or the correlation coefficient, which look at one or two variables at a time. (If you're unfamiliar with these and other tests mentioned in this chapter, you needn't worry about them now. There are non-technical descriptions of them in Norman & Streiner, 2003, and more detailed descriptions in Norman & Streiner, 2008.) However, it is now almost commonplace to find techniques such as factor analysis, discriminant function analysis, and multivariate ANOVA in papers. These techniques differ from the more widely known ones in that they can simultaneously examine a number of variables. In this paper, we will start to look at why these techniques are needed, what they can and cannot do, what the results mean, and some of their limitations. Let's start the discussion by exploring what we mean by "multivariate" and why these special techniques were developed.

The term *multivariate* in general simply means "many variables." In statistical jargon, however, it has a more specific meaning: many dependent variables (DV). In fact, to statisticians, any number of DVs greater than one is referred to as "many," so multivariate statistics are used whenever there is more than one DV. (This is why correlations are called "bivariate" rather than "multivariate"; neither variable is considered to be a dependent variable.) For example, if we did a study to determine whether or not the combination of cognitive behaviour therapy (CBT) and tricyclic antidepressants (TCAs) was more effective for treating patients with panic disorder than either treatment alone, we might design the following study. Patients would be randomly assigned either CBT or some form of attention placebo therapy. One-half of the patients in each of these groups would also receive either a TCA or a drug placebo. So, there would be four groups – CBT plus TCA, CBT plus drug placebo, therapy placebo plus TCA, and therapy placebo plus drug placebo. Our measure of outcome would be the number of panic attacks experienced during a one-week period, eight weeks after therapy began.

In this study, we are dealing with three variables: the presence or absence of CBT, drug or no drug, and the number of panic attacks. However, we would not need to use a multivariate test to analyse the results. Two of the variables – the presence or absence of the different treatments – are independent variables that we are manipulating to see their effects on panic attacks. Since there is only one outcome variable – the number of panic attacks – univariate statistics are sufficient (in this case, a 2 × 2 factorial ANOVA). If we were to add more DVs, such as a fear questionnaire or a depression inventory, then we would need to use some form of multivariate analysis.

The question that arises is why do we need a new class of statistical tests merely because we have more DVs? Why couldn't we simply run two or three ANOVAs, one for each of the outcomes? There are two reasons, which appear on the surface to be somewhat contradictory. First, if we used a number of univariate analyses, then the likelihood of finding a difference just by chance (a Type I or α-type error) increases to an unknown degree (the reason for which the amount is unknown will be explained in the next section). Second, it's possible that univariate analyses will not find statistically significant differences between the groups when they actually exist (a Type II or β-type error). How can these opposite effects come into play at the same time?

Advantages of Multivariate Statistics

Control over the Type I Error Rate

We'll start off by looking at the greater probability of a Type I (or α) error. This is the probability of finding a statistically significant result, given that the null hypothesis is correct (that is, there is no difference between the groups; this is explained in greater depth elsewhere:

Table 9.1 The eight possible outcomes, and their probabilities, of three tests with an α level of 5%

Panic attacks*	Fear*	Depression*	Probability
D	D	D	(0.05) × (0.05) × (0.05) = 0.000125
D	D	N	(0.05) × (0.05) × (0.95) = 0.002375
D	N	D	(0.05) × (0.95) × (0.05) = 0.002375
D	N	N	(0.05) × (0.95) × (0.95) = 0.045125
N	D	D	(0.95) × (0.05) × (0.05) = 0.002375
N	D	N	(0.95) × (0.05) × (0.95) = 0.045125
N	N	D	(0.95) × (0.95) × (0.05) = 0.045125
N	N	N	(0.95) × (0.95) × (0.95) = 0.857375

*D = significant difference; N = no difference.

Streiner, 1990, and Chapter 4). If we set α at 0.05, then this will occur 5% of the time. Now let's assume that the null hypothesis is correct, and that we have three DVs: panic attacks, a fear questionnaire, and a depression inventory. Each has a 5% chance of a Type I error and a 95% chance of yielding the correct result (no between-group difference). Thus, there are eight possible outcome combinations of true findings (there is no difference) and false findings (there is a difference), which are shown in Table 9.1.

To determine the probability of any test being statistically significant, we would add up the probabilities of all the lines that have at least one D (significant difference). But there's a short cut: because the sum of all eight lines has to be 1.0 (indicating that there is a 100% probability that one of these alternatives will occur), it is easier to subtract the value of the one line with no Ds (0.8574) from 1.0, yielding 0.1424. What we did was to turn things around and say that the probability of at least one Type I error is the complement of no Type I errors. We can write this as

$$Pr \text{ (at least one Type I error)} = 1 - Pr \text{ (no errors)}, \qquad [1]$$

where Pr means the probability. In our example:

$$Pr \text{ (at least one Type I error)} = (1.0 - 0.95^3) = 0.1424. \qquad [2]$$

If we had five DVs, then there would be a $(1.0 - 0.95^5) = 0.2262$ chance of at least one result being significant by chance alone.

This would be true if all of the DVs were completely independent, that is, if each one correlated about 0.0 with every other one. However, because all of the tests are correlated to varying degrees, then we have no idea what our Type I error rate would be. The result is that if we had k DVs, our nominal Type I error rate would be somewhere between 5% and $(1 - 0.95^k)\%$, but exactly where is unknown. (If you're a clinician, remember this lesson well – it also applies to diagnostic tests. Run five tests on a perfectly healthy person, and there's a 23% chance that one of the tests will yield a result outside the normal range.)

A number of techniques have been developed that try to keep the level at 0.05, such as the Bonferroni inequality (Pocock, Geller, & Tsiatis, 1987). However, all of these procedures are approximations, at best, and the Bonferroni correction itself is overly conservative, yielding a nominal α level of much less than 5%. However, multivariate procedures are designed so that the Type I error rate remains at 0.05, irrespective of the number of DVs. So, the first raison d'être of multivariate statistics is to prevent inflation of the study's nominal α level.

Detection of Patterns among Dependent Variables

The second reason that multivariate statistics are required is that they can find relationships that are not apparent when the DVs are analysed individually; that is, they can look at the patterns among the variables. Again, let's use an example to illustrate the points. For the sake of simplicity, we will consider just two groups – a treatment group and a control group, each with 20 subjects; and two DVs – scores on a depression inventory and on a fear questionnaire. The raw (fictitious) data are given in Table 9.2.

On a simple examination of the means, it appears as if the groups are quite similar. In fact, if we were to plot the distributions of scores for each of the variables, as we have done in Figure 9.1, it is apparent that there is considerable overlap between the two groups.

We can go further and run two *t*-tests (even though we have just said that we shouldn't). Not surprisingly, neither one even approaches statistical significance. To milk these data as much as we possibly can, we could correlate each variable with the grouping variable (1 for the treatment group, 2 for the control). We would find a correlation of −0.12 for the fear questionnaire and 0.10 for the depression inventory; these values don't statistically differ from zero. So, we would conclude from

Table 9.2 Data for two variables for two groups

	Treatment group		Control group	
	Fear	Depression	Fear	Depression
	9	18	8	24
	12	23	10	23
	9	22	12	26
	15	24	9	28
	13	25	12	30
	16	28	13	33
	11	27	16	32
	19	32	18	33
	15	33	15	34
	12	32	19	38
	21	35	16	39
	17	36	13	37
	15	40	19	40
	23	42	16	42
	21	45	23	47
	19	44	19	46
	25	46	18	45
	19	48	21	48
	23	52	18	49
	26	54	23	50
Mean	17.00	35.3	15.90	37.20
SD	5.15	10.64	4.36	8.58

Fig. 9.1 Distributions of anxiety and depression scores for the two groups separately

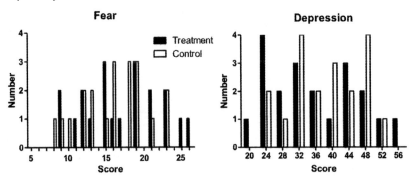

Fig. 9.2 Scatter plot of anxiety and depression scores for the two groups together

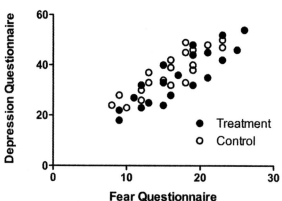

all of our univariate analyses that the treatment did not have an effect on our two outcomes.

Now, let's analyse the data properly, using one multivariate analysis of variance (MANOVA). We would find that the Group effect (that is, treatment versus control) is statistically significant ($p = 0.04$). Figure 9.2, which is a scatterplot of the two variables, helps explain why the univariate tests were not significant, but the multivariate one was. Although there is some overlap between the treatment and control data points, there is, in fact, a difference in terms of where they are located; the treatment group tends to be higher on the fear questionnaire and lower on the depression scale than the control group. We can confirm this by comparing the means of the two groups for these variables. The MANOVA detected that the pattern of the scores is different for the two groups. The univariate tests could not "see" this pattern, since, by definition, they look at the results one variable at a time. The second advantage of multivariate tests, then, is that they can detect differences between or among groups in terms of the patterns of the DVs, while univariate statistics cannot.

Drawbacks of Multivariate Statistics

Needless to say, the added advantages of multivariate statistics come at a cost. These are (1) greater complexity, (2) decreased power in some situations, (3) the availability of many ways of analysing the same data, and (4) ambiguity in the allocation of shared variance. We will discuss each of these points in turn.

Increased Complexity

Many univariate tests can be worked out on the back of an envelope or with a simple hand calculator, using nothing more than the four basic arithmetic operations – addition, subtraction, multiplication, and division (or, as Lewis Carroll called them, ambition, distraction, uglification, and derision). This is not the case with multivariate statistics, all of which require a more complex form of mathematics called matrix algebra. Before the days of computers, it was not unusual for graduate students to labour all summer performing one factor analysis, with no guarantee that they had not made some simple mistake in calculation somewhere along the way.

Computers have taken care of this portion of the work. However, there is still the problem that, because multivariate statistics are dealing with a number of DVs simultaneously, the level of complexity of the results increases considerably. For example, one of the assumptions underlying an ANOVA is that all of the groups have comparable variances. Its multivariate analogue, the MANOVA, differs in the following ways: first, an assumption that all of the variables have similar variances across groups; second, an added assumption that the relationships among the variables (similar to their correlations) are equivalent from one group to the next (that is, the pattern of correlations among the variables is the same from one group to another). On the interpretation side, continuing with the MANOVA example, there is an overall test of significance, which takes into account all of the variables and all of the groups. If the result is significant, we now have to perform an ANOVA on each variable, to see if any of them is individually significant. If so, these ANOVAs must in turn be followed up with other tests to see which group differences are responsible. Consequently, it is not unusual for the output from a multivariate analysis to run into dozens of pages.

Power

Power is the ability of a statistical test to detect a difference when that difference actually exists. It is defined as $(1 - \beta)$, which means that it is the complement of the Type II error (Streiner, 1990; see Chapter 4).

The answer to the question "are multivariate tests more or less powerful than univariate tests?" is "yes." That is, under some circumstances, multivariate analyses are more powerful, while under other conditions, they are less powerful. Unfortunately, it is often difficult to know ahead of time which they will be. In the univariate case, power is a function of the Type I and II error rates, the sample size, and the effect size, which also play a role in the multivariate situation; however, the number of DVs and the correlations among them also affect the power. Because of the large number of factors that affect the power, the unfortunate situation is that, at the present time, we can calculate it a priori for only a limited number of multivariate tests and, even then, only in some situations (Stevens, 1980).

Alternative Approaches

In the univariate realm, a given set of data can usually best be analysed with one specific statistical technique. For example, if we were comparing the age of onset of schizophrenics with positive symptoms versus those with negative symptoms, we would use a *t*-test; to study the relationship between the severity of the symptoms and length of time in hospital, we would run a correlation. With multivariate statistics, however, we often have a number of possible methods to examine the same data. In most cases, the various techniques yield comparable results, but this is not always the case. For example, if we had two groups and five DVs, we could analyse the data using a MANOVA, a discriminant function analysis, or a logistic regression approach. The first two methods would produce identical results, but the third might not, since it makes different assumptions about the data.

Furthermore, once a specific approach is chosen, there are many steps along the way where the data analyst must choose from different alternatives, depending on assumptions he or she is making about the data. So, even if two researchers decide that the appropriate method to use on a data set is a technique called factor analysis, they may differ in their selection of the exact procedures to be used at each step (see Chapter 10). In the end, it's possible that they could reach very different conclusions about the nature of the data, and there are few criteria we can use to say that one method is more valid than the other.

We need to consider the implications of having many possible methods. First, with multivariate tests, the user must be more aware of the underlying assumptions than is necessary with univariate statistics.

Second, it sometimes makes sense to analyse the data in two or three ways, not so much to select the test that leads to significance (and perhaps a publication), but to see if any difference in findings may temper our conclusions. Last, readers must be somewhat cautious in accepting the results of multivariate procedures and should look for justification of the approach taken.

Assignment of Shared Variance

Let's assume we are interested in studying the predictors of long-term compliance with lithium therapy in patients with a bipolar disorder. To keep the study simple, we will start off by looking at only one predictor variable: the number of previous episodes. If we found a correlation of 0.50 between the number of previous episodes and an index of compliance (such as the proportion of pills taken), we could say that 25% (that is, 0.50^2) of the variance between patients' compliance scores is explained by the number of episodes each patient has had.[1]

For the next step, we will add a second predictor variable: age. If the correlation between compliance and the two variables together is now 0.60, then we have explained 36% (0.60^2) of the variance. Can we say that 25% is due to the number of episodes and the other 11% is due to age? The answer is "no." Age and number of episodes are correlated, in addition to being correlated with compliance, as in Figure 9.3.

The amount of variance in compliance explained by the number of episodes is the overlap between the compliance and episodes circles (the areas labelled A and B in Figure 9.3). Similarly, the variance in compliance explained by age is the area enclosed by B and C; that is, the area in common for the compliance and age circles. The problem is area B, which is "claimed" by each of the two predictor variables. The overlap between the age and episodes circles is the result of the correlation between them (that is, if age and episodes correlated 0.0, there would be no overlap between their respective circles, and area B would disappear, whereas a higher correlation would result in

---

1 Any set of scores will show some degree of variability from one subject to the next. The amount of this variability can be expressed by a number called the variance (which is the square of the standard deviation). *Variance explained* is the proportion of variance that can be attributed to, or is caused by, another variable. In this example, 25% of the variability among patients' compliance scores is due to the number of previous episodes; therefore, 75% is unexplained and due to other factors.

Fig. 9.3 Illustration of shared variance

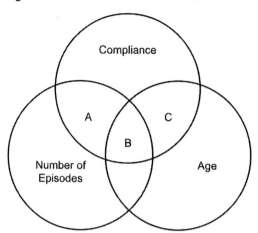

a greater degree of overlap). Which predictor variable should be "credited" with this variance?

There are a number of solutions. First, the shared variance could be assigned to neither variable. That is, we would say that number of episodes accounts for the variance in A and age for the variance in C; when both variables are considered together, they explain the variance in A, B, and C. A second approach would be to divide the shared variance in proportion to the variance explained by each variable. Yet a third possibility would be to determine which variable is the better predictor and then "give" the shared variance to that variable.

Needless to say, while all of these approaches account for the same amount of variance in total, they can lead to very different interpretations of the results. If, say, number of episodes correlated 0.50 with compliance and age correlated 0.49, then the first two techniques – crediting neither variable or dividing the variance proportionately – would lead to the conclusion that both variables contribute approximately equally. The technique of giving all the shared variance to the variable that individually accounts for most of the variance is the one used by "stepwise" or "hierarchical" solutions (terms we will explain in greater depth in a later chapter; see Chapter 11). In this case, the approach would result in assigning the variance in B to number of episodes, since that variable accounts for 25% of the variance, whereas age explains "only" 24%. This could lead the naïve user to believe that number of episodes is far more important than age, when, in fact, there is little difference between them. However, this approach would be particularly useful if we were trying to find the smallest number of predictor variables and eliminate redundant ones. Thus, there is no "correct" answer to how shared variance should be apportioned; it is dependent upon how and why the statistics will be used.

Summary

Multivariate procedures are far more complicated than univariate ones. This complexity and the availability of different ways of answering the same question put greater demands on users and require more sophistication from those who analyse their data using these techniques and those who read the results of the studies. Counterbalancing this, however, are the many advantages that multivariate statistics offer, primarily the ability to see relationships among variables, which would not be apparent using the simpler univariate procedures.

ACKNOWLEDGMENT

The author wishes to express his deep appreciation to Dr. Marilyn Craven for her excellent suggestions in the preparation of this manuscript.

REFERENCES

Norman, G.R., & Streiner, D.L. (2003). *PDQ statistics*. (3rd ed.). Shelton, CT: PMPH USA.

Norman, G.R., & Streiner, D.L. (2008). *Biostatistics: The bare essentials*. (3rd ed.). Shelton, CT: PMPH USA.

Pocock, S.J., Geller, N.L., & Tsiatis, A.A. (1987, Sep). The analysis of multiple endpoints in clinical trials. *Biometrics, 43*(3), 487–498. http://dx.doi.org/10.2307/2531989 Medline:3663814

Stevens, J. (1980). Power of the multivariate analysis of variance tests. *Psychological Bulletin, 88*(3), 728–737. http://dx.doi.org/10.1037/0033-2909.88.3.728

Streiner, D.L. (1990, Oct). Sample size and power in psychiatric research. *Canadian Journal of Psychiatry, 35*(7), 616–620. Medline:2268843

TO READ FURTHER

Grimm, L.G., & Yarnold, P.R. (1995). *Reading and understanding multivariate statistics*. Washington: American Psychological Association Press.
Grimm, L.G., & Yarnold, P.R. (2000). *Reading and understanding more multivariate statistics*. Washington: American Psychological Association Press.
Norman, G.R., & Streiner, D.L. (2008). *Biostatistics: The bare essentials*. (3rd ed.). Shelton, CT: PMPH USA.
Tabachnick, B.G., & Fidell, L.S. (2007). *Using multivariate statistics*. (5th ed.). Boston: Allyn & Bacon.

10 Figuring Out Factors: The Use and Misuse of Factor Analysis

DAVID L. STREINER, PH.D.

Canadian Journal of Psychiatry, 1994, *39*, 135–140

In a previous chapter (Streiner, 1993; see Chapter 9), we explored the rationale behind multivariate statistical procedures in general. This chapter will take a closer look at what is probably the most widely used of these techniques: factor analysis. To provide a context, imagine that we are conducting a study to examine more closely the phenomenology of people diagnosed as borderline personality disorders. We cast our net of possible variables fairly widely, since we're not sure ahead of time which ones best describe these patients. In the end, we come up with the 15 variables listed in Table 10.1. Some reflect demographic characteristics, some are ratings completed by the therapists, and yet others are paper-and-pencil tests filled out by the patients themselves.

One question that we can ask is whether we are measuring 15 different attributes or if there is a smaller number of underlying traits that could account for the values a person has for these variables. Simply looking at the names of the variables, we might suspect a priori that some of them will be related; for example, therapist-rated and self-reported depression would likely go together and both may also be correlated with morale. Similarly, age at first contact, age at first hospitalization, and number of admissions all may be related, but none of them would necessarily be correlated with the depression variables.

One approach to determining the number of underlying factors would simply be to correlate all these variables and look for patterns: are there some groups of variables that have a high correlation with each other and low correlations with the other variables? If we had

Table 10.1 Variables used in the study*

Variable	Abbreviation	How measured
Age at first psychiatric contact	AGE1CONT	Record
Age at first hospitalization	AGE1HOSP	Record
Number of psychiatric admissions	NOADMISS	Demographic
Self-rated depression	SELFDEPR	Questionnaire
Therapist-rated depression	TPSTDEPR	Questionnaire
Impaired morale	MORALE	Questionnaire
Number of suicidal attempts	SUICIDE	Self-report
Extent of social network[†]	SOCLNETW	Questionnaire
Impulsivity	IMPULSIV	Questionnaire
Tolerance for isolation[†]	ISOLATIN	Questionnaire
Therapist rating of anger	ANGER	Record
Number of police contacts	POLICE	Questionnaire
Stability of relations[†]	STABRELT	Questionnaire
Affective stability[†]	AFECSTAB	Questionnaire
Therapist rating of self-mutilation	MUTILATE	Questionnaire

*None of these variables refers to actual scales.
[†]Higher scores reflect greater pathology.

only a few measures, this might be feasible. However, with 15 variables, relying on "eyeball" judgments may be quite difficult. To begin with, there are a large number of correlations. The number of unique correlations is $[n \times (n - 1)/2]$, where n is the number of variables. In this case, it is $15 \times (14)/2 = 105$. Some of these may behave as we would like them to: (i) to correlate close to $+ 1.00$ or -1.00 with a few of the variables; and (ii) to hover around 0.00 with the remaining ones. However, this is rarely the case. It is more common for the correlations to be within a narrower range, meaning that it is harder to spot variables that are closely related and those that may be unrelated or related to a lesser degree.

What we need is a statistical method that can assess which variables "hang together" and how different this group of variables is from other sets. The technique to do this is called factor analysis. Now it's called *exploratory* factor analysis, or EFA, to differentiate it from another variant, called confirmatory factor analysis, or CFA, which we'll discuss in Chapter 17. (In contrast to psychoanalysis, you do not have to undergo personal factor analysis before you can use this technique.) To understand what it does and why, it's necessary to take a short detour and discuss what is meant by the term "factor." Factor is the statistical jargon for what psychologists refer to as a *hypothetical construct*. It may not seem as if we've made much progress, replacing one incomprehensible term with another. However, psychologists and psychiatrists are more likely to have encountered the latter phrase within the context of personality theory, but not to have recognized the fact that they are similar concepts. Attributes such as depression, anxiety, or intelligence are called hypothetical constructs because we cannot see or measure them directly. What we observe are discrete signs or symptoms, which we assume are manifestations of the construct. That is, we do not *see* "depression"; we may note that the patient has lost her appetite, shows less interest in sex, has sleep maintenance problems, is pessimistic about things getting better in the future, has thoughts of suicide; and so on. Our theory of psychopathology then leads us to say that these symptoms occur together because all reflect the underlying problem, that of depression. Therefore, depression is used as a hypothetical construct to account for the association among these variables and at the same time to explain why they would not necessarily be correlated with other variables such as social avoidance or compulsivity.

In the same way, the purpose of factor analysis is to determine if a small number of underlying factors can explain the pattern of scores obtained on a battery of tests. Returning to our example, we may expect that some of the variables together would reflect mood instability, others would tap problems with interpersonal relationships and self-image, and others might indicate difficulties in expressing anger. If we are correct (that is, if our conceptualization of the borderline disorder is accurate and if our scales indeed measure what we think they do), then each of these underlying problems would show up as a factor. Similarly, test developers use factor analysis to see if the items on one specific test cluster together in meaningful ways. So, for example, a test of anxiety should have one set of items tapping signs of autonomic hyperactivity, another group reflecting apprehensive expectations, a third indicating motor tension, and so on.

Figure 10.1 shows a simplified view of what we've been discussing. Here, we have just two factors (A and B) and four variables. In this highly idealized picture, variables one and two are associated with Factor A and the values of variables three and four are determined by Factor B. The absence of any arrows between Factor A and the bottom two variables and between Factor B and the top two indicates that each variable can be accounted for by one and only one factor; we will see later what happens when we relax this condition.

Fig. 10.1 Two factors, each consisting of two variables

Factor   Variable   Uniqueness

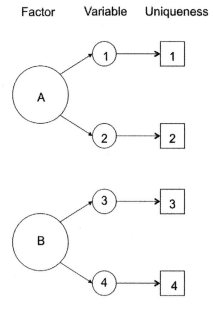

If the values of the variables (be they scales or individual items) are determined solely by the factors, then variables one and two should be identical, as would be three and four, and there would be no reason to include the second variable for each factor. However, hopelessness and depression, for example, are related but not identical concepts. Although scales tapping these traits would be correlated relatively strongly (which is a manifestation of the factor underlying both of them), each scale would also tap something unique that the other scale misses. This is what is meant by the circles and boxes in Figure 10.1; each variable is composed of two parts – what it has in common with all of the other variables associated with the factor (the *communality*) and what is unique to that particular variable (its *uniqueness*).

The first step of factor analysis consists of deriving these factors. Strictly speaking, this phase is referred to as Principal Components Analysis (PCA). However, since the primary use of PCA nowadays is as the first step in factor analysis, most people use the latter term to describe the entire procedure. If we start out with 15 variables, we'll initially end up with 15 factors. Each factor looks like a multiple regression equation (Norman & Streiner, 2003) with each variable (X_1, X_2, ... X_{15}) multiplied by some weight (w_1 through w_{15}); so, for Factor 1:

$$F_1 = w_1 X_1 + w_2 X_2 + \cdots + w_{15} X_{15}. \qquad [1]$$

There is a similar equation for each of the other 14 factors; they differ from one another in the fact that each equation uses a different set of weights. Again, it may not seem as if we've come very far; we've simply replaced 15 (readily understandable) variables with 15 (much harder to interpret) factors.

The potential gain comes from the manner in which these 15 equations were derived and their relationship to one another. The weights for the first factor were selected so that this factor explains (or accounts for) the most variance among the scores. The second factor is then derived so that it explains the maximum amount of the remaining variance, and so on through to the last factor, which explains the least amount of variance. The hope is that the first few factors explain a significant proportion of the total variance and the remaining factors account for relatively little variance. Thus, if we drop the last 10 or so factors, we may sacrifice only a small amount of the variance we are able to explain.

Introducing a bit more statistical jargon: Factor 1 will have the largest *eigenvalue*, Factor 2 the next largest, and Factor 15 the smallest. Very roughly, the eigenvalue is a measure of the variance accounted for by that factor, and it can be thought of as the contribution of the factor. The total amount of variance in the data set is equal to the number of variables. So, if the eigenvalue of the first factor turns out to be 5, it will account for $5/15 = 33\%$ of all of the variance.

The other important characteristic about the factors is that they are uncorrelated (the statistical term is *orthogonal*). That is, a person's score on one factor is independent of his or her score on the other factors. This means that, once we figure out what the various factors represent (a point that we will discuss shortly), then we are able to talk about a person's score on one factor without having to take into account his or her scores on the other ones.

At this point, the first, and perhaps most important, issue the factor analyst has to confront is how many of the factors to retain and how many can be discarded without sacrificing too much in explanatory ability. Almost all computer programs by default use the Kaiser criterion, which is also known as the eigenvalue-one rule (named after

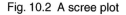

Fig. 10.2 A scree plot

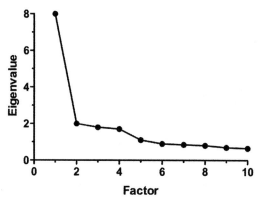

the statistician, Henry Kaiser, not the German leader with the funny pointed helmet). It is based on the belief that (1) since each variable adds 1 to the total amount of variance, and (2) since we want to end up with fewer factors than variables, then (3) each factor should explain at least as much variance as a single variable. Although this is by far the most commonly used criterion, it is not necessarily the best one. In many cases, it results in too many factors being retained – too many in the sense that, if the study were replicated with a new group of subjects, the first few retained factors may be the same both times, but the weaker ones (those with eigenvalues just over 1) would likely differ from one replication to the next. Also, this arbitrary cut-off point means that a factor with an eigenvalue of 1.01 will be retained, but one whose eigenvalue is 0.99 will be dropped. In fact, both of these values are equivalent, and the difference is likely due simply to sampling error.

Another criterion for determining how many factors to keep is called the *scree test*. Here, the eigenvalues for each factor are plotted in order on a graph, and we look for a break in the distribution where the line flattens out, as in Figure 10.2. Ignoring the break after the first factor (we will see later why it is almost always there), we see that the next one comes after the fourth factor, so we would retain the first four factors and discard the remaining ones. Had we used the eigenvalue-one criterion, we would have kept the fifth factor, too.

Retaining one extra factor may not appear to make much of a difference, but it may, in fact, drastically alter how we would interpret the factors. Making life somewhat more difficult for us, there are no accepted mathematical tests to determine where the break is. For this reason, we often have to run the computer program twice: once to produce the scree plot and then, after using our calibrated eyeball to determine how many factors there are, a second time where we limit the number of factors.

Recently, a number of other approaches have been proposed, such as parallel analysis (Hayton, Allen, & Scarpello, 2004) and the MAP test (Velicer & Jackson, 1990). However, these methods aren't widely used yet, because they haven't been implemented in the most commonly used computer programs.

At this point, the computer will produce a *factor-loading matrix*, similar to the one in Table 10.2. Each row reflects one of the variables, and each column represents one of the four factors. In keeping with how the factors were derived, Factor 1 has the highest eigenvalue and Factor 4 the lowest of the retained factors. The numbers inside the table are the factor loadings themselves; they can be thought of as Pearson correlations, showing the strength of the relationship between a variable and a factor. (For the technically minded, the squared loadings in each column will sum to the eigenvalue for that factor; the sum of the squared loadings in each row will yield the communality of the variable.) Like correlations, factor loadings can range between +1.0 and −1.0. Now, what does this table tell us?

First, if we adopt the somewhat arbitrary rule of looking only at loadings with absolute values greater than 0.30, we see that all of the variables load on the first factor. This result is quite common when we are dealing with personality variables; people tend to be consistent, and their responses on one scale are often correlated with those on other scales. Depending on your point of view and what you want to find out from your study, this can be seen either as showing that there is a general factor which permeates everything the person does, or it is a "garbage" factor, which tells you nothing that you didn't know before. (This debate is still raging in the area of intelligence, for example: is there one general factor that influences all aspects of intelligent behaviour or are there a number of different uncorrelated traits?) This correlation among variables also explains why the scree plot showed a definite break after the first factor, since it is far stronger than the other factors. The second point that emerges is that most of the loadings are of moderate size; few are close to 1 (or −1) or 0.

The third thing this table tells us is that many of the variables are factorially complex in that they load on more than one factor. Variable 1, for

Table 10.2 Initial factor-loading matrix

Variable	Factor			
	1	2	3	4
AGE1CONT	0.536	0.542	−0.228	−0.429
AGE1HOSP	0.552	0.557	−0.346	0.024
NOADMISS	0.648	0.177	−0.379	0.199
SELFDEPR	0.693	−0.457	0.104	−0.236
TPSTDEPR	0.710	−0.427	−0.052	−0.319
MORALE	0.708	−0.338	−0.021	−0.259
SUICIDE	0.694	−0.104	−0.058	0.205
SOCLNETW	0.690	0.194	−0.069	−0.243
IMPULSIV	0.447	0.049	0.584	−0.014
ISOLATIN	0.724	−0.284	−0.114	−0.095
ANGER	0.404	0.170	0.623	0.112
POLICE	0.523	0.303	0.465	0.020
STABRELT	0.448	−0.296	−0.068	0.605
AFECSTAB	0.584	−0.085	−0.177	0.531
MUTILATE	0.544	0.410	0.160	0.230

example, loads strongly on the first, second, and fourth factors. Mathematically, there is nothing wrong with this. However, factorial complexity makes it more difficult to understand what constructs are tapped by this variable and what each factor means. Last, factors 2 through 4 have both positive and negative loadings. Again, this is fine from a statistical viewpoint, but makes interpretation of the factor quite a bit harder, since it means that the factor is composed of high scores on some variables and low scores on others.

We can visualize these issues in the left side of Figure 10.3, which shows the 15 variables plotted against the first two unrotated factors. All four problems can be seen: (1) all of the variables load on Factor 1; (2) none of them is near the intercept or the extreme end (which would be the case if the loadings were near 0.0 or 1.0); (3) some of the variables are below the horizontal line, reflecting a negative loading on Factor 2; and (4) many of the variables have moderate loadings on both factors (they fall in the centre of the quadrant).

Now, what happens when we rotate the factors? By *rotation*, we mean that the axes are kept at right angles and turned in space. (We will see shortly that we don't have to keep them at right angles, that is, *orthogonal*, although it is the most commonly used approach.) Since we have four factors in this example, there are four axes, which are rotated in

Fig. 10.3 The 15 variables plotted against the unrotated and rotated factors

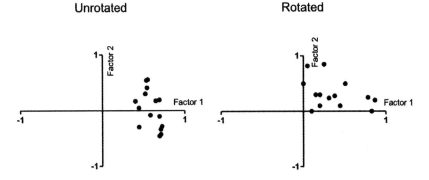

four-dimensional space. This does not make sense if we try to visualize the entire image at once, but we can do it mathematically without any difficulty. The factors are rotated in such a way that they are as close as possible to the points, each point representing one of the variables. The right side of Figure 10.3 shows the variables plotted against the first two rotated factors. (The pattern of points would look identical, offset only by the amount of the rotation, if we were dealing with only two factors. In fact, since we are dealing with four factors rotated simultaneously, graphing only two of them at a time distorts the picture to some degree.) With this manoeuvre, most of the problems disappear (they are not gone completely, since we're not considering the other two factors in this figure). Not all variables load on the first factor; the points are closer to the extremes; there are no significant negative loadings on Factor 2; and the variables seem to load on either the first or the second factor (or neither, if they load on Factors 3 or 4), but not both. This improvement is even more striking when we look at the rotated factor matrix, shown in Table 10.3. It differs from Table 10.2 in that it shows the loadings of each variable with the rotated factors, whereas Table 10.2 indicated the loadings with the unrotated ones. We have simplified the table by grouping the variables by the factor they load highest on, rank ordering them within the factor, and not printing out loadings that are less than 0.3 (most programs can do this for us).

Now it is clearer what the factors represent. The first appears to be a depressed mood factor, consisting of patient- and therapist-rated depression, impaired morale, number of admissions, limited social network, number of suicide attempts, and, to a lesser degree, social isolation. We

Table 10.3 Rotated loading matrix

Variable	Factor			
	1	2	3	4
TPSTDEPR	0.867			
SELFDEPR	0.829			
MORALE	0.784			
AGE1CONT		0.847		
AGEIHOSP		0.819		
NOADMISS	0.508			
STABRELT			0.778	
AFECSTAB			0.762	
ISOLATIN	0.311		0.688	
SOCLNETW	0.446		0.560	
ANGER				0.760
POLICE				0.699

can go through the other factors in the same way, trying to determine what construct ties the variables together. The naming of the factors is subjective, and another person, looking at the same table, may come up with a different set of labels. Ideally, though, the labels should represent similar constructs.

The table also shows that the rotation was not completely successful. Four of the variables load on two factors and one loads on three. We have a few choices we can make at this point. The easiest option is to simply assign a variable to whichever factor it loads highest on and ignore the fact that it also loads on other factors. This is done, in fact, if there is a large difference in the magnitude of the loadings, as in the case of the variable ISOLATIN (0.688 versus 0.311). When the loadings are more similar, for example, in NOADMISS (0.567 versus 0.508), we are deceiving ourselves, and perhaps misunderstanding the data, if we ignore the secondary loadings. Another option would be to simply drop that variable. This would probably be a wise choice for MUTILATE; it loads on three factors with almost equal strength, so we are not sure exactly what construct it is tapping. Dropping a variable is possible when there are three or more other variables that load on a factor. If dropping that variable means that only two variables define the factor, then it may be better to use the third option, that is, replace the variable with another that may perhaps tap the construct more directly. Thus, we may look to replace the scale used to measure SOCLNETW with a different index of social network.

Of course, this assumes that we are in a position such that we can repeat the study with new variables. Which option we take depends on the alternatives open to us: Can we replicate the study? Are there enough other variables defining the factors? How different are the loadings? And so on.

Orthogonal rotations are the most commonly used ones, for the reasons mentioned earlier; primarily that we can discuss each factor without regard to the others. However, it is often more realistic to assume that the factors themselves are correlated to some degree. Thus, a depression factor and a social isolation factor may be related, reflecting the fact that depressed mood can result in withdrawal from social contact, or vice versa. We can model this by using an *oblique* rotation, that is, not insisting that the factors remain orthogonal when we rotate them. The trade-off is between a more accurate reflection of the phenomenon versus greater difficulty in explaining the pattern of factor scores.

Although rotation is quite useful, it is somewhat controversial. The reason is that there are an infinite number of ways to rotate the axes, each of which yields a different factor matrix. Which rotation is "best" is a purely subjective judgment, based on our feeling about which one is most informative. Many traditional statisticians are uncomfortable with this lack of objectivity; they would prefer that any two people, starting out with the same data, always end up with identical conclusions. Those who use factor analysis, though, appreciate this subjective element and see it as a way of better understanding their data.

We have seen that we can use factor analysis to (1) search for underlying patterns among items or variables; (2) confirm a model (there are actually somewhat different programs that perform highly sophisticated *confirmatory factor analyses*; e.g., Loehlin, 1987; Streiner, 2006; see Chapter 17); and (3) look for variables that may be superfluous or may not perform as expected. A fourth use is to improve the ratio of subjects to variables. Most multivariate procedures require at least 10 subjects for every variable analysed. If we did a study that involved these 15 variables, plus another 20 or so lab tests, we would need over 350 subjects in order to use any of these tests, which likely is infeasible. However, we can now reduce the 15 variables to 4 factor scores, based on the factor analysis we just ran. If we run a factor analysis on the laboratory results, we may end up with a total of only 8 or 10 factor scores, rather than 35 raw scores, resulting in a proportionate reduction in the required sample size.

This chapter can give only a brief introduction to factor analysis. For those who want to delve into the topic in greater depth, look at the books listed below under "To Read Further." However, we will end with a series of recommendations which should be followed by anyone running a factor analysis or (if you are reading an article which used factor analysis), should have been used. These are presented somewhat dogmatically and inflexibly; as is the case in all multivariate procedures, though, the guiding motto is "It all depends." Norman and Streiner (2008) give justifications for these rules and the consequences if you ignore them.

Sample size. There should be an absolute minimum of five subjects per variable, with the proviso that there are at least 100 subjects. If there are fewer than 100, then the ratio should be closer to 10:1.

Eigenvalues. The eigenvalues of the retained factors must be reported. The sum of these eigenvalues should account for at least 50% of the variance. If this sum is not reported, you can figure it out yourself by remembering that the total variance is the number of items or variables.

Retention of factors. The criterion used to determine how many factors to retain must be given. If the eigenvalue-one test was used, there may be too many (and to complicate matters, sometimes too few) factors. The ideal procedure would be to replicate the factor analysis on another sample; barring that, the *scree test* is often a better criterion than the eigenvalue-one test, and parallel analysis and the MAP test are even better.

Rotation. If a rotation was performed, the type (for example, varimax, oblimin) should be specified.

Number of variables per factor. Each factor should be composed of a minimum of three variables; if there are fewer, the factor should be discarded or ignored.

Types of variable. Since the first step in factor analysis consists of calculating a matrix of correlations among all of the variables, then only interval or ratio data should be used. However, correlations are fairly robust (that is, they can tolerate deviations from normality), so even ordinal scales with at least 5 points can be included. However, unless fairly specialized and sophisticated techniques are used, dichotomous variables (true-false or yes-no) should never be factor analysed.

REFERENCES

Hayton, J.C., Allen, D.G., & Scarpello, V. (2004). Factor retention decisions in exploratory factor analysis: A tutorial on parallel analysis. *Organizational Research Methods, 7*(2), 191–205. http://dx.doi.org/10.1177/1094428104263675

Loehlin, J.C. (1987). *Latent variable models*. Hillsdale, NJ: Lawrence Erlbaum Associates.

Norman, G.R., & Streiner, D.L. (2003). *PDQ statistics*. (3rd ed.). Shelton, CT: PMPH USA.

Norman, G.R., & Streiner, D.L. (2008). *Biostatistics: The bare essentials*. (3rd ed.). Shelton, CT: PMPH USA.

Streiner, D.L. (1993, Feb). An introduction to multivariate statistics. *Canadian Journal of Psychiatry, 38*(1), 9–13. Medline:8448733

Streiner, D.L. (2006, Apr). Building a better model: An introduction to structural equation modelling. *Canadian Journal of Psychiatry, 51*(5), 317–324. Medline:16986821

Velicer, W.F., & Jackson, D.N. (1990). Component analysis versus common factor-analysis: Some further observations. *Multivariate Behavioral Research, 25*(1), 97–114. http://dx.doi.org/10.1207/s15327906mbr2501_12

TO READ FURTHER

Kim, J.-O., & Mueller, C.W. (1978). *Introduction to factor analysis: What it is and how to do it*. Beverly Hills: Sage.

Norman, G. R., & Streiner, D. L. (2008). *Biostatistics: The bare essentials*. (3rd ed.). Shelton, CT: PMPH USA. Chapter 19.

Weiss, D.J. (1970). Factor analysis and counseling research. *Journal of Counseling Psychology, 17*(5), 477–485. http://dx.doi.org/10.1037/h0029894

11 Regression in the Service of the Superego: The Dos and Don'ts of Stepwise Multiple Regression

DAVID L. STREINER, PH.D.

Canadian Journal of Psychiatry, 1994, 39, 191–196

When reading the "Results" section of a research paper, we often encounter a phrase like "a stepwise procedure was used," usually in the context of a multiple regression, a logistic regression, or a discriminant function analysis. This paper explores three questions: (1) What is meant by "stepwise" procedures? (2) Why are they used? and (3) When should and should they not be used?

To provide a context for our discussion, we'll use a study by Stewart and Cecutti (1993). They collected data on 548 pregnant women including, among other factors, whether or not they had been physically or sexually abused during pregnancy; the amount they smoked, drank, or used licit or illicit drugs; various demographic variables; and the results of some scales, such as the General Health Questionnaire (GHQ; Goldberg, 1972) and the Fetal Health Locus of Control scale (Labs & Wurtele, 1986). They used a linear regression (LR) to see if there was a relationship between the GHQ and a number of other variables. We'll explore how the results may differ when various stepwise procedures are used.

What Is Meant by "Stepwise"?

All types of regression boil down to solving an equation that looks like this one:

$$\check{Y} = \beta_0 + \beta_1 X_1 + \beta_2 X_2 + \cdots + \beta_k X_k + \varepsilon, \qquad [1]$$

Table 11.1 The independent variables and their correlation with GHQ

Variable	Abbreviation	Correlation
Age	AGE	−0.235
Number of cigarettes per day	NUMCIG	0.412
Use of prescription medication	RXMED	−0.279
Use of non-prescription medicine	NONRX	−0.245
Number of ounces of alcohol per week	ALCOHOL	0.226
Fetal Health Locus of Control – Powerful Others	FHLCPO	−0.211
Fetal Health Locus of Control – Chance	FHLCC	0.163
Fetal Health Locus of Control – Internal	FHLCI	−0.395
Education	EDUC	−0.240
Physical problems	PHYSPROB	−0.157
Emotional problems	EMOTPROB	−0.347
Healthy diet	DIET	0.283
Married/single	MARRIED	0.289

where the Xs are the independent or predictor variables, the βs (the Greek letter beta) are weights, and ε is the error term. In multiple regression Y is a continuous variable, such as the score on some scale, while in logistic regression and discriminant function analysis it is a categorical variable, such as group membership. In each case, the purpose of the technique is to find the best set of βs, where "best" is defined as the estimated value of Y for each person (written $\hat{Y}$ and pronounced "Y-hat," where the "hat" indicates that it is an estimate) that is closest to the actual value, Y. In the example being used, Y is the GHQ score, and the independent variables are listed in Table 11.1.

The equation can be solved in a number of ways. In the full rank (that is, non-stepwise) method, all of the variables are entered into the equation simultaneously; the results are shown in Table 11.2 (for now, we'll ignore the R^2 and adjusted R^2 at the bottom of the table).

There is one very important and often forgotten point about the βs: the fact that they are *partial* weights. That is, the β for the first variable gives us the contribution of AGE *over and above the contribution of all of the other variables*. In other words, it is the unique contribution of the woman's age on GHQ. The difficulty is that the β weights are hard to interpret once we have more than two predictor variables. If the variables are correlated (and they most often are in psychiatric research), then, taken together, the predictors may yield a high value of R (the multiple correlation), but each one's unique contribution may be quite low. We can see this when we compare Tables 11.1 and 11.2: a

Table 11.2 Results of the full-rank solution

Variable	β	t	p level
AGE	0.042	0.453	0.651
NUMCIG	0.161	1.710	0.089
RXMED	−0.125	1.606	0.110
NONRX	−0.038	0.478	0.634
ALCOHOL	0.013	0.168	0.867
FHLCPO	−0.151	1.792	0.075
FHLCC	0.040	0.498	0.616
FHLCI	−0.060	0.595	0.553
EDUC	−0.082	0.887	0.376
PHYSPROB	−0.038	0.509	0.611
EMOTPROB	−0.037	0.376	0.707
DIET	0.160	2.030	0.044
MARRIED	0.121	1.461	0.146

Note: Multiple $R = 0.533$; $R^2 = 0.284$; Adjusted $R^2 = 0.224$.

few variables correlate quite well with GHQ (for example, NUMCIG, FHLCI, and EMOTPROB), but only one variable is statistically significant (DIET). Overall, R is 0.533 (not great, but respectable). In fact, it is possible that no single variable is statistically significant, even though the independent variables are clearly related to the dependent variable. The higher the correlations among the predictors, the more likely it is for this to happen. So, just to reinforce the notion: the β weight and its associated significance level tells us about the unique contribution of a variable, once the contributions of the other variables are taken into account, not about how strongly it is associated with the dependent variable.

Another technique we can use to solve the equation is called *hierarchical regression*. In the most common variant of this approach, variables or groups of variables are entered in succeeding steps. The purpose of this technique is to "control" for the variables entering in earlier steps; that is, we now capitalize on the fact that the βs for subsequent variables will reflect their contributions after we have controlled for the previously entered ones. As an example, imagine that we want to examine whether alcohol abuse, on its own, is associated with a low score on the GHQ. If we suspect that alcohol consumption is related to the use of illicit drugs, then simply looking at drinking does not allow us to disentangle the effects of alcohol from the effects of abusing other substances. To control for this factor, we would enter the use of street drugs on the first step and only on the second step enter alcohol abuse as a predictor. Using the terminology of analysis of variance, drug use has been treated as a covariate, and we have looked at drinking after covarying it out. When we enter only the number of drinks per week into the equation, its β weight is 0.183, which is statistically significant; when we use street drugs as a covariate, the β weight for drinking falls to 0.063, which is much lower and not significant. Therefore, whereas we first would have said that drinking was significantly related to the GHQ score, we would now say that its contribution, independent of the effect of drug abuse, is relatively small.

In another example, Arthur, Garfinkel, and Irvine (1999) wanted to see if their new measure of hostility was related to the degree of coronary artery stenosis (it was). A clinician, though, may want to know whether or not it is worthwhile to administer the test, or whether or not the same information about stenosis can be gotten through routinely collected data. Here the hierarchy consisted of three steps: first, all demographic variables (for example, age, sex, smoking history); then the results from the cardiac workup; and finally the scores from the hostility test. The question is whether the scale added predictive power, after the demographic and cardiac variables were taken into account. (Of course, they could also have turned this question around and asked if the cardiac variables added anything after the less invasive hostility questionnaire was factored in.)

Another approach, called *forward stepwise regression*, allows the computer program to select the order in which the variables are selected. In this case, the program first chooses the one variable which best predicts GHQ; here, it was NUMCIG. At Step 2, it adds the variable which, in combination with NUMCIG, now best estimates GHQ; it was DIET. The third step, in an analogous manner, adds the variable which, along with NUMCIG and DIET, best predicts GHQ. This continues until (1) adding another variable does not improve the predictive power of the equation, or (2) all of the variables have been used. The results of running the analysis this way are shown in Table 11.3.

A variant of forward selection is called *backward selection*. Not surprisingly, it differs from forward selection in that it begins with all of the variables and then removes them, one at a time, until the next variable it would remove would produce an unacceptably large drop in predictive ability. The results of doing the calculations this way are slightly different from the forward method; the variable FHLCPO was

Table 11.3 Results of a forward-selection procedure

Variable	β	t	p level
NUMCIG	0.283	3.754	0.0002
DIET	0.165	2.345	0.0202
RXMED	−0.159	2.253	0.0256
MARRIED	0.149	2.042	0.0428

Note: Multiple $R = 0.501$; $R^2 = 0.251$; Adjusted $R^2 = 0.232$.

also included in the equation (that is, it showed a five-variable solution, with an R^2 of 0.268). Statisticians usually prefer to use forward rather than backward procedures, since there is less chance of an important variable being missed. In most cases, though, the results from these two types of solution are quite similar.

However, there is a potential flaw in these last two approaches. Using the example of forward selection, we have seen that, once NUMCIG was in the equation, the next variable added was DIET. Then, given the fact that these two variables were included, the next one entered was RXMED, followed by MARRIED (see Table 11.3). But these four variables may not necessarily be the best combination of any four variables. In Table 11.4, we show the four best of the 715 possible combinations of four variables and their associated multiple correlations. As can be seen, the combination of NUMCIG, DIET, RXMED, and FHLCI was only marginally better than the next one; the one chosen by the forward selection procedure actually ranked fourth, and other combinations were nearly as good as the first ranked solution. The reason that some of these combinations were not tried is that the stepwise approach is constrained after the first step to try only dyads which include the first variable entered and, after the second step, to try those triplets involving the first two variables, and so on.

There are two ways to avoid this trap. The first is called *all-subsets regression*, which was what we used to produce Table 11.4. The first step is the same as it is in the forward selection method. The second step, though, is not constrained by the results of the first; all combinations of two variables are tried. Similarly, the third step consists of all combinations of three variables at a time, and so on. The drawback is that it requires considerable computing time; if there are 8 predictor variables, then the first step would involve 8 possible solutions, the second step 28, and so on, for a total of 255. (In general, if there are p variables, then

Table 11.4 Multiple correlations for various combinations
of four predictor variables

Variables	R
NUMCIG + RXMED + FHLCI + DIET	0.5063
NUMCIG + RXMED + FHLCI + MARRIED	0.5055
NUMCIG + RXMED + EMOTPROB + DIET	0.5021
NUMCIG + RXMED + DIET + MARRIED	0.4960

there are $2^p - 1$ combinations). Computing power is not much of an issue now, with the ready availability of computers and efficient programs which do not try unpromising combinations, but be sure you have plenty of paper in the printer for the reams of output.

In addition to removing the constraints imposed by earlier calculations, the all-subsets approach has another advantage. For instance, it showed in this example that, while the variable NUMCIG was involved in all of the best equations, the other variables were not as consistent; FHLCI, for example, showed up in the best two equations, but then dropped out of the next two. This may serve as a warning signal that the first solution is not unique and one should not make pontifical and absolutist statements regarding the predictors of GHQ or of any variable in general.

The second way around the constraints imposed by the stepwise method is called *forward-backward selection*, which is what is usually implemented in computer programs. This method follows the general logic of the stepwise approach in terms of building on the results of the previous step. However, it adds an additional calculation at each step: seeing if any variables now in the equation can be removed without too much loss in predictive ability. So, for instance, after adding MARRIED to the equation, the program backtracks to see if the β weights for NUMCIG, DIET, and RXMED are still significant (they were in this case). When people say that they used "stepwise selection," this is most often the approach they used, not necessarily because it is the best, but rather because it is the default option for many programs and the easiest to select if you do not know what you are doing.

Note the major difference between hierarchical and stepwise procedures. In the former, the researcher selects the order in which variables enter into the mix. In the latter approach, the computer's (extremely primitive) brain takes over the role of the researcher's (hopefully more advanced) brain.

Why Stepwise Procedures Are Used

Stepwise solutions, which were made possible by the wide availability of computers, were devised to fill a need. In this section we'll discuss four of these reasons and later we'll discuss which ones are more perceived than real.

The accuracy with which the βs are estimated is dependent, among other factors, on the ratio of the number of subjects to the number of variables. In multiple regression, this is captured in the concept of *shrinkage*. In the current example, using the full-rank solution, we found a squared multiple correlation (R^2) of 0.284 between the GHQ score and the 13 predictor variables. (We generally use R^2 rather than R, since it expresses the percent of variance in the dependent variable explained by or predicted by the independent variables.) Now, if we were to draw another random set of pregnant women and plugged their values on the same variables into the equation derived from the first sample, what would R^2 be for them?

We don't know definitely; we do know, though, that it would be less than 0.284. The reason is that the regression equation based on the first sample derived the β weights so that they explained the maximum amount of the variance in that data set. Some of this variance was "real," reflecting true differences among people; but some was error variance, caused by unreliability in our measuring instruments, fluctuating attention levels of the subjects, recording mistakes, and other factors. The women in the new sample should have the same true variance (assuming that the two studies used truly random selection) but the error component will be different. Consequently, the equation will not accurately capture this, and the R^2 will suffer accordingly.

There are a number of equations which can be used to estimate the degree of shrinkage (referred to as the adjusted R^2) but they all take the general form:

$$\text{Adjusted } R^2 = R^2 - \frac{p\,(1-R^2)}{N-p-1}. \qquad [2]$$

The important point is that p, the number of variables, plays a greater role in the numerator than in the denominator, meaning that the more variables there are in the equation relative to N (the number of subjects), the greater will be the reduction in R^2. In this case, we can see in Table 11.2 that the adjusted R^2 is 0.224. When we used only four variables in the stepwise solution in Table 11.3, R^2 was lower (as we would expect with fewer independent variables), but the adjusted R^2 did not shrink as much and was actually somewhat higher (0.232) than when the 13-variable solution was used. So, the first reason stepwise procedures are used is to improve the subject-to-variable ratio and thereby the accuracy of the equation when it is used to make statements about people in general (not just those on whom the equation was derived).

A second reason for using stepwise procedures is equally pragmatic. In trying to understand a phenomenon, it is far easier to wrap our minds around three or four independent variables than a dozen or so. In fact, there is reason to believe that the upper limit of our ability to keep different facts in mind simultaneously is "the magical number seven, plus or minus two" (Miller, 1956). A third reason is related to this: parsimony. If our goal is to come up with a set of variables that predicts some phenomenon (for example, how well a person will do in therapy), then we do not want to inflict unnecessary tests on our patients. Why have the person complete (and our secretary score) 15 questionnaires when we can do almost as well with only four or five? In this case, we are using stepwise procedures to select a smaller subset of variables to be used subsequently.

Last, some people use stepwise procedures to reduce the effects of *multicollinearity*. As shown in the next section, though, this use has been called "misguided" by some (Fox, 1991); it is discussed here because examples of the misuse of stepwise procedures for this purpose are abundant in the literature.

Multicollinearity exists when there are high correlations among the independent variables. In fact, the concern here is not only with the correlations among pairs of variables but also with the situation where any one independent variable has a high multiple correlation with any subset of the other independent variables. For example, if the data included a person's Full Scale (FS), Verbal, and Performance IQs, then the first can be very accurately predicted from the latter two. Thus, multicollinearity may not be apparent by just looking at the matrix of pair-wise correlations. To see why it's a problem, remember that the βs are partial weights; that is, they show the effect of the variable after controlling for the other variables. Now, since FSIQ is strongly correlated with the combination of Verbal and Performance IQs, then once we have partialled out the effects of the latter two variables, there may be little or no variation left in FSIQ. It is shown in another chapter (Streiner, 1993a; see Chapter 22) that the reliability of an instrument (and here a variable can be considered to be an instrument with one item) depends on its ability to discriminate among objects or people. If FSIQ is left with little variability, then its reliability suffers accordingly and this is reflected in an imprecise estimate of its β weight. Thus, the hope (unfounded as it may be) is that stepwise procedures will keep FSIQ out of the equation and that the remaining βs will therefore be accurate. However, as we'll see in the next section, all that will happen is that we'll end up with an equation that is hard to interpret.

When Should Stepwise Procedures Be Used and Not Be Used?

Implicit in what we've said, we can use multiple regression for three different purposes: (1) predicting how a new group of people will score on some outcome; (2) finding out which variables explain or predict the dependent variable; and (3) selecting the best subset of independent variables. Stepwise solutions have a very legitimate place in the first instance and can do more harm than good in the latter two.

The goal in prediction, as in the example of the success of patients in therapy, is to find the smallest number of variables which do the job. The reasons here are twofold: to increase the ratio of subjects to variables and hence the accuracy of the equation and to reduce the amount of work required by the subjects, the person scoring the tests, and the one entering the data into the equation. At the extreme, we do not really care *why* this subset of variables works, only that it *does* work. There are a number of examples of this in medicine, for example, predicting which patients with chest pain should be admitted because of a possible heart attack or which ones who have had accidents should have an X-ray (e.g., Stiell et al., 1992). This is similar to using specific symptoms to make a diagnosis: we may use head-banging as a pathognomonic sign of autism without understanding why the child does this or what it says about the nature of autism.

The situation is very different, though, when we try to use the equation to *understand* the determinants of a phenomenon. We discussed the reason for this in a previous chapter in this series (Streiner, 1993b; see Chapter 9). Briefly, it has to do with the assignment of shared variance when the independent variables are correlated (that is, under conditions of multicollinearity). To show this more clearly, let's use an artificial example, which predicts the Volume (V) of a box from its Width (W), Length (L), and Height (H). As you remember from high school, the relationship among the dimensions is $V = W \times L \times H$, so we know

Table 11.5a Predicting the volume of a box from its height,
width, and length: full-rank solution

Variable	β	t	p level
Height	0.322	1.309	0.215
Length	0.320	1.407	0.185
Width	0.340	1.058	0.311
(Constant)		5.106	< 0.001

Notes: Multiple $R = 0.947$; $R^2 = 0.897$; Adjusted $R^2 = 0.871$.

Table 11.5b Predicting the volume of a box from its height,
width, and length: stepwise solution

Variable	β	t	p level
Width	0.930	9.463	< 0.001
(Constant)		4.688	< 0.001

Notes: Multiple $R = 0.930$; $R^2 = 0.865$; Adjusted $R^2 = 0.855$.

beforehand what the regression equation should look like. The problem
has also been designed so that there is a high correlation among L, W,
and H.

If we run a full-rank solution, we will get the results shown in the
top part of Table 11.5. As you can see in the column labelled "Beta,"
the three independent variables have similar weights, showing that
each variable's unique contribution to predicting volume is about the
same as those of the others' contribution. (The t-tests are not significant,
although the overall equation is, which is a common problem when
there is multicollinearity, as we discussed earlier).

Now let's use a stepwise procedure. We find that the R for Width is
0.930 – only a slight reduction from 0.947 using all three variables – and
Length and Height do not even enter into the equation. Why is β_{Width} so
much higher now than previously? The reason is that in the full-rank
solution, the variance the variables share with each other and with
Volume is not "credited" to any of the them, although it is reflected
in the size of R^2. In the stepwise solution, though, since Width had a
slightly higher correlation with Volume (0.930) than did Length (0.902)
or Height (0.907), it entered the equation first, and is credited with
its unique variance plus the variance it shares with Volume and the
other variables. Because the unique variances of Length and Height

add relatively little in relationship to the amount of variance already explained, they do not enter into the equation. It is not a coincidence that the β weight for Width with the stepwise solution (0.930) is almost the same as the sum of the three β weights in the full-rank solution (0.982), since the two equations must predict the same thing: how much the Volume changes in response to a change in one unit among the independent variables.

The problem arises if we now try to interpret this equation as explaining the major correlates or predictors of Volume. We would be grossly misinterpreting both the equation and reality if we say that Width is strongly related to Volume, but that Length and Height are not. We can say that with our (admittedly contrived) set of data we can predict Volume almost as well using only Width as we can using all three dimensions, but that is as far as we can go. We cannot say that Height or Length are not related to Volume, or even that Width is "more important" than the other two variables.

As is the case with other sets of (real) data, we cannot say that variables are unimportant simply because they do not enter into a stepwise solution. If multicollinearity is present (and it is always present to some degree), then which variables enter the equation and the order in which they enter are influenced by the correlations among the independent variables. We have also seen how very slight differences among the correlations of the predictor variables with the dependent variable affect which variables enter; if these correlations are changed just a little (as would happen with a new group of subjects or even if a few subjects were added to existing groups), the stepwise solution could result in a completely different set of variables.

Now let's discuss the third issue, that of selecting the ideal subset of variables. Implicit in what has been said so far is that stepwise approaches do not always come up with the "best" subset (where "best" may be defined as maximizing R^2 or by some other criterion). We saw this in the comparison of the all-subsets solution with the set of four variables chosen by the stepwise procedure, which has been recognized as a problem for nearly 40 years (Hauser, 1974). In fact, some simulations have shown that under certain (not unreasonable) conditions, up to 75% of the variables chosen by stepwise procedures may be "noise" or "garbage" variables, not related to the dependent variable at all (Derksen & Keselman, 1992). Even when the best equation is found, many other solutions may be almost as good (Henderson & Denison, 1989).

The Bottom Line

We can draw some conclusions from the foregoing.

1. When the researcher determines the order in which the variables enter into the equation, hierarchical methods are very useful in controlling for the effects of covariates.
2. Stepwise procedures can be used to derive a subset of variables to efficiently predict a dependent variable.
3. The order in which variables enter into a stepwise solution, or even which variables are included, does not tell us anything about the relative importance of those variables in explaining the dependent variable.
4. In a full-rank solution, the β weights reflect the unique contribution of a variable. If there are two or more independent variables, the βs cannot be interpreted as reflecting the relative importance of each variable.

The question, then, is how can we evaluate which variables are important and which are not? The answer is: only with great difficulty. It's been seen that looking at the βs does not work. For the same reasons, determining how much each variable adds to R^2 has serious drawbacks: because of multicollinearity, R^2 cannot be uniquely allocated among the independent variables (Leigh, 1988). Some authors (e.g., Darlington, 1990) have advocated using the correlation of each variable with the dependent variable after partialling out the effects of the other variables (that is, the semipartial correlation). However, this suffers from the same problems as does β: it gives only the unique contribution of a variable and it is very dependent on the other variables that are in the equation.

Perhaps the best that can be done is to choose an ideal (or almost ideal) subset of variables. As more variables are added to the equation, the value of R^2 goes up. But, as we've shown, the adjusted R^2 is dependent on the number of variables and may actually decrease when more variables are added. Thus, one approach which has been advocated by some authors (e.g., Neter, Wasserman, & Kutner, 1983) is to run all possible subsets and choose the one (or ones) with the highest adjusted R^2. If the computer program doesn't print the adjusted R^2, then an equivalent test would be to look at the mean square (error) for each possible subset and choose the one with the lowest value.

The best advice, though, is not to rely on stepwise solutions at all when looking for a subset of variables. The ideal approach is to rely on theory and a knowledge of the phenomenon, or, as Henderson and Denison (1989) put it, *"prior specification by a substantive expert is the preferred method of selecting predictor variables"* (p. 255; italics in original).

In conclusion, then, multiple regression and the various stepwise procedures are very useful and powerful techniques. However, users of them must be aware of what they can do and, even more important, what they cannot do.

ACKNOWLEDGMENT

I would like to thank Dr. Donna Stewart for allowing me to use her data.

REFERENCES

Arthur, H.M., Garfinkel, P.E., & Irvine, J. (1999, May). Development and testing of a new hostility scale. *Canadian Journal of Cardiology, 15*(5), 539–544. Medline:10350663

Darlington, R.B. (1990). *Regression and linear models.* New York, NY: McGraw-Hill.

Derksen, S., & Keselman, H.J. (1992). Backward, forward and stepwise automated sublet selection algorithms: Frequency of obtaining authentic and noise variables. *British Journal of Mathematical and Statistical Psychology, 45*(2), 265–282. http://dx.doi.org/10.1111/j.2044-8317.1992.tb00992.x

Fox, J. (1991). *Regression diagnostics.* Newbury Park, CA: Sage Press.

Goldberg, D. (1972). *The detection of psychiatric illness by questionnaire.* London: Oxford University Press.

Hauser, D.P. (1974). Some problems in the use of stepwise regression techniques in geographical research. *Canadian Geographer, 18*(2), 148–158. http://dx.doi.org/10.1111/j.1541-0064.1974.tb00116.x

Henderson, D.A., & Denison, D.R. (1989). Stepwise regression in social and psychological research. *Psychological Reports, 64*(1), 251–257. http://dx.doi.org/10.2466/pr0.1989.64.1.251

Labs, S.M., & Wurtele, S.K. (1986, Dec). Fetal health locus of control scale: Development and validation. *Journal of Consulting and Clinical Psychology, 54*(6), 814–819. http://dx.doi.org/10.1037/0022-006X.54.6.814 Medline:3794026

Leigh, J.P. (1988). Assessing the importance of an independent variable in multiple regression: Is stepwise unwise? *Journal of Clinical Epidemiology, 41*(7), 669–677. http://dx.doi.org/10.1016/0895-4356(88)90119-9 Medline:3397763

Miller, G.A. (1956, Mar). The magical number seven plus or minus two: Some limits on our capacity for processing information. *Psychological Review, 63*(2), 81–97. http://dx.doi.org/10.1037/h0043158 Medline:13310704

Neter, J., Wasserman, W., & Kutner, M.H. (1983). *Applied linear regression models.* Homewood, IL: Richard D. Irwin.

Stewart, D.E., & Cecutti, A. (1993, Nov 1). Physical abuse in pregnancy. *Canadian Medical Association Journal, 149*(9), 1257–1263. Medline:8221480

Stiell, I.G., Greenberg, G.H., McKnight, R.D., Nair, R.C., McDowell, I., & Worthington, J.R. (1992, Apr). A study to develop clinical decision rules for the use of radiography in acute ankle injuries. *Annals of Emergency Medicine, 21*(4), 384–390. http://dx.doi.org/10.1016/S0196-0644(05)82656-3 Medline:1554175

Streiner, D.L. (1993a, Mar). A checklist for evaluating the usefulness of rating scales. *Canadian Journal of Psychiatry, 38*(2), 140–148. Medline:8467441

Streiner, D.L. (1993b, Feb). An introduction to multivariate statistics. *Canadian Journal of Psychiatry, 38*(1), 9–13. Medline:8448733

TO READ FURTHER

Hauser, D.P. (1974). Some problems in the use of stepwise regression techniques in geographical research. *Canadian Geographer, 18*(2), 148–158. http://dx.doi.org/10.1111/j.1541-0064.1974.tb00116.x

Leigh, J.P. (1988). Assessing the importance of an independent variable in multiple regression: Is stepwise unwise? *Journal of Clinical Epidemiology, 41*(7), 669–677. http://dx.doi.org/10.1016/0895-4356(88)90119-9 Medline:3397763

12 Regression towards the Mean: Its Etiology, Diagnosis, and Treatment

DAVID L. STREINER, PH.D.

Canadian Journal of Psychiatry, 2001, 46, 72–76

Imagine this typical, open-label trial of a drug. People coming to psychiatrists' offices are screened for depression with the Hamilton Rating Scale for Depression (HRSD). Those who score 16 or more are started on an antidepressant and followed carefully for eight weeks. At the end of the two months, a second HRSD is administered. The investigators (and, needless to say, the drug company) are ecstatic that most patients now have scores within the normal range and claim that this new drug, which costs three times as much as existing ones, should be the treatment of choice .

In another study, patients with schizophrenia are selected if their scores on a measure of social functioning are below some criterion. They are entered in a program emphasizing social skills training, work-appropriate behaviour, and independent living. At the end of six months, most of the patients have significantly higher scores on the scale, and the investigators conclude that this intervention is highly successful with these people.

Are the researchers justified in their enthusiasm for these treatments? The answer is a resounding "no!" for a multitude of reasons. First, the natural history of the disorder may be such that positive change can be expected over the time course of the study, even in the absence of an intervention. This is more likely in the first example, but can never be completely ruled out in the second. A second possible alternative hypothesis is the so-called Hawthorne effect: simply paying attention to a subject in a study may produce positive changes. Although what actually happened at the bank-wiring plant in Hawthorne probably had nothing to do with the Hawthorne effect itself (Bramel & Friend, 1981; Jones, 1992), it serves as a handy label for describing the non-specific effects of filling out questionnaires, talking to clinical and research staff, and being treated in a different and special way. It is for these and other reasons that treatment studies should always have a control or comparison group in which it is expected that the natural history and Hawthorne effect will be comparable.

In this paper, though, I want to discuss a third possible explanation for the results, *regression towards the mean*. As we'll see, this does not mean reverting to an anal sadistic stage of development, but, more prosaically, it is a statistical concept relating to people's scores when they are tested on two or more occasions. It is a function of the tests themselves and, more particularly, the manner in which they are used to select subjects.

The Role of Tests in Regression towards the Mean

To understand regression towards the mean, it is necessary to take a brief detour into test theory. "Test," in this context, does not refer only to a paper-and-pencil instrument such as term finals or entrance exams for graduate and medical school; it includes any procedure that is used to classify someone or measure some attribute of a person. So, a "test" can be an unstructured diagnostic interview; the measurement of blood pressure, weight, or a serum level; or even an X-ray. To keep things simple, though, we'll restrict the discussion to only those tests that yield a number, such as the HRSD or a measure of social functioning. The number that we get at the end is called, for obvious reasons, the Observed score. According to classical test theory, this Observed score comprises two parts: a True score and an Error component:

$$\text{Observed score} = \text{True score} + \text{Error.} \qquad [1]$$

This means that we can never see the True score: it is always obscured to some degree by the Error. Where does the Error come from? Actually, from a multitude of sources, which can be grouped into three main categories: the person, the instrument, and the rater or recorder. Even in the simple case of a self-report scale, such as the Beck Depression Inventory, these three sources of error come into play. The person may deliberately lie about some symptoms, either to ensure that he or she will receive treatment or be discharged from hospital, may mean to circle a 2 for a specific item but circle a 3 by mistake, may over- or underestimate the magnitude of a symptom such as sleep disturbance, and so on. The instrument itself is not perfectly reliable: ambiguities in wording, for example, may lead a person to select a given response at one time but a different answer on a second occasion. Finally, the recorder may add the numbers incorrectly, or add them correctly but make a mistake transcribing the total. If the recorder is also the person who must observe and rate the symptoms, as is the case in the HRSD, then there is further room for observer error. (And if there is room, then it definitely will be occupied.)

But how does the fact that the observed score is composed of True and Error components contribute to regression towards the mean? One assumption of the Error term is that its mean value is 0. That is, sometimes the person will record a 2 when he or she means a 3, but just as often the opposite will occur. Over the long run (the person completing the test a number of times, or the scores averaged over many people, or the patient being observed by two or more raters), these errors will tend to cancel each other out; if they don't, then it is not error, it is a bias, but we won't look at that issue in this chapter. For example, most physicians and nurses (at least those who value accuracy and are aware of the limitations of a single measurement) take a person's blood pressure three or four times and use the average. They are capitalizing on the fact that any errors due to momentary changes in the actual pressure, inconsistencies with the cuff, and in hearing the Korotkoff sounds, will cancel each other out, and the more measurements that are taken, the more likely this will happen.

But let's see what happens when we select a person for a study based on one score being above some extreme value, such as an HRSD score of 16. (The same reasoning applies if we choose people based on scores below some criterion, as would be the case for social functioning, for example). Imagine that it were possible to actually know a person's True score. In that case, there would be four classes of people, defined by whether their True and Observed scores were above or below the cut-point, as seen in Table 12.1. Note in the column labelled "Decision" that two types of people are admitted to the study: those in Group C, whose True scores are 16 and above (and who therefore should be in the study); and those in Group B, whose members have True scores under 16 but for whom the Errors were in a positive direction and of such magnitude as to make their Observed score at least 16. Similarly, two types of people are excluded: those whose True scores are

Table 12.1 Decision rules to include or exclude persons from a study based on their True and Observed scores

True score	Observed score	Decision	On retest
A. Below criterion	Below criterion	Exclude	N/A
B. Below criterion	Above criterion	Include	Above criterion
C. Above criterion	Above criterion	Include	Above criterion
D. Above criterion	Below criterion	Exclude	N/A

below the criterion and who should not be in the study (Group A); and those in Group D, whose True scores qualify them for inclusion, but for whom the magnitude and direction of the Errors put the Observed scores under 16.

Let's assume that the intervention was totally useless. An interesting thing happens when the subjects are retested, which usually occurs at the end of the study. All of the people in Group C will continue to have True scores of at least 16, but, because of the assumption that the Errors have a mean value of 0, the Error scores of some of them will now result in their Observed scores being below the criterion (the last column in Table 12.1). In Group B, remember, the True score was below the criterion, but the Error component made the Observed score fall above it. To an even greater extent than in Group C, these people's Observed scores on retesting will fall below the cut-off. So, at Time 2, several people will now be in the "cured" range, even in the absence of an effect of the intervention. Similarly, the mean score for the group as a whole will fall to some degree.

One obvious question is why this reclassification of people into the "cured" range isn't counterbalanced by the increase in Error scores for the other people. The answer is that we excluded them from the study. People in Group D have True scores within the inclusion range, but were eliminated because their Observed scores were below the criterion. It is quite likely that about one-half of them would have higher scores if they were retested, because the Error scores would go in the positive direction the second time around. But we'll never see this; these people weren't included in the study, so they won't be tested again. Similarly, a small proportion of people in Group A may have positive Error scores large enough on the second testing to put them over the mark, but again, since they were excluded from the study, we won't see their scores. As a result, the people whose increased scores would have balanced out those whose Observed scores decreased aren't around to do so.

The Effects of Regression towards the Mean

Thus, the net effect of regression towards the mean is to shift a selected group's average (either high or low) closer to the mean of the entire population. This phenomenon was first described by Sir Francis Galton (1886), who noted that tall parents tended to have children who were shorter than they, albeit still above average height, and, conversely, that the children of short parents were still shorter than average, but taller than their parents. He called this effect "filial regression toward mediocrity" and attributed it to some biological force. He abandoned both the name (much to the delight of more "mediocre" people) and the explanation when he realized that, by using the same reasoning, it can be argued that short people have taller parents and tall ones shorter parents; it was difficult to maintain a biological explanation that worked backward in time (Campbell & Kenny, 1999).

In fact, as is apparent from the examples that opened the chapter, the effects of regression towards the mean are not limited to situations where biology can play a role. They occur any time a group of people is assessed on two occasions and the correlation between the two tests is less than perfect. Campbell and Kenny (1999) state that we can define it as

Regression towards the Mean = Perfect Correlation – Actual Correlation.   [2]

For those of a more mathematical bent, the actual degree of regression towards the mean using the same test on both occasions can be estimated by

$$T_2 = \overline{X} + r \ (T_1 - \overline{X}),$$ [3]

where T_1 is the person's score at Time 1; T_2 is the estimated score at Time 2; $\overline{X}$ is the common mean for Times 1 and 2; and r is the correlation between the tests. Equation [3] can be used either after the fact to determine how much of the change was due to regression or predictively if we have estimates of the common mean and the correlation from other studies. For the sake of illustration, let's assume that the common mean is 20 and the test-retest reliability is 0.8. If a person scores 20 at Time 1, then the estimated retest score is

$$20 + 0.8 \ (20 - 20) = 20.$$ [4]

This shows that scores at or near the mean at Time 1 change very little. But, if the person's score is 30, then the estimated score at Time 2 is

$$20 + 0.8 \, (30 - 20) = 28, \qquad\qquad [5]$$

or a two-point decline. So, the more the initial score deviates from the mean, the greater the regression towards it. If we stay with the same scores, but lower the reliability to 0.5, then the estimated score becomes

$$20 + 0.5 \, (30 - 20) = 25, \qquad\qquad [6]$$

illustrating that the lower the correlation between the two tests (or the lower the reliability), then the greater the regression.

So, two factors that affect the magnitude of regression towards the mean are (1) the amount that a score deviates from the mean, and (2) the (un)reliability of the test. In fact, though, regression can occur even with a test that has perfect reliability: anything that lowers the correlation between the test and retest will lead to regression towards the mean (Campbell & Kenny, 1999).

Sometimes, attempts to circumvent or detect regression towards the mean lead us into more difficulty. We may suspect that the amount that people change is related to their initial score; that is, someone near the top end of the scale has a long way to come down, whereas a person nearer the mean has less room to improve. This is likely why many studies of depression use the quite arbitrary criterion of "success," defined as a 50% reduction in initial HRSD score : a person with a score of 30 has to have a larger decrease than one whose initial score is 20 (15 points versus 10). However, employing this criterion in turn leads to other problems. First, it means that the definition of success is different for each person. More troubling, though, is that it assumes that the scale has interval-level properties; that is, that a change from 30 to 25 reflects the same decrease in depressive symptoms as a change from 15 to 10. This is almost never the case with scales used in psychiatry (Streiner & Norman, 2008).

A seemingly intuitive way to determine whether the degree to which people change is related to the severity of their disorder is to correlate the change score (that is, $T_1 - T_2$) with the initial score – intuitive, but wrong. The reason it is wrong is again based on regression towards the mean. Except under highly unusual conditions, the correlation can never be positive (the direction of change will never be towards the more extreme) and is rarely 0. In fact, the correlation of T_1 with $(T_1 - T_2)$ is approximately

$$-\frac{\sqrt{1-r}}{\sqrt{2}},\qquad\qquad [7]$$

even in the absence of an intervention. So, if the correlation between the pre- and posttests is 0.7, then we would expect that the correlation between the initial score and the change score would be $-\sqrt{0.3}/\sqrt{2} = -0.39$. That is, the change score is always related to the pretest value, and the correlation means not that sicker people benefit more, only that more extreme scores regress more. This equation also implies that the correlation of change with the posttest (T_2) score is always positive. The important point is that these are mathematical truisms and are not due to the efficacy (or lack thereof) of the intervention or to the initial degree of severity. So, a negative correlation merely tells us that the earth is turning on its axis as it should and reveals nothing about the data.

Detecting Regression towards the Mean

To avoid being misled by "effects" that are due to regression towards the mean, two things are necessary: (1) an acknowledgment that it can occur and, in fact, is fairly ubiquitous; and (2) some methods for seeing its effects. To expand somewhat on what we've said before, regression towards the mean will occur any time a person is assessed on two occasions and the measures used are correlated to some degree, either because the same test is used twice or because the measure used the second time is related to the one used first. Below are several examples of regression towards the mean, some of which are taken from the bible on this subject, Campbell & Kenny (1999).

- Rookies of the Year suffer a "sophomore slump" during their second year.
- Children of self-made millionaires are less successful than their parents.
- The offspring of university professors do less well on college entrance exams than did their parents.
- People who suffer from stuttering, pain, and other disorders improve "spontaneously."

- People who are chosen to be journal editors (or departmental chairs) "burn out" after their terms expire.
- High-users of medical services have fewer visits after even one session of psychotherapy.

In all of these cases, the people were selected because they were above the average in some regard – Rookies of the Year have among the highest batting averages or lowest ERAs in the league, chairs and editors are selected in part because of their large numbers of publications, millionaires are identified because they make much more money than authors of papers about research design, and so on. Consequently, it is not surprising – indeed, it is predicted by regression towards the mean – that a subsequent evaluation will show a decline. Note that in some of these examples (millionaires and university professors) the second measures are on different people: the offspring. However, because traits such as intelligence are correlated across generations, the same arguments apply. A second point to note is that this phenomenon operates at the level of the group, not the individual. That is, a specific tall parent may have an even taller child, but tall parents, as a group, have children shorter than themselves.

So, one easy way to detect regression effects is simply to look at the mean scores on the two occasions; they will be closer to the mean the second time. This works, though, only if members of the group are initially selected because of their extreme score the first time. If the full range of scores is used (that is, correlating incomes of parents and children for all social classes), then the means will be similar, because those below the mean will increase, and those above the mean will decrease. A very good way to visualize whether regression towards the mean has occurred is to use a *Galton squeeze diagram*, which was developed by Campbell and Kenny (1999). An example of such a diagram is shown in Figure 12.1. For each value of the pretest (plotted on the left), the mean posttest score is plotted on the right, with a line connecting them. For example, to make this figure, I generated data for 500 people on a "test" with a mean of 10, a standard deviation of 3, and a correlation between the pretest and posttest of 0.63, comparable to many scales used in psychiatry. To simulate an extreme group, I selected only "people" who had an initial score over 13 – one standard deviation above the mean. The 42 cases with an initial score of 13 had a mean posttest score of 11.62, the 39 cases who scored 14 on pretest had a mean of 12.87 on posttest, and so on. The "squeeze" towards the mean is obvious. Had

Fig. 12.1 Example of a Galton squeeze diagram

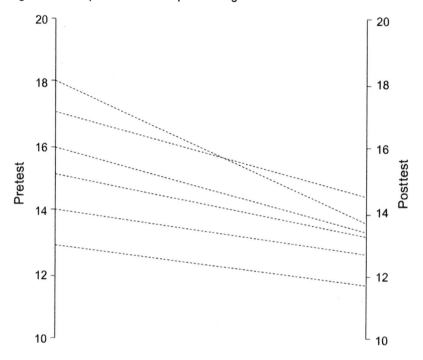

the full range of values been plotted (3 to 18), then the lines for initial scores below the mean would have sloped upwards.

What to Do about It

The best defence against regression towards the mean is a good offence – minimize it happening or be aware that it can occur. First, an extreme group should never be selected on the basis of a single test score. In much the same way that patients are selected for trials of antihypertensive agents only if they are above a criterion on three successive readings, patients in psychiatric trials should have test scores above the cut-point on three occasions. This will minimize (although not eliminate) the possibility that they are in the extreme group because their Observed score is above the criterion, while their True score is below it. Even with this precaution, regression will occur because they are in an extreme group. This effect cannot be eliminated, but we can compensate for it with a control group – one that went through an equivalent screening process and had similar scores, but was not given the intervention. Since regression effects will affect both groups to the same degree, the difference between the groups at the end will in dictate whether the intervention worked.

Conclusions

Regression towards the mean is a fact of life. But, as with other facts of life, we often avoid the ugly details, are embarrassed to talk about it in front of others, and are surprised at its powerful effects. We can, though, approach it like mature, responsible adults. First, we must recognize that it exists and can rear its head in a wide range of circumstances. Second, if we want to eliminate the negative consequences, we must use appropriate and effective precautions: adequate pretesting and control.

REFERENCES

Bramel, D., & Friend, R. (1981). Hawthorne, the myth of the docile worker, and class bias in psychology. *American Psychologist, 36*(8), 867–878. http://dx.doi.org/10.1037/0003-066X.36.8.867

Campbell, D.T., & Kenny, D.A. (1999). *A primer on regression artifacts.* New York: Guilford Press.

Galton, F. (1886). Regression towards mediocrity in hereditary stature. *Journal of the Anthropological Institute of Great Britain and Ireland, 15,* 246–263. http://dx.doi.org/10.2307/2841583

Jones, S.R.G. (1992). Was there a Hawthorne effect? *American Journal of Sociology, 98*(3), 451–468. http://dx.doi.org/10.1086/230046

Streiner, D.L., & Norman, G.R. (2008). *Health measurement scales: A practical guide to their development and use.* (4th ed.). Oxford: Oxford University Press.

TO READ FURTHER

Campbell, D.T., & Kenny, D.A. (1999). *A primer on regression artifacts.* New York: Guilford Press.

McDonald, C.J., Mazzuca, S.A., & McCabe, G.P., Jr. (1983, Oct–Dec). How much of the placebo 'effect' is really statistical regression? *Statistics in Medicine*, 2(4), 417–427. http://dx.doi.org/10.1002/sim.4780020401 Medline:6369471

Morton, V., & Torgerson, D.J. (2003, May 17). Effect of regression to the mean on decision making in health care. *BMJ (Clinical Research Ed.)*, 326(7398), 1083–1084. http://dx.doi.org/10.1136/bmj.326.7398.1083 Medline:12750214

Vollmer, W.M. (1988). Comparing change in longitudinal studies: Adjusting for initial value. *Journal of Clinical Epidemiology*, 41(7), 651–657. http://dx.doi.org/10.1016/0895-4356(88)90117-5 Medline:3397761

13 Stayin' Alive: An Introduction to Survival Analysis

DAVID L. STREINER, PH.D.

Canadian Journal of Psychiatry, 1995, 40, 439–444

In what is perhaps the most common experimental design used in psychiatry, we usually form two groups, measure them on some characteristic, give an experimental intervention to one of them, and use the other as a control group. Then, at the end of some period, we measure them again, and hope that the two groups have changed to different degrees. Most drug trials, for example, use this design: groups are assessed at baseline to test for comparability; one is given the new drug and the other a placebo or an older drug; and then, after some months, the groups are tested again to see if the new drug produced a greater reduction in symptoms or fewer adverse reactions.

In some circumstances, though, we are interested not so much in how much a group may change because of some intervention, but rather in how long it takes for people to reach some end-point. The primary aim of many community psychiatry programs, for instance, is to increase the time between admissions. For a substance abuse program, the time would be until the patient resumes drug use or drinking. For prison-based skills development programs, the time would be the period between incarcerations. The original studies of this type looked at various interventions to increase the life expectancy of cancer patients, where the outcome of interest (at least to the investigators) was time until death. As a result, they are still called *survival studies*, even though we may not be interested in issues of living or dying. What remains the same is (1) the outcome of interest is time and (2) the target event is binary: either it occurs or it does not.

In addition to differing in terms of what is measured (time until some event occurs rather than a score on some scale), survival studies also differ from more traditional designs in three other respects: recruitment of subjects into the study, the length of the follow-up, and loss of subjects. Because of the limited capacity of most programs, it is often the case that these survival-type intervention trials do not have enough people at any one time that half could be assigned to one group, half to the other, and all the people entered into the trial simultaneously. Rather, it is more common that subjects are recruited into the trial over a period of months, or even years. As we'll see later, this introduces some issues about the consistency of the program over time. It also affects the length of time that different individuals in the study can be followed up. For example, assume it takes two years for the program to discharge enough patients to do a proper study, and we want to follow the people for a minimum of three years after discharge. This means that the last subject recruited into the study will be at risk for relapse for a maximum of three years, the first subject can be at risk for up to five years, and the other subjects will have risk periods between these extremes.

This long duration of the study, in turn, leads to the third problem, which is the loss of subjects. Attrition is a problem in most studies where people are tested more than once: subjects die, move out of the area, refuse to continue to participate, or simply forget to show up for their appointments. The longer the duration of the study, the greater this problem becomes. However, there is an additional problem in survival studies. Unfortunately, no study is funded forever. At some time, we have to shut it down and move on to other things, which means that we will have to stop collecting data before all patients reach the end-point. Even after 5 years, some people may not have been readmitted to hospital, resumed drinking, or been arrested. They may experience the target event one minute after we stop collecting data, or go on for another 5 years or 10 years without relapsing, but we'll never know. For reasons that will become apparent shortly, we refer to this as *right censoring* of the data. Thus, in more traditional studies, there are two possible outcomes: (1) we have a final measure on a subject; or (2) he or she dropped out (died, refused, and so on). In survival studies, though, there are three possible outcomes for each subject: (1) the target event occurred, (2) the person was lost to follow-up, or (3) the study ended before either of these took place (his or her data were *right censored*). Figure 13.1 illustrates what we've discussed so far, for a fictitious study with 12 subjects and a 3-year follow-up interval. Each horizontal line represents a different subject, where the left end indicates when the follow-up period began. The right end of each line is labelled with one of three letters, showing what

Fig. 13.1 Outcomes of 12 people followed up to 36 months

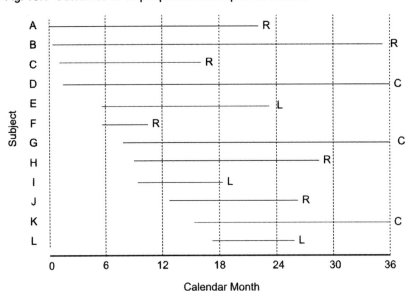

happened to that person: an R if the person relapsed, an L if he or she was lost to follow-up, and a C if the data were censored (that is, no event occurred by the time the study ended). We can also see why it's called right censoring, since the line is terminated at the right side of the graph.

Calculating the Risk of Relapse

The problem is how best to summarize these results. Two ways appear obvious but, as we'll see, they can lead to wrong conclusions and do not make full use of all the data. Once we've discussed these approaches, we'll describe a third method, which avoids such problems. The first (wrong) method is called *mean survival*. With this technique we take only those subjects for whom we have complete data and calculate how long, on average, they survived until they suffered a relapse. Two problems are immediately apparent. For one thing, we'd be able to use the data only for subjects A, B, C, F, H, and J, which would be, in essence, to throw out half of the people, even though they can provide useful information. For another, we are loading the dice against ourselves, since the people who are most successful, and do not suffer a relapse, are never included in the average.

The second (still wrong) method, called the *survival rate*, attempts to minimize these problems by calculating the proportion of people who have not relapsed as of a certain time after discharge. This, in fact, is what is often done in reporting the consequences of different types of cancers and their treatments: the five-year survival rate. The first problem with this approach is that again we would be tossing out subjects – those who were lost to follow-up or censored before their five-year anniversary. The second problem is why five years? Why not two years, or ten years, or seven years and three months? The point is that any fixed time is arbitrary, even if it has the blessing of the consensus of clinicians.

The third (and, finally, correct) method is called *survival analysis* or *life table analysis*. The key is that we shift our focus from looking at people to looking at time. That is, we calculate how many people are still surviving (in our example, have not relapsed) at the end of each week, month, or year. The length of the interval is arbitrary and depends on how often relapses occur: if they are infrequent, it may make sense to look at the data every three months, whereas, if the study consists of a large number of people and relapses occur often, a weekly interval may be more appropriate. We begin by redrawing the figure (at least in our minds, if not on paper) to look like Figure 13.2. What we have done is simply to shift each line to the left, as if all the subjects began follow-up at the same time. Notice, though, that the name of the X-axis has changed, from calendar month (reflecting the date when follow-up began for each person) to months of follow-up (indicating how long he or she was in this phase of the study).

From this figure, we can construct a table summarizing what has occurred during each time period. The first column of Table 13.1, called "Number of months in study," simply labels each interval which, to make this example easier, is six months long. The second column is called "Number at risk," and indicates the number of subjects who are still in the study at the start of the interval (that is, the number of horizontal lines which cross the left boundary of the interval). The third column, called "Number relapsed," and the fourth column, called "Number lost," count the number of people who relapsed and were lost to follow-up during that interval. The fourth column also includes those people whose data were censored, since, for the purposes of the analysis, the result is the same: we don't know what happened to them.

What we would like to do is figure out the *hazard* for each interval, which is the probability of relapsing for people who were at risk. This would be straightforward if the only alternatives were survival or

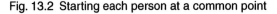

Fig. 13.2 Starting each person at a common point

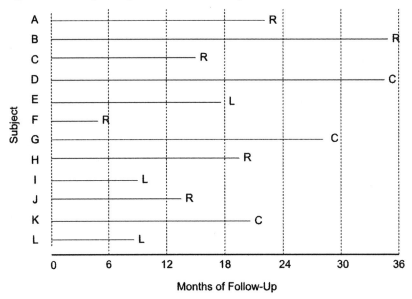

relapse; we would simply calculate the number who relapsed divided by the number at risk. The problem is what to do with the people who were lost during the interval. If we include them in the denominator (that is, the number at risk), we are assuming that they were at risk for the entire interval and survived it, which would result in an underestimate of the hazard. Conversely, if we omit them from the denominator, we are not crediting them for having survived the previous interval, and thus we would overestimate the hazard during that time. In the true spirit of compromise, we assume that they were at risk for half of the interval (or equivalently, that half of those lost were at risk for the entire interval). Over the long run, this does not introduce any bias, because if people drop out at random times, this will average out to being lost to the study halfway through the time period. Thus, we can calculate the *hazard*, or probability of relapsing, for each interval as

$$\text{Hazard} = \frac{\text{Number who relapsed during the interval}}{\text{Number at risk} - \dfrac{\text{Number lost}}{2}}. \tag{1}$$

Table 13.1 Outcome of 12 subjects in a relapse follow-up study

Number of months in study	Number at risk	Number relapsed	Number lost
0–6	12	1	0
6–12	11	0	2
12–18	9	2	1
18–24	6	2	1
24–30	3	0	1
30–36	2	1	1

Let's work this out for the third interval (12 to 18 months), where we have both patients who relapse ($n = 2$) and dropouts ($n = 1$). The hazard for this time period is

$$\text{Hazard} = \frac{2}{9 - \frac{1}{2}} = 0.2353. \qquad [2]$$

Now we can derive three numbers for each interval: the *probability of relapsing*, the *probability of surviving* (which is simply 1.0 minus the probability of relapsing), and the *cumulative survival probability*. If we do this for the data in Table 13.1, we will end up with Table 13.2. The only column which requires some explanation is the last one, the cumulative probability. For the first interval, the probability of surviving and the cumulative probability of surviving are the same. For the second interval, the cumulative probability is the probability of surviving that interval (1.0000) times the cumulative probability of the previous interval (0.9167). Similarly, for the third interval the cumulative survival probability is the probability of surviving interval three (0.7647) times the cumulative probability for the second interval (0.9167), or 0.7010, and so on for the remainder of the table. The third column reflects the probability of survival for people who have lasted up to that time, while the last column is the probability of surviving since the follow-up began. So, staying with the third interval, people who have survived to 12 months have a probability of 0.7647 of surviving until 18 months. The probability is 0.7010 that, starting at day 1, a person will last for 18 months. The last column goes by the formal name of the *survival function* and is shown graphically in Figure 13.3, where it is known as the *survival curve*.

The approach to survival analysis we have been discussing so far resembles what insurance actuaries do; given that you have reached

Table 13.2 Life table based on Table 13.1

Number of months in study	Probability of relapse	Probability of survival	Cumulative probability of survival
0–6	0.0833	0.9167	0.9167
6–12	0.0000	1.0000	0.9167
12–18	0.2353	0.7647	0.7010
18–24	0.3656	0.6344	0.4461
24–30	0.0000	1.0000	0.4461
30–36	0.6667	0.3333	0.1487

your 30th birthday, what are the chances that you will die by the age of 65 and they will have to pay your relatives? That is, they calculate the odds at fixed time points. Consequently, this method is referred to as the *actuarial method* of analysis. It is most useful in situations where we gather data on patients at fixed intervals, say every month or half-year. If the person relapses or is lost, we may not know the exact date, though we might know that these events occurred at some time between one follow-up visit and the next.

In some situations, though, we may have access to the exact date of the target event through hospital records, death notices, and the like. In that case, we are not limited to calculating the survival probability only at the end of the interval. Rather, we can determine how it changes every time an event occurs. This approach is called the *Kaplan-Meier* method of survival analysis. Some people prefer the Kaplan-Meier approach when there are fewer than 50 subjects because of its greater efficiency (since we do not have to assume that all losses occurred exactly halfway through the interval), and the actuarial method when there are more than 50 subjects because it makes better use of the data from the drop-outs. In most cases, though, the two techniques yield similar results (Norman & Streiner, 2008).

Looking at More Groups

The real power of survival analysis becomes even more apparent when we compare two or more groups. Does our intervention in fact result in longer survival times than result from conventional therapy or no therapy? If we did such a study, we would end up with two or more survival curves, and the question is whether or not they would differ significantly from one another. If we were interested in the difference at

Fig. 13.3 The survival function for the 12 people

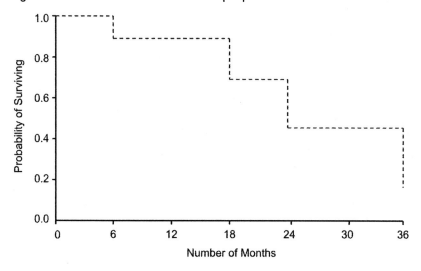

only one specific time, as are the oncologists, and had only two groups, we could calculate a z-test using the equation

$$z = \frac{P_1 + P_2}{\sqrt{[SE(P_1)] + [SE(P_2)]}},$$ [3]

where P_1 is the cumulative probability of surviving at that time for the first group, and P_2 the probability for the second group. The standard error (SE) for Group 1 is defined as

$$SE = P_1\sqrt{\frac{1 - P_1}{R_1}},$$ [4]

where R_1 is the number of people at risk at that time; the SE for the second group is computed the same way. As with all z-tests, a value of 1.96 or greater shows that the results are significant at the 0.05 level. We can also calculate the *Relative Risk* (RR) of surviving this interval as

$$RR = \frac{1 - P_1}{1 - P_2}.$$ [5]

As we discussed previously, though, there are limitations to calculating the significance or RR at any one point: the time chosen is arbitrary, and a lot of useful information is discarded. A better method is to calculate the difference at the end of every interval and then combine these results into one global test of significance. This method is called the *Mantel-Cox chi-squared*. As is true with other versions of chi-squared tests, it involves calculating how many relapses would be expected in each group at each time, under the assumption that the intervention does not work (the null hypothesis), and then seeing how much the observed data deviate from these expected values. It is usually too laborious to figure out by hand, although a small example is worked out in Norman and Streiner (2008) for those whose masochistic tendencies run in the direction of doing slowly what a computer can do quickly. Similarly, the overall relative risk is calculated using the observed and expected relapses and would be too time-consuming to compute using pencil and paper.

Cox Proportional Hazards Model

We began by looking at a group and then expanded the discussion to consider two (or more) groups. Let's add a final modification of survival analysis, which is adjusting for covariates. We may be interested in covariates for two reasons. It is possible that the time to relapse is affected by some other factors, such as gender, age, or number of previous admissions. One question we may wish to ask is the degree to which these variables affect the overall survival rate. The second reason for being interested in them is that the groups may differ on one or more key background variables. Even if the differences are not significant, we can sometimes achieve greater precision in our estimate of the RR if these factors are considered. This is similar to what is seen in another technique, Analysis of Covariance; adjusting for even small baseline differences between the groups may result in statistical significance, which would not be achieved without the adjustments (Norman & Streiner, 2008).

The mathematics of this approach, which is called the *Cox proportional hazards model*, are beyond the scope of this paper. Interested readers can look at the books and articles listed under "To Read Further." Suffice it to say that, with the results of the computer output in front of us, we would be able to determine the degree to which these other variables affect the survival rate. The major assumption of this model, and the reason that the term "proportional" is included in its name, is that the effect of the covariate does not change over time. What this means is that, for any given value of the covariates (for example, males with three previous admissions), if the hazard for the control group is twice that of the experimental group at Time 1, it remains twice as high for every other time. In other words, the hazard functions are proportional to each other over time. What this also means is that we can sometimes do an "eyeball" test to see if the data meet the assumption of proportional hazards. If the two survival curves ever cross, then the assumption is not met, since the ratio of the hazards is obviously different before and after the point of crossover.

Assumptions, Sample Size, and Other Issues

If, after reading this chapter, you decide that survival analysis is the only way to fly, there are a few assumptions and requirements you should be aware of.

- *There must be an identifiable starting point.* All patients have to enter the trial at an equivalent point. If it is when they are discharged from a program which has a defined termination criterion, then allocation is fairly straightforward. Sometimes, though, the situation can be more problematic. Inpatient units, for example, may send a person home directly, keep another person on leave of absence for 30 days before finally discharging him or her to see how he or she does in the community, or send a third person to a halfway house for a few months so he or she can readapt slowly to independent living. These cannot be considered equivalent points, since the patients' conditions at entry into the follow-up portion of the trial may be very different.
- *There must be a common end-point.* Like the starting point, the end-point has to be consistent for all people. Again, readmission to hospital may be simple, but what is "relapse" in an alcohol treatment program: when the person has a first drink, passes out for the first time, is arrested for being drunk and disorderly, or something else? Any of these criteria may be appropriate, but whichever one is chosen, it must be used for all subjects.

One consequence of these first two constraints is that, for any subject, once you're out, you're out. That is, if a person experiences the target event, he or she cannot be re-enrolled in the program to await a second event, since his or her starting point and ending point would now be different from those of other subjects.

- *Loss to follow-up must be unrelated to the outcome.* When we calculate the hazard, the people who are lost to follow-up are put in the denominator of the equation, indicating that they were at risk for at least a portion of the time; they are not put in the numerator, indicating that they did not relapse. If they were lost for some reason related to the outcome, then we would be underestimating the risk. If many people were lost for these reasons, the underestimate could be quite serious. For example, if we were evaluating some form of therapy to treat depression, where relapse was defined as rehospitalization, we could not blithely assume that those who dropped out of sight did so for trivial reasons unrelated to their condition. There is a very real possibility that their loss might be due to an unreported suicide, which is quite different from simply moving out of the area. If a large number of subjects were still lost after strenuous attempts were made to determine their status, a conservative approach would be to analyse the data twice: once by treating the subjects as lost, and again by assuming the worst and treating them all as "relapsers." If the results were about the same with both analyses, you could be fairly confident in them. However, if a significant outcome becomes non-significant on re-analysis (or, even worse, significant in the opposite direction), then your findings would, at best, be considered equivocal.
- *There must be no secular trend.* We are not suddenly injecting religion into the discussion at this point; "secular trend" refers to change over time. We mentioned in the beginning that trials that extend over long periods of time have some associated methodological problems, and this is the major one. We assume that, over the course of the recruitment and follow-up intervals, diagnosis, the criteria used for admission into the program, the treatment itself, and the criteria for the outcome event have not changed. If they have changed, then patients who entered the study towards the beginning may be quite different, or have been treated quite differently, from those recruited last; or what is termed an event may vary between those who relapse early versus those who relapse later. This would tend to act against us, since it would (1) introduce

greater variability among the subjects, (2) mean that fewer subjects were exposed to effective treatment than our sample size would lead us to believe, and (3) make interpretation of any significant findings problematic.

Finally, how many subjects are required for a survival analysis? As is usual with any sample size determination, we have to make a few assumptions and guesses. The easy ones are the alpha (α) and beta (β) levels; by tradition, we set the first to 0.05 and the second to 0.15 or 0.20. More difficult to estimate is delta (δ), which is the ratio of the expected hazards of the two groups at the end of the study. Once we estimate this ratio, we can plug the values into the equation:

$$d = \frac{2(Z_\alpha + Z_\beta)^2}{\log_e \delta},$$ [6]

where d is the number of events in each group; Z_α is 1.96 for $\alpha = 0.05$; and $Z_\beta = 0.84$ for $\beta = 0.20$. So, if we expect that the relapse rate in the treated group will be 50% by the end of the follow-up period, then we would have to multiply d by 2 (that is, $1/0.5$) to determine how many subjects to enter into each group. In other words, if the equation tells us that we need 20 relapses and the expected relapse rate is 50%, we would have to enrol 40 subjects to test for this difference. Sample size tables are provided in Norman and Streiner (2008) and George and Desu (1974).

In conclusion, survival analysis is a very useful technique when the outcome of interest is the time until some event happens. It is often more powerful than simply counting how many events occur in each group and provides useful information about the course of a disorder.

REFERENCES

George, S.L., & Desu, M.M. (1974, Feb). Planning the size and duration of a clinical trial studying the time to some critical event. *Journal of Chronic Diseases*, 27(1–2), 15–24. http://dx.doi.org/10.1016/0021-9681(74)90004-6 Medline:4592596

Norman, G.R., & Streiner, D.L. (2008). *Biostatistics: The bare essentials.* (3rd ed.). Shelton, CT: PMPH USA.

TO READ FURTHER

Lee, E.T., & Wang, J. (2003). *Statistical methods for survival data analysis*. (3rd ed.). New York: Wiley.

Norman, G.R., & Streiner, D.L. (2008). *Biostatistics: The bare essentials*. (3rd ed.). Shelton, CT: PMPH USA.

Tibshirani, R. (1982). A plain man's guide to the proportional hazards model. *Clinical and Investigative Medicine. Medecine Clinique et Experimentale, 5*(1), 63–68. Medline:7116716

14 Life after Chi-squared: An Introduction to Log-Linear Analysis

DAVID L. STREINER, PH.D., AND ELIZABETH LIN, PH.D.

Canadian Journal of Psychiatry, 1998, 43, 837–842

One of the most widely used (and abused) of the statistical procedures is the chi-squared (χ^2) test. In its simplest and most familiar form, it examines if there is any relationship between two categorical variables (that is, those that consist of discrete categories, such as gender or diagnosis, as opposed to continuous variables, such as degree of anxiety, which are measured on continua). To illustrate its use, let's examine the possible causes and correlates of that dread disorder, photonumerophobia (PNP). As explained in a previous chapter in this book (Streiner, 1998; see Chapter 6), PNP was first described by Norman and Streiner (2008) and is a condition in which patients are fearful that their fear of numbers will come to light. Imagine that we survey an undergraduate class of 3000 university students. We gather some basic demographic information and administer a fear of numbers questionnaire. We have a hunch that the prevalence of PNP is different for males and for females, based on the politically incorrect notion that men focus on quantity, women on quality. So, we arrange our findings in a 2 × 2 (or fourfold) table, like Table 14.1. The actual numbers we *observed* (O) are arranged as follows: Cell A is the number of males with PNP; Cell B the number of non-phobic males; Cell C the number of phobic females; and Cell D the number of non-phobic females.

The question is whether our observed values are different from what we would expect, under the null hypothesis that gender and PNP are not related. How do we determine what would be expected? Of the 3000 students one-third are men and two-thirds are women. If the two variables – gender and phobia – are unrelated, we would expect that

Table 14.1 Cross-classification of gender and photonumerophobia (PNP);
O = observed, E = expected

	PNP	No PNP	Total
	A	B	
Male	$O = 36$	$O = 964$	1000
	$E = 62$	$E = 938$	
	C	D	
Female	$O = 150$	$O = 1850$	2000
	$E = 124$	$E = 1876$	
Total	186	2814	3000

these proportions would be the same in both diagnostic groups. So, of the 186 phobic patients, we would expect that one-third, or 62, would be male and two-thirds, or 124, would be female. Similarly, 33.3%, or 938, of the 2814 non-phobic people would be men, and 66.7%, or 1876, would be women. These are the *expected* (*E*) frequencies in Table 14.1, or, calculated another way, since 6.2% of the sample are phobic, then 6.2% of the 1000 males should be phobic, and so on for the other cells. In all cases, the expected frequencies will be the same. To summarize, to compute the expected frequency for Cell A, we find the proportion of the sample that is male, multiply this by the proportion of the sample that has PNP, and then multiply by the sample size, so that we end up with an actual count, rather than a proportion.

$$\text{Expected (Cell A)} = \frac{1000}{3000} \times \frac{186}{3000} \times 3000 = \frac{1000 \times 186}{3000} = 62. \quad [1]$$

We want to see if the differences between the O and E frequencies in each cell are greater than we would expect by chance. The more they differ from each other, the greater the probability that the null hypothesis is wrong and that gender and PNP are related. We cannot simply subtract the two values and sum over the four cells, since the result will always be 0. To avoid this outcome, the value $(O - E)$ is squared for each cell. But even if the null hypothesis were true, O and E would still differ from each other because of random sampling error. Consequently, we compare our findings with naturally occurring variation. In parametric tests, such as the t-test or Analysis of Variance, this index of variability is the standard deviation or variance within each group. When the data consist of counts of people instead of a continuous score, as is the case here, the measure of variance is the expected frequency for each cell. (Why this is the case is beyond the scope of this chapter, but see Norman & Streiner, 2008, for an explanation.) Finally, we end up with the formula for the chi-squared test:

$$\chi^2 = \sum \frac{(O-E)^2}{E},$$ [2]

where the Greek capital sigma (Σ) means to sum over all the cells in the 2×2 table. In this case, we find that

$$\frac{(36-62)^2}{62} + \frac{(964-938)^2}{938} + \frac{(150-124)^2}{124} + \frac{(1850-1876)^2}{1876} = 17.44.$$ [3]

If we now look at a table of the critical values of the chi-squared test found in the back of a statistics book or the computer output, we will see that this is significant ($p < 0.0001$), indicating that there is a relationship between gender and PNP.

So far, we have been discussing a simple 2×2 case. However, in real life we are seldom content to leave things that uncomplicated. Suppose that, in addition to having a hunch that gender and PNP are related, we also think that birth order plays a role, based on casual observations that younger children are often helped in math by their older siblings. We could do a $2 \times 2 \times 2$ chi-squared, but we would run into the problem that the calculations become very laborious and, more important, difficult to interpret. Even if the results were significant, it becomes hard to tease apart exactly where the significant differences are. This problem worsens as we add more variables (for example, whether or not either parent is numerophobic) or look at more levels of each variable (for example, rating the PNP as mild, moderate, or severe).

There are two options: stop asking complicated questions or find some other way of analysing these data. Since the first choice is highly unlikely, let's discuss an alternative to chi-squared tests for looking at cross-classified data (in which people are assigned to cells in a table on the basis of their values on two or more variables). This approach is called *log-linear analysis*. Rest assured that it is a statistical technique, not a way of determining if trees are straight.

To understand log-linear analyses, we must introduce (to people who do not frequent racetracks) the concept of *odds*. Imagine that the names of the 3000 people in our sample were put in a hat and you drew one name at random. The odds that the person whose name you drew is male are (1000/2000), or 0.50 to 1.00, or 1 to 2 (usually written 1:2), since for every male student there are two female students. (Note that the odds of drawing a male's name are different from the chance of drawing a male: the chance [or probability] of drawing a male is 1000/3000 or 0.33.) Conversely, the odds that the person is female are 2000/1000 = 2.00 or 2:1, which is the reciprocal of 0.50 (that is, 1/0.50 = 2.00; and 1/2.00 = 0.50). Similarly, the odds that the person has PNP are 186/2814, or 0.066:1, and that the person is not phobic are 2814/186, or 15.129:1. So, odds of 1.00 means that the probability is 50%, or 0.50; odds less than 1.00 mean a probability of less than 0.50; and odds above 1.00 reflect a probability of over 0.50.

Let's look at men and women separately. For women, the odds of being phobic are 150/1850, or 0.081; for men, they are 36/964, or 0.037. These are referred to as *conditional* odds, since they are the odds of being phobic conditional on gender. In fact, we can now take the ratio of these odds to determine if men or women are more likely to have PNP. Not surprisingly, this is called the *odds ratio* (OR), and in our example it is

$$OR = \frac{150/1850}{36/964} = \frac{0.081}{0.037} = 2.171, \qquad [4]$$

which means that women are more than twice as likely as men to be photonumerophobic. Conversely, conditional on being phobic, the odds that the person is female are 150/36 = 4.167; conditional on not being phobic, the odds that the person is female are (1850/964) = 1.919. The ratio of these two odds is 2.171, exactly what we found before. So, we can say either that the odds that a phobic person is female as opposed to male is 2.171 to 1, or that the odds a female is phobic as opposed to a male being phobic is 2.171 to 1. Both conclusions are equally valid interpretations of the OR.

However, there are two problems with odds. First, although their lower limit is 0.0, their upper limit can, in theory, approach infinity, making it difficult to compare relative magnitudes of odds. Second, we saw that the odds for the phobic person being female are 2.171:1, while the odds that the person is male are the reciprocal, or 0.461:1. It is not intuitively obvious that these two numbers reflect the same relationship from opposite directions. We can solve both of these difficulties by using the *logarithm* of the odds. For females, the log odds are the log (to the base e) of 2.171, or 0.775; for males, the log odds are the log of 0.461, or −0.775. Three things are immediately apparent. First, odds greater than 1.0 result in positive log odds, and odds less than 1.0 have negative log odds. Second, log odds of 0.0 mean odds of 1.0, an equal probability of being in one or the other group. Last, an odds and its reciprocal have exactly the same log odds, differing only in being a positive or a negative value.

Now, let's calculate the expected, or E, value for each cell (which we will call E_{ij}) in Table 14.1, using the concept of odds. In a completely analogous way to the method we used in Equation [1], it is the odds of being either male or female (λ_G for the gender odds) times the odds of being phobic or not (λ_P, for the phobic odds) times some value related to the sample size in each cell, Θ (theta). So, we end up with

$$E_{ij} = \theta \times \lambda_G \times \lambda_P. \qquad [5]$$

We can express the O values the same way. As we said, if there is no relationship between gender and diagnosis, then the O and E frequencies would be the same, within the limits of sampling error. In other words, both O and E would have the same value as the right-hand side of Equation [5]. However, if there *is* a relationship, we would expect a significant gap between O and E, indicating that the variables represented by the rows and columns (in this case, gender and PNP) affect or "interact" with each other. So, we simply add a term to reflect this interaction to Equation [5] resulting in

$$O_{ij} = \theta \times \lambda_G \times \lambda_P \times \lambda_{GP}. \qquad [6]$$

The question is, now, how well do these equations fit the data? By definition, Equation [6] fits them perfectly, since it models exactly what we observed. The issue is whether it is any better than Equation [5], which does not include the interaction term. If it is not any better, then this term is not needed, and we would conclude that there is no relationship between gender and phobia. If it is better (that is, if Equation [5] does not fit the data very well), then we would conclude the opposite: the interaction term is necessary, and there is an association present in the data. Before we go any further, let's simplify our lives a bit. People find it easier to add than to multiply and much easier to understand additive relationships than multiplicative ones. We can simplify Equation [6] by taking the log of each side, since we can multiply two numbers by adding their logs (this also makes it easier to figure out the log odds). Equation [5] becomes

$$\log E_{ij} = \log \theta + \log \lambda_G + \log \lambda_P, \qquad [7]$$

and Equation [6] results in

$$\log O_{ij} = \log \theta + \log \lambda_G + \log \lambda_P + \log \lambda_{GP} \qquad [8]$$

and gives rise to the name of the procedure: it is a *linear model* (that is, there are no multiplication terms) based on the *logs* of these parameters. (In mathematics, we usually denote log to the base e as ln; we're using log instead, just to simplify matters, although some may dispute this assertion.)

Let's simplify even more. Rather than writing out these equations in full every time we want to refer to them, we can write Equation [7] as {G}{P} to indicate that it is a function of gender and phobia; and Equation [8] becomes {G}{P}{GP} to show that it includes the interaction term. We can simplify the notation once more. In hierarchical models (which is what we will discuss here), the presence of the interaction term means that the lower-level terms must be present, too, so {G}{P}{GP} can be written simply as {GP}, which implies that {G}and {P} must be present. To rephrase the question using our simplified notation, our task is to determine if the model without the interaction – {G}{P} – is sufficient, or whether we need the full model – {GP}, referred to as the *saturated* model – to explain the results. ("Saturated" means simply that all possible terms – main effects and interactions – are present in the equation. The saturated model always fits the data perfectly.)

How do we determine which model to choose? We use some statistic similar to the chi-squared (variously called G^2, or the likelihood ratio chi-squared), which tells us the goodness of fit for each model, that is, how well each equation models the data. For our example, the model without the interaction term, {G}{P}, has a G^2 value of 19.04, which, with one degree of freedom, is highly significant. To understand what this means, we have to think in a somewhat backwards fashion. Chi-squared increases when there is a large discrepancy between the observed and the expected data. Analogously, G^2 increases if there is a large difference between the observed and the modelled data. So, the significant value of G^2 means that {G}{P} does not fit the data well (there is too much differ-

Table 14.2 Cross-classification of gender, photonumerophobia (PNP), and birth order

	First or only child			Second or later child		
	PNP	Not PNP	Total	PNP	Not PNP	Total
Male	15	330	345	21	634	655
Female	85	420	505	65	1430	1495
Total	100	750	850	86	2064	2150

ence between the "reduced" model and the actual data), and therefore the model with the interaction term, {GP}, is necessary.

Not surprisingly, this is exactly what we found when we used a simple chi-squared: there is an interaction of gender with PNP. So why go through all of these gyrations? The log-linear model becomes useful when we want to add more variables, such as birth order, which we will designate with the letter B. If we were to write out the saturated model in full, it would read

$$\{G\}\{P\}\{B\}\{GP\}\{GB\}\{PB\}\{GPB\}, \qquad [9]$$

where there are three first-order interactions (GP, GB, and PB) and one second-order interaction term (GPB). Chi-squared can tease apart these interactions only with the greatest difficulty, while it is very straightforward to do so with log-linear analysis. To illustrate, we'll use the data in Table 14.2. The log odds of being phobic for men and women, conditional on birth order, are shown in Figure 14.1, which comes directly from the table. The log odds are negative, because even in the highest-risk group (women who are firstborn or only children), most women do not develop PNP, so the odds are less than 1.0, and the log odds are therefore negative. (To test your understanding of these concepts, see if you can derive the log odds shown in Figure 14.1 from the data in Table 14.2; the answers are in Table 14.3.)

Looking at Figure 14.1, we see clearly that women are at a higher risk of PNP than men and that being an only or a firstborn child puts one at higher risk than being born later in the sib line. The question is whether there is an interaction between gender and birth order. One positive indication is shown in the graph; the slope of the line for females is steeper than that for males, which may show that the difference in the likelihood of PNP between firstborn versus later-born may be greater for women than for men. We can actually calculate the OR for males (the log odds

Fig. 14.1 Log-odds of having photonumerophobia (PNP) for males and females, conditional on birth order

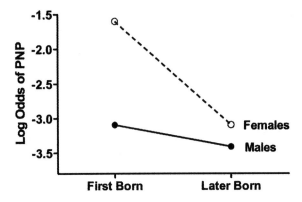

Table 14.3 Adding the odds and log odds for photonumerophobia (PNP)

	First or only child				Second or later child			
	PNP	Not PNP	Odds	Log odds	PNP	Not PNP	Odds	Log odds
Males	15	330	0.045	−3.091	21	634	0.033	−3.408
Females	85	420	0.202	−1.598	65	1430	0.045	−3.091

of PNP for later-born males divided by the log odds of PNP for firstborn males) and do the same for females. For males, it is −3.408/−3.091, or 1.103; and for females, it is −3.091/−1.598, or 1.934. This confirms what the graph shows: for men, being firstborn adds an additional 10.3% risk of PNP compared with being later-born; for women, being firstborn nearly doubles the risk. But, is this difference between the ORs for men and for women statistically significant? To answer that question, we use a log-linear analysis to select the correct model.

The logic of selecting the correct model is fairly straightforward. As we've said, by definition, the saturated model {GPB} fits the data exactly. If we eliminate the highest-order interaction, which is $G \times P \times B$, then we are left with a model that consists of the effects of each of the variables individually (the main effects) and the two-way interactions among them:

$$\{G\}\{P\}\{B\}\{GP\}\{GB\}\{PB\}. \qquad [10]$$

Table 14.4 Log-linear program output for photonumerophobia, gender, and birth order (Tests that k-way and higher interactions are zero.)

k	df	L.R. Chisq	Prob
3	1	9.421	0.0021
2	4	120.511	< .0001
1	7	3807.019	< .0001

If this model fits the data (that is, if G^2 is not significant), then we try to eliminate the next-highest interactions and so on, until we reach a point where the model doesn't fit the data very well, at which point we stop. Needless to say, every computer program presents the output somewhat differently, in a relatively successful attempt to confuse people, but most will have something that looks like Table 14.4.

Table 14.4 shows us, first, what the probability is that the three-way interaction contributes nothing (the line with $k = 3$); then, whether the two- and three-way interactions have any effect ($k = 2$); and finally, whether all of the terms have any effect. In the case of our data, if we remove the three-way interaction, the likelihood ratio chi-squared ("L.R. Chisq" in the table) is significant, meaning that there is a difference between the observed data and the values predicted from the model without the GPB term. Translated into English, it means that this interaction term is necessary to explain our findings and that birth order does affect the relationship between gender and PNP.

That was relatively easy. Now let's look at a different set of variables. Perhaps there is something in the "right-brain/left-brain" stuff, and left-handedness exacerbates the problems of PNP in females more than in males. Our new variables are thus PNP, gender, and handedness {H}. The output from the computer program is shown in Table 14.5, and the results are somewhat different from what we saw previously. The first line of the top part ($k = 3$) shows that the three-way interaction has no effect; that is, its removal would not affect how well the model fits the data The second line tells us that we need at least some of the two-way interactions, but we still need more information. There are several ways we can have significant two-way interactions: all three interactions – {GP}, {GH}, and {PH} – are needed; two of the three are needed; or only one is necessary. If only one or two are required to fit the data, we have the additional question of which one(s)? To answer, we must look a bit further at the computer output.

Table 14.5 Log-linear program output for photonumerophobia, gender, and handedness (Tests that k-way and higher interactions are zero.)

k	df	L.R. Chisq	Prob
3	1	0.809	0.3686
2	4	19.895	0.0005
1	7	5336.747	<0.0001

If deleted, simple effect is:	df	L.R. Chisq change	Prob
PHOBIA * HAND	1	0.030	0.9013
GENDER * HAND	1	0.026	0.8709
GENDER * PHOBIA	1	19.038	<0.0001

The bottom part of Table 14.5 shows what would happen if each two-way interaction were removed: not much if we dropped {PH} and {GH}, but there would be a significantly poorer fit if the {GP} interaction were eliminated. This confirms the results of the previous analysis, showing that there is an interaction between gender and phobia and also that handedness does not play any role.

Summary

So, the major advantage of log-linear analysis is that it allows us to look at the relationship among many categorical variables much more easily and meaningfully than does the chi-squared test. In theory, we could extend our analysis of the causes and correlates of PNP far beyond gender, birth order, and handedness. However, we have to exercise some degree of restraint; we could easily extend our list of possible causes far beyond both what the data would allow us to analyse (even with a sample size of 3000) and what could be easily interpreted. For example, we could extend the study to ask whether left-handed, firstborn females who were raised in a female-headed household are more at risk for PNP than other individuals. To test this question, however, we would have to examine a model that includes one five-way interaction (handedness, gender, birth order, type of household, and PNP), five four-way interactions, ten three-way interactions, ten two-way interactions, and five main effects. The problem isn't the statistics but "merely" our ability to make sense of what we find. Within these constraints, though, log-linear analysis is a powerful tool for examining relationships among categorical variables.

REFERENCES

Norman, G.R., & Streiner, D.L. (2008). *Biostatistics: The bare essentials.* (3rd ed.). Shelton, CT: PMPH USA.

Streiner, D.L. (1998, Mar). Let me count the ways: Measuring incidence, prevalence, and impact in epidemiological studies. *Canadian Journal of Psychiatry, 43*(2), 173–179. Medline:9533971

TO READ FURTHER

Agresti, A. (2007). *An introduction to categorical data analysis.* (2nd ed.). New York: Wiley. http://dx.doi.org/10.1002/0470114754

Christensen, R. (1997). *Log-linear models and logistic regression.* (2nd ed.). New York: Springer.

Knoke, D., & Burke, P.J. (1980). *Log-linear models.* Newberry Park, CA: Sage.

Norman, G.R., & Streiner, D.L. (2008). *Biostatistics: The bare essentials.* (3rd ed.). Shelton, CT: PMPH USA.

15 Confronting the Confounders: The Meaning, Detection, and Handling of Confounders in Research

ANNE E. RHODES, PH.D., ELIZABETH LIN, PH.D.,
DAVID L. STREINER, PH.D.

Canadian Journal of Psychiatry, 1999, 44, 175–179

What Is Confounding?

If you read enough about research, you will most likely have come across the term "confounding." Although you can easily find definitions in standard epidemiology textbooks (Kelsey, Whittemore, Evans, & Thompson, 1996; Kleinbaum, Kupper, & Morgenstern, 1982; Rothman, Greenland, & Lash, 2008; Schlesselman, 1982), the concept is by no means straightforward. To familiarize ourselves with confounding, let's begin with some examples. Say that we are interested in testing whether caring for an ill family member "causes" depression (Figure 15.1).

Our first step is to design a study. Ideally, we would conduct a randomized controlled trial in which one-half of our participants are assigned to caregiving and one-half are not. But who would agree to participate? We need to conduct an observational survey, such as a cohort, case-control, or cross-sectional study (Streiner & Norman, 2009). For this paper, we'll assume that the study has been well executed and that we have the data. Also, we'll assume that our results show an association between being a caregiver and depression, but that in reality there is no such relationship. Why would this happen? It's possible that another factor, such as gender, could produce a spurious association between being a caregiver and depression. Because we are not able to randomly allocate people to caregiving, we cannot prevent having unequal numbers of men and women among our caregivers. Because caregivers are often women (Mohide et al., 1990), more

Fig. 15.1 Relationship between caregiving and depression

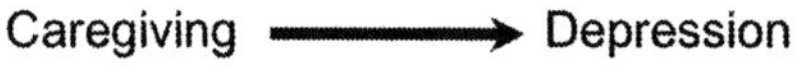

Caregiving ➞ Depression

Fig. 15.2 Gender as a confounder, leading to a relationship

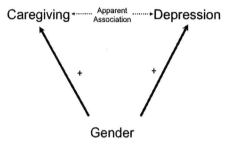

caregivers in our study will be women than men. Since women are also more likely than men to suffer from depression (Bland, 1997), our data will show that caregiving is related to depression, when really it is not (Figure 15.2). That is, the "real" association is between gender and depression, and any other variable that is correlated with gender, such as wearing skirts or putting the toilet seat down, will also be correlated with depression.

This example shows how a third variable can make two other variables appear to be associated when they are not. Conversely, sometimes a third variable can actually hide or mask a real association rather than produce a false one. For example, suppose we find in another study that gender is not associated with going to see a therapist. We are automatically suspicious, since many other studies have shown that women typically seek treatment more often than men (Lin, Goering, Offord, Campbell, & Boyle, 1996). When we look at the data more carefully, we find that in our sample there are many low-income women in comparison with men. (Our study design did not attempt to control for income differences.) Since people who have high incomes are more likely to see a therapist, the association between gender and going to see a therapist appears when we control for income. In this example, income actually hides a real association between gender and seeing a therapist, until we control for it (Figure 15.3). These examples show that sometimes there is a third variable, or a confounder, that hinders testing a hypothesis of interest. Let's see how it happens and what can be done about it.

Fig. 15.3 Income as a confounder, masking a relationship

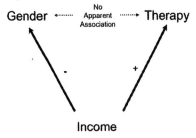

The Lurking Confounder

If we knew the literature well, we might suspect the confounders described in the above examples. But, as in real-life police work, capturing and disarming a confounder is more complicated than identifying a suspect from a line-up. We need to ascertain whether our suspect really is a confounder or is merely an innocent bystander.

In the depression and caregiving example our suspect, gender, is associated with depression and caregiving. So gender looks guilty because it keeps regular company with both depression and caregiving. In the gender and therapy-going example our suspect, level of income, is linked with both gender and therapy-going. The case against our suspects is building, but we don't yet have enough information to convict them. Determining whether a suspected variable is associated with both the independent and the dependent variables of interest is the first step in assessing confounding.

If the suspect is associated only with the dependent variable or only with the independent variable, but not with both, then it is not a true confounder. More subtly, the confounder must be related to the independent variable regardless of the dependent variable, and the confounder must be related to the dependent variable regardless of the independent variable. So, in the caregiving example, gender is related to being a caregiver in those who are depressed and in those who are not depressed. Also, gender is associated with depression in both caregivers and non-caregivers.

Often in our analyses, we come upon variables that are related to one another, and we are not sure which ones are independent variables and which ones might be confounders. The study's hypotheses and purpose are key to helping us decide. If our goal is simply to predict the

Fig. 15.4 Effects on behaviour of eating chips and drinking beer

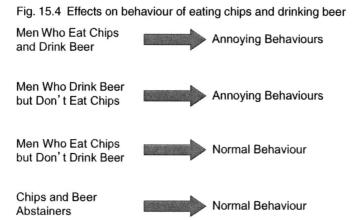

Men Who Eat Chips and Drink Beer	Annoying Behaviours
Men Who Drink Beer but Don't Eat Chips	Annoying Behaviours
Men Who Eat Chips but Don't Drink Beer	Normal Behaviour
Chips and Beer Abstainers	Normal Behaviour

dependent variable, then confounding is not an issue. We can happily proceed using stepwise regression (Streiner, 1994; see Chapter 11) or some other technique to select the best predictors. However, if our goal is to explain what causes the dependent variable, then we need to focus on a specific independent variable and worry about confounding.

Let's use an example to illustrate the difference between prediction and explanation. We have observed a strange neuropsychological phenomenon: on Monday nights, some men become loud and obnoxious. After further observation, we venture that this behaviour is connected to watching football. However, not all men who watch football act this way. After more study, we narrow our hypothesis to the association of two substances with this behaviour: potato chips and beer. We can stop here if we are not interested in what causes the behaviour; we just want to identify these men so that we can stay away from them! In this instance, whenever we see a man eating chips and/or drinking beer, we know we should head in the opposite direction. However, if we decide that we want to know why some men act this way in order to stop the behaviour, then we have to do a bit more detective work. It occurs to us that men who just eat chips behave acceptably. However, if men both eat chips and drink beer at the same time, they are troublesome. Come to think of it, they're a pain if they just drink beer and don't eat any chips. We begin to realize that potato chips, on their own, are not associated with annoying behaviours. They appear to be a problem only because they often accompany beer drinking (Figure 15.4).

Fig. 15.5 Social isolation in the causal pathway
between caregiving and depression

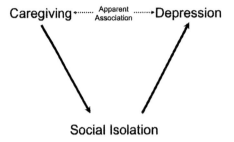

Social Isolation

Alcohol is the likely suspect causing the behaviour. This fits with
what we know about the effects of alcohol on the brain; after all,
when were we last warned not to eat potato chips and drive? So, to
return to our study goal, to explain the dependent variable – annoying
behaviour – we would focus on beer drinking rather than chip eating.
However, we need to consider whether eating chips is a confounding
variable. In this example it is not a confounder, because we find it is
related only to the independent variable (beer drinking), but not to the
dependent variable (raucousness), so we do not have to control for it. In
fact, we would be wise not to control for it. For example, if we put both
drinking beer and eating potato chips in an equation to explain annoying behaviours, eating potato chips would steal some of the thunder
(variance) from drinking beer because both activities are highly associated, and beer drinking would not look as important as it should.

Let's return to our caregiving and depression example. Because we are
interested in explaining why people get depressed, not simply who gets
depressed, we cannot shy away from the possibility that gender con-
founds the relationship between caregiving and depression. The next
step in our detective work requires some knowledge or theory about
the relationships between the variables under study. We are relatively
certain that caregiving does not cause gender (Figure 15.2). But, putting
gender aside for a moment, what if our suspected variable were social
isolation? It is quite possible that being a caregiver causes one to become
socially isolated and that social isolation causes depression. Here, being
a caregiver is an indirect cause of depression (Figure 15.5).

Although social isolation is related to both caregiving and depression in this example, social isolation is not a confounder, because it is in
the causal pathway between gender and depression; that is, caregiving

Fig. 15.6 Relationship between caregiving and depression using a continuous measure

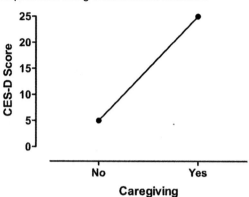

leads to isolation, which in turn leads to depression. We would not want to control for social isolation, because the association between caregiving and depression could disappear, leading us to think, incorrectly, that caregiving does not cause depression. We have just identified the second step in identifying a confounder. A confounder gets in the way of understanding relationships and must be controlled for; it is not part of a causal pathway (Rothman et al., 2008).

Our detective work is almost done. In the caregiving and depression example, gender meets the first two criteria for being a confounder (that is, it is related to both the dependent and independent variables, and it is not part of the causal pathway). The last step is probably the most difficult to comprehend. In our caregiving study, assume that we have measured depression using the Center for Epidemiologic Studies-Depression (CES-D) scale (Radloff & Locke, 1986), scores for which can range between 0 and 60. We find that the mean CES-D scores for caregivers in our sample is 25, whereas the mean score for non-caregivers is only 5. We are initially encouraged because this large difference fits our hypothesis that caregivers are more depressed (Figure 15.6). Next, we compare the mean CES-D scores for caregivers and non-caregivers, but now broken down by gender (Figure 15.7). In this graph, we see that women have higher mean depression scores than men, but that the difference between caregivers and non-caregivers, whether they are men or women, is small and constant, that is, 2 points. In fact, the two lines are parallel. A constant difference between the independent and

Fig. 15.7 Caregiving and depression by gender

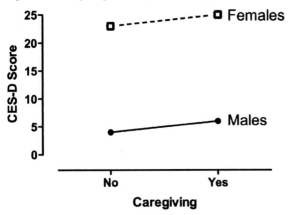

dependent variables at all levels of the potential confounder is the final piece of evidence we need to identify a true confounder.

If the difference were not constant (that is, the lines were not parallel), then this would be evidence of an *interaction* rather than of confounding. Here, the relationship between caregiving and depression would be different for men and for women; that is, the distance between the lines for caregivers and non-caregivers would not be the same for men and for women. Therefore, we would need to talk about the relationship between caregiving and depression separately for men and women. However, because the relationship is the same for men and women, we can remove these confounding effects (for more information about interactions, see Rothman et al., 2008). Since gender has met all three confounding criteria, we need to control for it to accurately estimate the true association between caregiving and depression.

In this example, we looked at differences between the means, because our dependent variable, the CES-D, is a continuous variable. For categorical dependent variables, the same rules apply, but the detection method differs. Suppose we were dealing with a dichotomous dependent variable, such as whether or not the person is diagnosed as having a mood disorder. Instead of examining the differences between the means, we would examine differences between measures of risk, such as the odds ratio or the relative risk (Streiner, 1998; see Chapter 7).

It should be amply clear now why confounding can be a confusing concept to the uninitiated. It is not an intuitive process; it requires some understanding of statistics – the specific criteria that distinguish a confounder from other types of relationships occurring among independent, dependent, and "suspect" variables (Kelsey et al., 1996; Kleinbaum et al., 1982; Rothman et al., 2008; Schlesselman, 1982) – as well as substantive knowledge of the clinical area being studied. Most of us would probably like to avoid confounding altogether. This would be a shame, though, because we would either restrict ourselves to prediction types of questions or conduct explanatory studies that would fall short by not controlling for confounding. So, read on.

Spotting a Confounder

Now that we've discussed what confounding is and when it matters, let's learn to recognize it. First and foremost, confounding can (and should) be considered at the design phase of a study. For example, in many observational studies, investigators use matching, stratification, or restriction of the study sample to control for confounders (such as age and gender). To avoid confounding, in clinical trials randomization attempts to make the groups as similar as possible on all variables that may be confounders. Multivariate analyses may also be used to control for confounding variables after the fact, that is, at the analysis stage (Kelsey et al., 1996; Kleinbaum et al., 1982; Rothman et al., 2008; Schlesselman, 1982).

During the analysis phase of the study, the assessment of confounding involves comparing the initial relationship between the independent variable and dependent variable (for example, caregiving and depression) with the relationship between caregiving and depression now controlled for the suspected confounder, gender. In Figure 15.6, the mean difference between caregivers and non-caregivers (crude relationship) was 20 points. In Figure 15.7, after controlling for gender, we found a constant difference of 2 points between caregivers and non-caregivers. The mean difference between caregivers and non-caregivers was reduced from 20 to 2 points once we controlled for gender. Since we feel that a distortion of 18 points with respect to the CES-D scale is quite important, we would need to control for gender.

When we have a dichotomous dependent variable (for example, the presence or absence of a disorder), we assess confounding by comparing the initial risk ratio with the risk ratio controlled for the potential confounder. A general rule is to control for confounding if the difference between these risk ratios is 10% or more (Maldonado & Greenland, 1993).

Note that we haven't mentioned statistical significance. This is because confounding is about distortions in the magnitude of a difference, whereas statistical significance is affected by the magnitude of a difference and the sample size (Rothman et al., 2008). We all know that if the sample is large, we can achieve statistical significance with puny differences. So, the moral of the story is that we should compare the initial estimates (crude estimates) and estimates controlled for the potential confounder (adjusted estimates), since these estimates give a direct measure of the magnitude of the difference (Elwood, 2007). Then a judgment can be made about whether the magnitude of the distortion is clinically relevant. Beware of studies that attempt to reassure the reader by saying, "We didn't need to control for variables X, Y, and Z, because none of them was statistically significantly related to the dependent variable." An association between an independent and a dependent variable can still be distorted by a third variable, even if none of these variables is related at a statistically significant level.

The examples we have given in this paper are (relatively) straightforward. In real life, there are often many confounders operating simultaneously. Some of these might be known beforehand, others might be suspected, and still others would be unknown. Thus, it is often a more complex job to detect and correct for them than has been presented here. But after all, that's what statisticians are paid for.

REFERENCES

Bland, R.C. (1997, May). Epidemiology of affective disorders: A review. *Canadian Journal of Psychiatry*, 42(4), 367–377. Medline:9161761

Elwood, J.M. (2007). *Causal relationships in medicine: A practical system for critical appraisal*. (3rd ed.). New York: Oxford University Press.

Kelsey, J.L., Whittemore, A.S., Evans, A.S., & Thompson, W.D. (1996). *Methods in observational epidemiology*. (2nd ed.). New York: Oxford University Press.

Kleinbaum, D.G., Kupper, L.L., & Morgenstern, H. (1982). *Epidemiologic research: Principles and quantitative methods*. New York: Van Nostrand Reinhold.

Lin, E., Goering, P., Offord, D.R., Campbell, D., & Boyle, M.H. (1996, Nov). The use of mental health services in Ontario: Epidemiologic findings. *Canadian Journal of Psychiatry*, 41(9), 572–577. Medline:8946080

Maldonado, G., & Greenland, S. (1993, Dec 1). Simulation study of confounder-selection strategies. *American Journal of Epidemiology*, 138(11), 923–936. Medline:8256780

Mohide, E.A., Pringle, D.M., Streiner, D.L., Gilbert, J.R., Muir, G., & Tew, M. (1990, Apr). A randomized trial of family caregiver support in the home management of dementia. *Journal of the American Geriatrics Society, 38*(4), 446–454. Medline:2184186

Radloff, L., & Locke, B. (1986). The community mental health assessment survey and the CES-D scale. In M. Weissman, J. Myers, & C. Ross (Eds.), *Community surveys of psychiatric disorders* (pp. 177–189). New Brunswick, NJ: Rutgers University Press.

Rothman, K.J., Greenland, S., & Lash, T.L. (2008). *Modern epidemiology.* (3rd ed.). Philadelphia, PA: Lippincott Williams and Wilkins.

Schlesselman, J.J. (1982). *Case-control studies: Design, conduct, analysis.* New York: Oxford University Press.

Streiner, D.L. (1994, May). Regression in the service of the superego: The do's and don'ts of stepwise multiple regression. *Canadian Journal of Psychiatry, 39*(4), 191–196. Medline:8044725

Streiner, D.L. (1998, May). Risky business: Making sense of estimates of risk. *Canadian Journal of Psychiatry, 43*(4), 411–415. Medline:9598280

Streiner, D.L., & Norman, G.R. (2009). *PDQ epidemiology.* (3rd ed.). Shelton, CT: PMPH USA.

TO READ FURTHER

Elwood, J.M. (2007). *Causal relationships in medicine: A practical system for critical appraisal.* (3rd ed.). New York: Oxford University Press.

Greenland, S., & Morgenstern, H. (2001). Confounding in health research. *Annual Review of Public Health, 22*(1), 189–212. http://dx.doi.org/10.1146/annurev.publhealth.22.1.189 Medline:11274518

16 Finding Our Way: An Introduction to Path Analysis

DAVID L. STREINER, PH.D.

Canadian Journal of Psychiatry, 2005, 50, 115–122

One of the first things we learn in Statistics 101 is that there are two types of variables – independent variables (IVs) and dependent variables (DVs). The distinction between them is, in most cases, relatively clear and straightforward: we want to see what effect the IVs (sometimes called *predictor* variables in multiple regression) have on the DV. For example, if we compare antidepressant medication to cognitive behaviour therapy to see which leads to greater remission in depressive symptoms, the IV is the type of treatment and the DV is, perhaps, the score on a depression scale. In selecting candidates for medical school, the DV would be successful graduation or not, and the IVs could be grade point average in university, a numerical grade assigned to letters of reference, qualifying examination scores, and so on.

Unfortunately, the real world refuses to fall into just these two categories of variables. Life insists on being more complicated, and there are situations in which, if we are asked if a certain variable is a DV or an IV, we would have to say "yes." Let's assume, for example, that we found that women with young children at home suffer more from depression than women matched for age and marital status who do not have children at home. One hypothesis is that children at home make women suffer more from depression, based on the well-known fact that children can drive us crazy. This is the model shown at the top of Figure 16.1: children at home have a direct effect on depression. However, another hypothesis is that staying at home leads to social isolation, and that the isolation leads to dysphoria; this is the model at the bottom of Figure 16.1.

Fig. 16.1 Two possible models of the effects of children at home
on depression

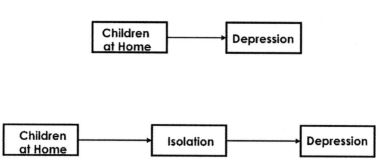

In both models, it is obvious that children at home is the IV and
depression is the DV. But what do we call isolation? It is a DV with
respect to children, but it is an IV as regards depression. In fact, the
problem goes beyond mere terminology; the deeper problem is how we
should analyse the lower model. The issue becomes more complicated
as our models become more complex. For example, we can posit that
other factors that may directly influence depression, such as hormonal
changes or past depression and family history of depression; that children at home cause other stresses that in turn affect the woman's mood;
and that there can be outcomes in addition to dysphoria. If we want to
look at all of these variables simultaneously, we need both new terminology and a new analytic strategy.

The name for the strategy comes from the pictorial representation of
the models themselves. At the bottom of Figure 16.1, we are describing a
path from children to isolation to depression. More complicated models
may have more paths, or paths that lead through more variables. Not
surprisingly, then, this technique is called *path analysis*. Path analysis
is an extension of multiple regression that allows us to examine more
complicated relationships among the variables than having several IVs
predict one DV and to compare different models to see which one best
fits the data. Before we begin, though, a disclaimer about both the statistic and the terminology. In the past (and occasionally now, among the
benighted), this technique was referred to as *causal modelling*, because it
was believed that it could be used to uncover causal pathways among
variables – which factors were responsible for which outcomes. As

we'll see later, this is a laudable goal, but one that cannot be solved by statistical methods, no matter how powerful. From a statistical vantage point, models that map out totally bizarre routes that can never exist in reality may look as good – or even better – than models that conform more closely to reality. Causality can be proven only through the correct research design (for example, longitudinal studies or experiments), and no amount of statistical legerdemain can pull cause and effect out of a cross-sectional or cohort study.

Some Terminology and Drawing Conventions

To return to the naming of the variables. In path analysis (and its more sophisticated counterpart, *structural equation modelling*, which is discussed in Streiner, 2006; see Chapter 17), we completely avoid the confusion around IVs and DVs by the simple expedient of not using those labels. Rather, we use the terms *exogenous* and *endogenous* variables.

- *Exogenous variables* have straight arrows emerging from them and none pointing to them (except from error terms).
- *Endogenous variables* have at least one straight arrow pointing to them.

The rationale for these terms is that the causes of (or factors that influence) exogenous variables are determined outside the model that we're examining, whereas the factors affecting endogenous variables exist within the model itself. In a moment, we'll see why there is that restriction on the shape (not the moral fibre) of the arrow. Thus, at the bottom of Figure 16.1, having children is an exogenous variable, and both social isolation and depression are endogenous ones. Let's take a look at some other possible models.

In Figure 16.2 (a), we are hypothesizing that exogenous variables of both having children and being isolated independently influence depression, and that children and isolation are not correlated. This would be called an *independent* model, reflecting the lack of correlation between the two exogenous variables. If we believe that the variables are correlated, we draw a curved, two-headed arrow between them, as in Figure 16.2 (b), where a curved, double-headed arrow reflects a correlation (or covariance, a term that will be defined shortly) between variables. This is the run-of-the-mill multiple regression model, although we often have more than two exogenous or pre-

Fig. 16.2 Some possible path models

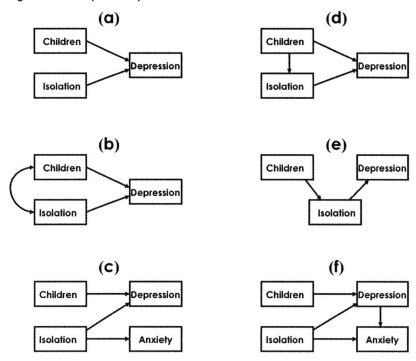

dictor variables. Also, because, as Meehl said, "everything correlates to some extent with everything else" (1990, p. 204), we customarily assume that the correlations are present, so I won't bother to draw the curved arrows (except when necessary). In Figure 16.2 (c), we are extending the model by looking at two endogenous variables, depression and anxiety. We are saying that having children affects only depression but not anxiety, while isolation influences both depression and anxiety.

The models on the right side of Figure 16.2 are called *mediated* or *indirect*, because the exogenous variables act on an endogenous variable, at least in part, through their influence on an intermediary (endogenous) variable. Thus, in Figure 16.2 (d), having children directly influences depression, as does isolation, but having children also affects isolation, which then acts on depression; in other words, being isolated would cause women to suffer from depression even in the absence of children,

Fig. 16.3 Adding disturbance terms and making the model non-recursive

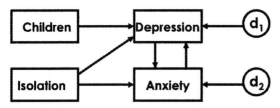

but the presence of children exacerbates this effect. This model is somewhat different from that of Figure 16.2 (e), which is the same as the bottom part of Figure 16.1 in that isolation is due solely to the rug rats and would not exist in women if not for them. Finally, in Figure 16.2 (f), we see that one final endogenous variable (depression) can also affect another one (anxiety). This by no means exhausts the possibilities. Paths can be much longer and involve more intermediate steps, and there could (and often are) more variables that are brought into the picture – both literally and figuratively.

There are two more terms that need to be introduced. In Figure 16.3, note that pointing towards the two endogenous variables are small circles with ds in them. The ds indicate *disturbance*, which in path analysis is similar to the error term tacked on the end of regression equations. Like the error term, the disturbance term captures two things: (a) imprecision in the measurement of the endogenous variable, because all of our measurement tools are subject to some degree of error; and (b) all the other factors that affect the endogenous variable that we didn't measure, because of oversight, lack of time, ignorance of their importance, laziness, or whatever. Because every endogenous variable must have a disturbance term associated with it, we often don't bother to draw it, to keep the drawing simpler, but, if it's not explicitly drawn, it's implicitly present.

Finally (yes!), Figure 16.3 differs from Figure 16.2 (f) in one subtle but important way. In Figure 16.2 (f), one endogenous variable (depression) affects a second (anxiety), which is logical, but the second does not affect the first. It likely makes more clinical sense for there to be a path in both directions; that is, depression affects anxiety, and anxiety in turn is depressogenic. The latter model, with a feedback loop, is called *non-recursive*, whereas path models that lead inexorably in one direction are referred to as *recursive*. (No, I didn't inadvertently reverse the terms. They are, for some unfathomable reason, utterly counterintuitive. You'll just have to live with that.) There is one cardinal rule for attempting to analyse non-recursive models: DON'T! Although they are often a more accurate reflection of the way things work in the real world, the analytic problems they produce are horrendous. Even more troubling, these problems are not immediately apparent from most computer printouts, especially to neophytes, so they are not aware that they are getting into a quagmire.

As we go through some examples, two other terms will keep appearing – *variances* and *covariances*. (Because they were probably first mentioned in introductory statistics, I'm considering them to be old terms, so I haven't violated my statement about the number of new ones I'm introducing.) Variance is simply the amount of variation in a variable from one person to another and, formally, is the square of the standard deviation (SD). A covariance is the first cousin of a correlation. A correlation tells us whether, if variable *A* goes up, variable *B* also goes up (a positive correlation), goes down (a negative correlation), or changes in a way unrelated to variable *A* (zero correlation). When we calculate a correlation, both variables are transformed into standard scores that have a mean of 0 and an SD of 1. Covariance is exactly the same thing, except that the variables aren't transformed but remain in their original units of measurement. For various arcane reasons, it is often better to calculate multivariable statistics by using the covariances among variables rather than their correlations. The reason for our obsession with them is that they are all we have to work with in determining how variables influence each other. When we've done a study measuring several variables on each person, what we end up with is a matrix consisting of the variances of each variable along the main diagonal (the cells running from the upper-left to the lower-right corners) and the covariances in all the cells off the main diagonal. The job of path analysis is to determine whether there are any meaningful patterns in these data.

A Multiple Regression Example

Let's begin to see what path analysis can do by using a different example and framing it first in multiple regression terms. In previous chapters in this book, you have been introduced to a disorder not yet found in the DSM – photonumerophobia, which is the fear that our fear of numbers will come to light. We may want to see whether a person's

Table 16.1 Means, SDs, correlations among the variables, and unstandardized and standardized regression weights for the relationship between photonumerophobia (PNP), anxiety (ANX), high school math grade (HSM), and income tax discrepancy (TAX)

	PNP	ANX	HSM	TAX	Mean	SD	b	β
PNP	1.000	0.509	−0.366	0.346	26.79	7.33	–	–
ANX	–	1.000	−0.264	0.338	20.33	5.17	0.414	0.292
HSM	–	–	1.000	0.260	74.69	5.37	−0.517	−0.379
TAX	–	–	–	1.000	1983.23	525.49	0.005	0.346

score on a scale of photonumerophobia (the PNP scale, which ironically is scored using numbers) can be predicted from three factors: overall level of anxiety (ANX), high school math grade (HSM), and the discrepancy between what the person estimated last year's taxes to be and what the tax people said it actually was (TAX). That is, we are hypothesizing that photonumerophobia is related to a person's overall anxiety level (we would expect a positive correlation) as well as to doing poorly in math class (a negative correlation) and to screwing up one's income tax returns (again a positive correlation: the more severe the phobia, the greater the mistake). If we wrote this hypothesis as a regression, it would look as follows:

$$PNP = b_0 + b_1 ANX + b_2 HSM + b_3 TAX + Error,$$ [1]

where b_0 is the intercept, and the other bs are the slopes for each IV. The means and SDs of the variables and the correlations among them are shown in Table 16.1, as are the unstandardized regression weights (b) and the standardized ones (β). (Very briefly, the b weights are used with the data in their original units of measurement; the β weights, after each variable has been standardized, have a mean of 0 and an SD of 1. For a more complete description of the difference, see Norman & Streiner, 2003, 2008). The multiple correlation, R, is 0.638; therefore, R^2 (the square of R, reflecting the proportion of variance in the DV accounted for by the equation) is 0.407.

In the conventions of path analysis, each IV or predictor variable (now called an exogenous variable) would be shown as a rectangle, with another rectangle for the DV, or endogenous variable, as in the left side of Figure 16.4. Because computer programs suffer from severe organic brain damage, it's necessary to draw the curved arrows reflecting correlations among the variables and the disturbance term. When

Fig. 16.4 Hypothesized model (a) and results (b) of the regression equation

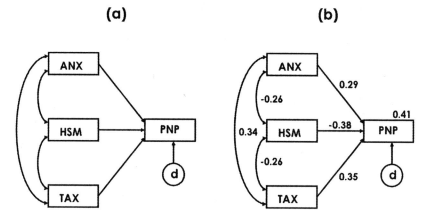

we run the program, we'll get reams of paper, but most of the results can be summarized in a diagram, shown on the right side of Figure 16.4. Very reassuringly, the correlations (next to the curved arrows) agree with the results from the regression analysis; as do the β weights, which are printed near the paths (the straight arrows). Finally, the number over the right side of PNP is the value of R^2, which again is identical to the results from the multiple regression. Also reassuring from a theoretical standpoint is that the signs of the paths correspond to what we hypothesized.

Let's review what we've accomplished so far. We've taken a problem that is easily handled with inexpensive, well-known, and widely available computer programs (those for multiple regression) and shown how we can get identical results by using an expensive and arcane one (for path analysis and structural equation modelling). If this is all there is, then it reflects progress that we can easily live without. Fortunately, though (especially for the purveyors of the software), path analysis can do much more. For example, we can postulate other hypotheses about the relations among the variables and see whether they are better or worse in accounting for the variance in the PNP scale. Two examples are shown in Figure 16.5. In Figure 16.5(a), it's hypothesized that, rather than the variables acting separately on PNP, there is truly a path where anxiety leads to poor math grades in high school, which results in mistakes in completing tax forms and culminates in photonumerophobia. In Figure 16.5(b), the hypothesis is that anxiety results in both poor

Fig. 16.5 Other possible models

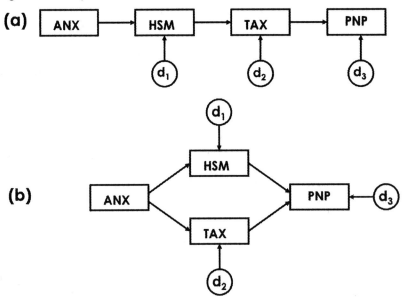

grades and computational errors in filling out tax forms and that both together lead to photonumerophobia.

Fitting the Model

The issue now is how to choose among the models. The first place to look is at the path coefficients themselves. As mentioned above, they are standardized regression weights, identical to the β weights of multiple regression. Their sign should correspond to what the model predicts. If we expect anxiety to be positively correlated with PNP, then a path coefficient with a negative sign would increase our own anxiety level, as well as lead to rejection of the model. Moreover, the β weight should be statistically significant. We aren't able to determine this from the diagram, but the accompanying printed output will tell us whether it's significant or not.

There are several (actually, myriad) fit indices that tell you how well the model fits the data. Because they are also used in structural equation modelling, and because of space limitations in this chapter, they will be discussed in the next one (Streiner, 2006; see Chapter 17).

Model Specification

What can account for a poorly fitting model? The most likely cause is *model misspecification*. This can occur in several ways: the inclusion of variables that are not related to any of the endogenous variables, the omission of crucial variables, and specifying paths that connect variables that are not, in fact, related to each other. Ideally, if an extraneous variable has been included, its path coefficient will be low and non-significant, signalling that the model should be rerun without that variable. The same situation should apply if a path is drawn between variables that aren't related to each other. Unfortunately, there is nothing that can tell us when we've omitted some crucial variable(s); further, if the omitted variables are correlated with some in the model, the fit indices can still be quite high (Tomarken & Waller, 2003). Protecting yourself against this error requires knowledge of the literature and a reasonable hypothesis regarding what can affect the outcomes.

If we attempt to apply these fit indices to the model in Figure 16.4, we'll see somewhat unusual results. All of the indices that should be above 0.90 are, in fact, 1.00 – a perfect fit! Moreover, the goodness-of-fit χ^2 (χ^2_{GoF}), which should be low, is as low as it can get: 0.00 (albeit with 0 degrees of freedom [df]). We know the model makes sense, but no prediction model is this good. Common sense would tell us that each of these variables is measured with some degree of error, so that even if the theoretical model were a perfect reflection of reality (in which case the next Nobel Prize would be mine), the match between the data and the model wouldn't be perfect. Moreover, the R^2 is only 0.41, so our "perfect" model isn't accounting for the majority of the variance in PNP. What's going on?

The problem has to do with the *identification* of the model. Identification refers to how many things we have to estimate (such as the path coefficients) in relation to how much information we can derive from the data, information in terms of the observed variances of the variables and the covariances among them. In this regression model, the amount of information is exactly equal to the number of paths we have to estimate; it is *just-identified*. We can see this from the fact that, as noted in the previous paragraph, $df = 0$. So, let's see what's meant by *identifying* the model. We'll start off with a simple example: what are the values of the unknown terms in the following equation?

$$A + B = 10. \qquad [2]$$

The answer is indeterminate, in that there are an infinite number of possibilities. *A* can be 10 and *B* can be 0; or *A* can be 9 and *B* can be 1; or *A* can be 938 and *B* can be −928; and so on, ad infinitum. We do not have enough information to solve the equation, so we say that it is *under-identified*; in other words, we cannot derive unique values for the two unknowns (and, by analogy, the various parameters in this model). If we know that *A* = 7, then there is only one possible solution, and the model is said to be *just-identified*, which is good. Even better is an *over-identified* model: we have more information than we need (for those who remember high school math, analogous to having more simultaneous equations than unknown variables), so we can test different models against one another. Equally important, we have seen that we cannot get any fit indices from models that are just-identified but we can with over-identified models.

How many parameters can we estimate in a model? If there are *k* variables, then we have *k* variances and $[(k^2 - k)/2]$ covariances, for a total of $[(k^2 + k)/2]$ pieces of information. In Figure 16.4, there are four variables, so we can estimate a maximum of $[(4^2 + 4)/2] = 10$ parameters. The next question, then, is how many parameters do we *want* to estimate in this model? To begin with, there are the three paths from the exogenous variables (ANX, HSM, and TAX) to the endogenous one (PNP). Next, there are three covariances (or correlations) among the exogenous variables. Then, there is the variance of the disturbance term (*d*). Finally, there are the variances of the exogenous variables themselves, for a total of 10. The *df* is the difference between the number of parameters we *can* estimate and the number of parameters we *want* to estimate. Note that *df* is not related to the number of subjects in the study; simply increasing the sample size will not solve the problem of a model that is under- or just-identified (although it does have other benefits, which I'll discuss later).

Two questions arise from this. First, why don't we want to estimate the variance of PNP (or any other endogenous variable, for that matter)? The answer is that the purpose of path analysis is to find out what affects the endogenous variable; that is, how the exogenous variables work together (their covariances) and which paths are important (determined in part by the variances of the exogenous variables). Because the model postulates that the endogenous variables are determined or influenced solely by the exogenous ones, they are not free to vary on their own, but to vary only in response to the exogenous variables. Consequently, we are not concerned with estimating PNP's variance. In general, then, we want to estimate (a) the paths, (b) the covariances among the exogenous variables, and (c) the variances of the exogenous variables, but not the variances of the endogenous ones.

Types of Path

The second question is "how can we increase the *df* to turn an under-identified model into an over-identified one?" The answer arises from the fact that paths come in two flavours: *free* and *fixed*. What we've been looking at so far are free paths, that is, paths free to take on any value that best fits the data; in most cases, this is what we are most interested in. We can increase the *df* by setting various paths to some predefined value; in other words, to *fix* them so that the program won't have to estimate them from the data. The most efficient way is to set some paths equal to zero, that is, to simplify the model by dropping some of the hypothesized links. Depending on the variable that's dropped from the model, this can sometimes increase *df* by two or more, since it is not necessary to estimate either the path or the variance of the term, and there may be fewer covariances to estimate. Needless to say, this can be a draconian method if all of the variables and paths are deemed to be essential to the model, but it may at times be necessary. For example, in the discussion about Figure 16.4, I said that we should not have anxiety influencing depression and depression influencing anxiety, logical as it may seem, because that would result in a non-recursive model. Deciding which arrow to eliminate may be based on our theories of anxiety and depression or, perhaps, on research that may indicate which condition is generally present first or, in the absence of these, on just a guess – not an ideal situation by any means, but one imposed by the technique.

The need for parsimony should also serve as a warning, which I'll return to later: path analysis is a model-*testing* approach, not a model-*building* one. You should not throw in any variable that's available and draw every conceivable path, just to see what comes out. There should be a sound rationale for the model, based on theory and research, or even a strong hunch. But don't be scared off by the term "theory." The rationale does not have to rival Einstein's theory of general relativity in its complexity or degree of development. A postulate as simple as "isolation leads to dysphoria" is a theory, albeit not one that will immortalize its developer.

Another technique to reduce the *df* is to fix the value of a path to be equal to 1. For example, the paths from the disturbance terms to the endogenous variables are automatically fixed by the program to be 1. (This is because we do not have enough information to estimate both the variance and the path coefficient of the *d*s, for the same reason, explained above, that we have difficulty when trying to estimate the values of *A* and *B* to add up to 10. Because we are usually more interested in the magnitude of the error, as reflected by its variance, than we are in the path coefficient, the latter is fixed, although we can overrule the program if we wish.)

Sample Size

As we just mentioned, the *df* depends solely on the number of variables and parameters in the model, not on the number of subjects. An under-identified model will remain under-identified even if we use 10 times the number of people. The sample size becomes important in accurately estimating the values of the paths, variances, and covariances. Because all of these are parameters, there is a standard error (SE) associated with each one, as well as a z-test, which is the ratio of the parameter to the SE. If the sample size is too small, the estimates of the parameters are unstable, reflected in large SEs and non-significant z tests for the significance. Klein (2010) recommends a minimum of 10 cases for every parameter that's estimated, and 20 if you can find them; 5 are too few. Don't forget that there are two or three parameters for every variable, so path analysis is much hungrier for subjects than other multivariable techniques, such as multiple regression or factor analysis, which usually require "only" 10 subjects per variable.

Assumptions

Because path analysis is an extension of multiple linear regression, many of the same assumptions hold for the two techniques. First, as the name implies, the relationships among the variables must be linear. Second, there should be no interactions among the variables (although we can add a new term that reflects the interaction of two variables). Third, the endogenous variables must be continuous (although you can get away with a minimum of five categories if you have ordinal data) and relatively normally distributed, with skewness and kurtosis coefficients below 1. Fourth, it is assumed that the covariances among the disturbance terms are zero (equivalent to the assumption of uncorrelated errors among the predictor variables in regression), although more advanced variants of path analysis can deal with violations of this assumption. Finally, as mentioned previously, path analysis is quite sensitive to the specification of the model; including irrelevant variables or, more seriously, omitting relevant ones, can drastically affect the results.

Interpretation and Model Building

As I mentioned above (but cannot mention too often, although you may dispute this), path analysis is a technique for testing models, not for building them. It does not make sense to draw all possible paths, close your eyes, and press the "compute" button. You may get results (assuming your model isn't under-identified), but it would be fatuous to believe them, or even to hope that they would be replicated. Similarly, most computer programs for path analysis can print out *modification indices* that tell you how the model can be improved, for example, by including covariances between variables or error terms, or by including paths between variables that weren't specified in the model. The major criterion for accepting or rejecting the suggestions is your theory. If the changes make theoretical sense, try them out; if there is no theoretical justification for them, ignore them. Changing your model simply to increase the fit may result in a model that is neither sensible nor reproducible.

Finally, having a model that fits the data doesn't prove that the model is correct. There may be better models that you haven't tested. More important, often changing the direction of an arrow, or even a series of arrows, may result in models that are statistically equivalent. For example, if we ran the model shown in Figure 16.5(b), we would find that R^2 was 0.434 (admittedly with not-too-impressive fit statistics). Changing the direction of the arrow between ANX and TAX (and moving the disturbance term as required) results in an identical value for R^2 and all the fit indices. Obviously, both cannot be correct; they simply fit the data equally well. This fact also illustrates the point that path analysis cannot be used to establish causality; that is done through the design of the study, not its analysis.

Following in the Paths of Others

Assuming that the readers of this chapter will more likely be consumers than doers of path analysis, the following are points to bear in mind, akin to the Convoluted Reasoning and Anti-Intellectual Pomposity (CRAP) detectors in *PDQ Statistics* (Norman & Streiner, 2003).

1. Are the signs of the paths correct, and are they statistically significant? Don't be fooled by pretty diagrams and the bottom line; each element of the model has to make sense.

2. Does the final model presented in the paper make sense? That is, does it appear as if the model were derived from some coherent theoretical and (or) empirical base, or could the paths have been drawn simply to improve the fit of the model?
3. Was the sample size sufficient? Add the number of paths, the number of curved arrows, the number of exogenous variables, and the number of disturbance terms, and multiply by 10. If the sample size is less than this, interpret the results with a considerable degree of scepticism.

Summary

Path analysis is a powerful statistical technique that allows for more complicated and realistic models than multiple regression, with its single dependent variable. However, the increased sophistication places additional demands on users. Mastering a new computer program and new terminology is perhaps the easiest part; the more demanding requirement is that far greater attention must be paid to the underlying model, in terms of including as many relevant variables as possible, weeding out irrelevant ones, and specifying relations among the variables. This requires a solid knowledge of the literature and a model that makes clinical and theoretical sense. However, the rewards are being able to test these models and to compare different models against one another. Path analysis also provides a stepping stone to an even more sophisticated and useful technique – structural equation modelling – which is discussed in Streiner (2006; see Chapter 17).

REFERENCES

Klein, R.B. (2010). *Principles and practice of structural equation modeling*. (3rd ed.). New York: Guilford.
Meehl, P. (1990). Why summaries of research on psychological theories are often uninterpretable. *Psychological Reports, 66*, 195–244.
Norman, G.R., & Streiner, D.L. (2003). *PDQ statistics*. (3rd ed.). Shelton, CT: PMPH USA.
Norman, G.R., & Streiner, D.L. (2008). *Biostatistics: The bare essentials*. (3rd ed.). Shelton, CT: PMPH USA.
Streiner, D.L. (2006, Apr). Building a better model: An introduction to structural equation modelling. *Canadian Journal of Psychiatry, 51*(5), 317–324. Medline:16986821

Tomarken, A.J., & Waller, N.G. (2003, Nov). Potential problems with "well fitting" models. *Journal of Abnormal Psychology, 112*(4), 578–598. http://dx.doi.org/10.1037/0021-843X.112.4.578 Medline:14674870

TO READ FURTHER

Klein, R.B. (2010). *Principles and practice of structural equation modeling.* (3rd ed.). New York: Guilford.

Norman, G.R., & Streiner, D.L. (2008). *Biostatistics: The bare essentials.* (3rd ed.). Shelton, CT: PMPH USA.

Olobatuyi, M.E. (2006). *A user's guide to path analysis.* Lanham, MD: University Press of America.

17 Building a Better Model: An Introduction to Structural Equation Modelling

DAVID L. STREINER, PH.D.

Canadian Journal of Psychiatry, 2006, *51*, 317–324

In a previous chapter in this book, I discussed a powerful analytic technique called *path analysis* (Streiner, 2005; see Chapter 16). Very briefly, path
analysis is an extension of multiple regression that allows us to consider
more than one dependent variable (DV) at a time and, more important,
allows variables to be both DVs and independent variables (IVs). In other
words, it permits us to consider chains of association, such that Variable
A can influence Variable *B*, and *B* in turn can affect *C*. To avoid confusion
about what to call Variable *B* – it is a DV because it is affected by *A*, but it
is also an IV because it is a predictor of *C* – we avoid those terms entirely.
Instead, we substitute the terms *exogenous variables* for those that aren't
influenced by any other variable in the model, and *endogenous variables* for
those that are. (And this was supposed to *reduce* confusion?)

However, one limitation of path analysis is that it can handle only
variables that are observed. At first glance, this hardly seems like a limitation; after all, if we can't observe a variable, we surely can't measure
and analyse it. It has the flavour of the "ether" that supposedly permeated all of space, but had the unique properties that it couldn't be seen,
tasted, felt, or perceived in any other way, which led scientists down
the garden path for centuries.

In fact, though, we deal with unobservable variables all the time,
although we use other terms for them. In personality theory and test
construction, they are called *hypothetical constructs*; in factor analysis
they are referred to as *factors*; and in structural equation modelling
(SEM), the technique we will be considering here, they are known as
latent variables. So much for the use of consistent terminology to explain

exactly what we mean. Whatever they're called, though, they refer to the same thing – variables that we cannot observe directly, but know about through their purported effects on phenomena we can observe. This would apply to concepts such as intelligence, anxiety, depression, quality of life, coping style, schizophrenia, locus of control, and hundreds of others we encounter every day in psychiatry and psychology. Let's use anxiety as a model, recognizing that the principles apply equally well to the other constructs.

According to one theory (Antony, 2001), anxiety consists of four facets – cognitive, affective, behavioural, and physiological – which themselves are unobservable hypothetical constructs. When we say that a person is anxious, what we mean is that he or she is showing observable behaviours that are manifestations of one or more of these facets. In the physiological realm, for instance, there may be tachycardia, shortness of breath, and sweatiness (all of which are measurable); while in the cognitive realm, there may be decreased ability to concentrate and hypersensitivity to perceived threats (again measurable). We postulate that the reason that these manifestations tend to occur together is that they all are produced by the anxiety. In other words, "anxiety" is something we hypothesize to tie together observable phenomena that are correlated to some degree. In a similar way, we do not see schizophrenia or intelligence; we see only a constellation of observed behaviours that tend to occur together and that we postulate are caused by some underlying mechanism.

SEM is an extension of path analysis that allows us to examine the relationships among both measured and latent variables. (To add to the confusion, SEM is also used as an abbreviation for the *standard error of the mean* and the *standard error of measurement*; its meaning is usually clear from the context.) It does this by combining path analysis with a form of factor analysis called *confirmatory* factor analysis (CFA), so it is probably easiest to begin with a discussion of CFA and how it differs from the more commonly encountered forms of factor analysis. (A reminder for those from the Maritime provinces of Canada: CFA does *not* stand for "Come from Away," or visitors from the rest of Canada – as one anonymous reviewer suggested.)

Confirmatory Factor Analysis

Until about 20 years ago, if someone said "factor analysis," there would be relatively little ambiguity about what he or she meant (Streiner, 1994; see Chapter 10). It is a technique that is used when we have many items or variables and want to see if they can be explained by a smaller number of factors. We enter the data, close our eyes, press the "compute" button, and see what comes out. That is, we don't have any a priori hypotheses regarding which variables or items will cluster on the same factor. Even if we did have some hunches (for example, if we were analysing a questionnaire we developed, and have some idea of which items should tap the same construct), there was no way to tell this to the computer program ahead of time. All we can do is look at the output and say that the results are pretty close to what we expected, or we can go back to the drawing board and rewrite the items in the hope that the next iteration will give us results that are more to our liking. When CFA came upon the scene, there had to be some way to differentiate it from the more traditional form, so the older method was renamed *exploratory factor analysis* (EFA) in recognition that we use it when we're simply examining the data.

As its name implies, CFA is used when we do have a priori hypotheses about which items or variables are grouped together as manifestations of an underlying construct, and we wish to test how well our data match – or "fit" – this model. As in path analysis, it is very helpful to draw the hypothesized relationships in a diagram, particularly as the most commonly used computer programs, such as LISREL (SSI, Lincolnwood, IL), AMOS (SPSS, Somers, NY), EQS (Multivariate Software, Encino, CA), and MPlus (Muthén & Muthén, Los Angeles, CA), accept these diagrams as input – it's not necessary to specify the relationships mathematically. So, let's begin by drawing our theory of anxiety, which is shown in Figure 17.1.

If you recall the diagrams that were used with path analysis, you'll remember that there were two types of symbols: rectangles to represent the measured variables, both endogenous and exogenous, and circles to show the disturbance, or error, terms. In SEM (of which CFA is a subset), a third symbol is used: ovals, to depict the latent variables. Thus, Figure 17.1 shows that there's a latent variable, anxiety, which in turn is composed of four latent variables: cognitive, behavioural, affective, and physiological. These give rise to several measured variables, each with an associated disturbance, or error, term. The figure shows that all four latent variables have three measured variables, but this was done simply because it was easier to draw it this way. In reality, each latent variable can have any number of measured variables, although, as I'll discuss later, there should ideally be at least three.

Fig. 17.1 A structural equation model of anxiety, with its four subcomponents and their measured variables

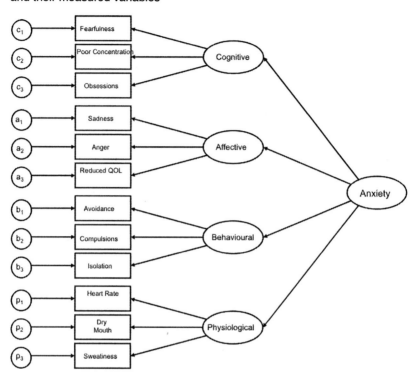

The directions of the arrows is important, not only for the analyses, but as a reflection of the underlying theory of latent variables, CFA, and SEM in general. The arrow from anxiety to the other latent variables, and from those four to the measured variables, means that anxiety leads to four areas of involvement, and that each of those gives rise to the observed variables. That is, if it weren't for the underlying construct of cognitive changes, for example, the observed behaviours would not be correlated. Of course, they would exist in people, but there would be no reason to expect that fearfulness and obsessions would go together were it not for the fact that both were outward manifestations of anxiety.

I mentioned in the chapter on path analysis that it is a model *testing* procedure and should not be used for model *building*. The same injunction applies to SEM in general and CFA in particular, which is reflected in what CFA tells us, in contrast to what we are told in the output from the exploratory form of factor analysis. In EFA, the program may say that Variables A, C, and F, for example, belong together in Factor Y; and Variables B, D, and E load most highly on Factor Z. Even if we hypothesized a different combination of variables clustering, EFA would simply go with the math and show the "best" configuration (where "best" may be defined differently in the various forms of EFA).

When we do a CFA, though, we stipulate where we think the variables should load, and the program tells us simply whether or not the model fits the data. If the model doesn't fit, there are few clues to guide us in how to shuffle the variables to make the model better fit the data. Further, even if the model does fit, that doesn't guarantee that some other way of arranging the variables (that is, a different model) would not lead to an even better fit. Thus, our guide to the model is our theory, knowledge, or previous research, rather than reliance on statistical criteria.

CFA by itself is an extremely powerful and useful tool. For example, when validating a scale, EFA must rely on post hoc reasoning: "yes, these results seem to make sense and more or less conform to what I had expected." With CFA, though, the hypotheses must precede the data analysis, so that a good fit is even stronger evidence that the scale is structured as predicted.

Let's take a look at some (fictitious) results to see what CFA can tell us. After specifying the model, the computer will print a diagram similar to Figure 17.2. (I will not go into the messy details of how to specify the model, because it varies from one program to the next and can become somewhat technical. With uncharacteristic modesty, let me recommend the chapter on SEM in *Biostatistics: The Bare Essentials* [Norman & Streiner, 2008] as a place to start.) To simplify matters, Figure 17.2 shows only two of the four components of anxiety. Above each arrow from a latent variable to a measured or another latent variable is a number, called the *path coefficient*. This is equivalent to the factor loadings in EFA, so it can range from -1.0 to 1.0, higher numbers (positive or negative) showing a stronger association. As can be seen, Obsessions doesn't fit very well with the Cognitive trait, and the variable Anger doesn't seem to fit the Affective component. The numbers over the variable names are the *squared multiple correlations* (SMRs), which are simply the squared values of the path coefficients; they are interpreted in the same way as R^2 in multiple regression – how much of the variance in one variable is explained by, or has in common with, the other variable. Finally, the numbers over the arrows between the error terms

Fig. 17.2 A subset of Figure 1, showing the path coefficients, squared multiple correlations, and error variances

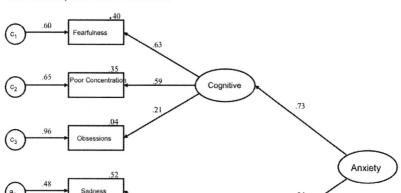

and the variables are the variances of the errors. You'll note that the sum of the SMR plus the error variance for each variable is 1.0; that is, all of the variance of a variable is divided between that shared with the latent variable and error. This is equivalent in EFA to the communality (that portion of the variable's variance explained by the factors) and the uniqueness (what's left over); again, same concepts, different terms. At a higher level, note that in this example, the Cognitive domain is correlated more highly with the latent trait of Anxiety than is the Affective realm, as reflected in their respective path coefficients.

Another use of CFA is to compare the psychometric properties of different versions of a scale, or to determine whether it performs the same way with different groups. For example, to see if men and women respond similarly to the items on a test, we can begin by doing an exploratory factor analysis on the women's data. The results of this EFA then constitute the model against which we test the data from the men. Then, we can run the CFA in several ways, each time imposing stricter and stricter criteria for similarity. In our first run, we can simply see whether or not the same items load on the different factors. If this model fits, we can then add the restriction that the magnitudes of the factor loadings must be the same in both groups. If there is still a good fit, we would go the final step and see whether the variances of the items are also similar across groups. Once a scale has passed these three increasingly more rigorous tests, we can be fairly confident that it is performing in an equivalent manner across groups. The same approach is used in assessing a translated form of a scale: it is compared against the factor structure in the original language. A nice example was done by Furukawa et al. (2005).

Structural Equation Modelling

With this background to CFA and the previous paper on path analysis (Streiner, 2005; see Chapter 16), it is a relatively easy step to structural equation modelling (SEM). Instead of being limited to drawing paths among the measured variables, as we were when using path analysis, we can draw paths among the latent variables, too. Each of the latent variables has at least two (and ideally three or more) associated measured variables, so that each latent variable becomes a small CFA in its own right. In fact, we'll use the same example – trying to predict a person's degree of photonumerophobia (PNP; the fear that our fear of numbers will come to light) on the basis of anxiety (ANX), high school math scores (HSM), and tax return errors (TAX). Now, though, we'll treat each of these three as if it were a latent variable, as shown in Figure 17.3. In keeping with the convention, what were squares in the original figure in the previous paper are now ovals, and each has a number of measured variables associated with it.

Here, ANX is measured by three different scales. Instead of using the marks from only one school year to measure HSM, we will use grades from three years and, similarly, look at errors for the past three years to measure TAX. PNP is a bit more difficult, because we have only one scale to measure it. For reasons that will be explained shortly, we randomly divide the scale into two parts, treating each as if it were a separate scale.

This step in SEM is called the *model specification* stage. Although no mathematics is involved, it is probably the most difficult – and most important – part. It is the most difficult because it requires the most thought and understanding of the theoretical model of the purported influences on PNP. No computer program can help us at this

Fig. 17.3 A structural equation model of the factors associated with photonumerophobia

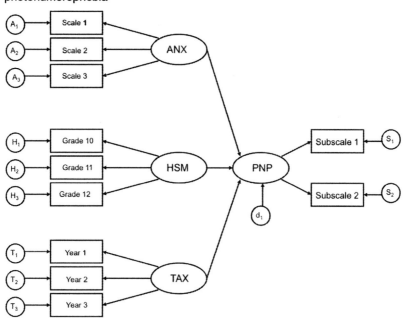

stage – only our knowledge of the field. It is the most important step because everything depends on how well we specify the model. The computer programs may help us in determining whether some variables aren't important, and, as I explained in Chapter 16, we can play with different paths to see if they improve the model. However, the primary cause of poorly fitting models (not only in SEM, but in path analysis and multiple regression, too) is the omission of crucial variables, and there are no programs in the world that can help us in this regard. For example, if the prime determinant of PNP is actually the PNP level of one's parents (because of either genetics or learning), and if this isn't correlated with any of the other variables we're examining, our model will explain little of the variance, and we will never know why.

The next step is relatively easy; we simply run the computer program. Because our model is complex, so is the output. In essence, we are specifying five separate models: four CFAs (one for each of the latent variables), as well as the one that ties them all together. Before looking at the

Table 17.1 Correlations among two scales of anxiety
(A_1 and A_2) and two scales of introversion (I_1 and I_2)

	A_2	I_1	I_2
A_1	0.74	0.49	0.42
A_2	1.00	0.45	0.40
I_1		1.00	0.70

overall fit of the model, we should look at each of the CFAs. The main focus is on the paths – from the latent variable to the measured variables and from that latent variable to the next one in the path. Do they all have the right sign? Are they significant? If the answer to either question is "no," it may be best to respecify the model by dropping non-significant variables and (or) seeing if there are others in the data set that should be included.

Here, it is worthwhile mentioning another advantage of CFA and why we prefer to deal with latent variables with two – and ideally more – measured variables associated with them, rather than simply measured variables, as in path analysis. To keep the example simple, we'll deal with only two variables, anxiety and introversion, and – for reasons that will become obvious shortly – measure each with two scales (A_1 and A_2 for anxiety; and I_1 and I_2 for introversion). The usual way to test the hypothesis that the constructs are correlated is to give the scales to a group of people and use Pearson's correlations. Table 17.1 presents the (again fictitious) results for 200 people.

As can be seen, the correlation of the two anxiety scales is 0.74; and the correlation of the two introversion scales is 0.70. The correlations between the anxiety and introversion scales range between 0.40 and 0.49, which is in the moderate range.

The problem, though, is that the magnitude of the correlations between the anxiety and introversion scales is affected by three factors: the degree to which these two constructs are actually related, the reliabilities of the anxiety scales, and the reliabilities of the introversion scales. Because the reliability of any scale is less than 1.0, the correlation that we find always underestimates the true correlation between the variables. We can get a better estimate of the true correlation if we *disattenuate* the variables – that is, if we compensate for the lack of perfect reliability (Streiner & Norman, 2008) – but, how do we know what the reliability is? By using several indices (or splitting each index in half, as we did with PNP), we can treat them as parallel forms of the same scale. In this example, even though they are different, each of the anxiety scales could be seen as (imperfect) measures of the trait of anxiety (and similarly for introversion). The degree to which the correlations between the two scales of a construct are less than 1 reflects the magnitude of this imperfection, that is, their parallel form reliability. In SEM, this is taken into account when the correlations among the latent variables are examined, hence reflecting their "true" correlation.

When we rerun this problem, looking at the correlation between the *latent* variable of anxiety (measured with the two scales) and the *latent* trait of introversion with its two scales, we find a correlation of 0.62. This result is considerably stronger than the 0.40 to 0.48 we found previously and better reflects the actual relationship between the traits.

Now let's return to the SEM example. Once we have cleaned up the model by pruning non-contributory paths, we can examine the fit of the overall model. The most common index of how well the data match the model (although not necessarily the best) is the χ^2_{GoF} (the chi-squared Goodness of Fit). Actually, the name is somewhat of a misnomer: it's actually a *badness* of fit test. Usually, we want χ^2 to be statistically significant; in path analysis and SEM, though, we want χ^2_{GoF} to be *non*-significant. Why our change of heart? In general, χ^2 tests how much our data deviate from some hypothesized model. In the usual case that we're familiar with from introductory statistics, the model is that the variables are independent of one another, and we are delighted when we can reject this null hypothesis and conclude that the variables are, in fact, related. However, when we use the χ^2_{GoF} test in path analysis (or with other statistical tests), our hypothesized model is the one we have drawn (as opposed to the null hypothesis that nothing is related). If χ^2_{GoF} is statistically significant, that means that the data differ from (that is, do not fit) the model, which is *not* what we want. Thus, we want a path model that results in a non-significant χ^2_{GoF}. The good news is that all programs print out the results, and that the χ^2_{GoF} test, in contrast to the tests I'll discuss next, has a probability level associated with it. The bad news is that we can't fully trust the results, because they are highly dependent on the sample size. If the study has relatively few subjects (fewer than 75 or so), then χ^2_{GoF} may be non-significant even with a patently ridiculous model, simply because there isn't enough power to reject the null hypothesis. Conversely, with a very large sample size (over 400), even minor and trivial deviations of the data from the model can result in statistical significance. So, we should keep the results of the χ^2_{GoF} test in mind, but not be overly influenced by it.

Another fit index is called the Root Mean Square Error of Approximation (RMSEA), which is a variant of the χ^2_{GoF} test, in that it sees how much the data deviate from the model. Values over 0.10 are considered to be a bad fit, those less than 0.08 reflect a reasonable fit, and those less than 0.05 indicate a good fit.

There are myriad other fit indices, all of which can be interpreted as measures of association or effect size (Norman & Streiner, 2008). They can be grouped into four main categories (the fact that there are four categories gives some indication of just how many individual indices there are and that none has been accepted as the gold standard). The *comparative fit indices* represent one type; these generally yield scores between 0 and 1. As the name implies, they show how good the model is, compared with some alternative. Most often, the alternative model is that all of the variables are independent of one another; that is, that all of the correlations (more accurately, the covariances) are zero. Because this is highly unlikely – let's not forget Meehl (1990), who said that everything is correlated with everything else – it's not surprising that 0.90 is the minimally acceptable value, 0.95 being the minimum if the χ^2_{GoF} test is significant (Klein, 2011). The second class of fit indices, which also have values between 0 and 1, reflects how much of the variance in the data can be accounted for by the model; again, 0.90 (or 0.95, if χ^2_{GoF} is significant) is the absolute minimum.

For both of these classes, there are modifications of the basic indices, reflecting their *parsimony*. These are based on the fact that two things happen as we add more variables. First, the amount of variance accounted for by the model increases, with rare exceptions. At the same time, each new variable also adds more error variance. Statistical techniques, though, cannot differentiate between true variance and error variance, so they find the best model that fits all of the variance. The problem this introduces is that, if we were to measure identical variables on a new sample of people, the true variance should be the same, but the pattern of the error variance would be quite different, since we assume that error is random. Consequently, the original model won't fit the new data as well. The parsimony indices penalize us for adding more variables, much as the adjusted R^2 in multiple regression imposes a penalty proportional to the number of variables in the model.

Unfortunately, we can interpret the RMSEA and the other fit indices (with the exception of the χ^2_{GoF}) only by using rules of thumb (under

0.08 for RMSEA, over 0.90 for the others if χ^2_{GoF} isn't significant, over 0.95 if it is). There are no statistical tests of significance for them.

These techniques of path analysis, CFA, and SEM ask a lot from both the user and the reader. They introduce new terms for new concepts (for example, endogenous and exogenous variables and recursive and non-recursive models), replace terms we know (construct or factor) with novel ones for the same concept (latent trait), and require specialized computer programs. What they give us in return, though, are more powerful ways of thinking about and analysing our data – ways that more closely approximate the real world of many variables that interact in a complex fashion and that don't neatly fit into cause-effect relationships.

Summary

In a previous chapter in this book (Streiner, 2005; see Chapter 16), we saw how path analysis extended multiple regression by allowing chains of association between variables; for example, we saw how variables *A*, *B*, and *C* could affect variable *D*, which in turn would influence variable *E*. A seemingly very different technique, exploratory factor analysis (EFA), was explained in a different chapter (Streiner, 1994; see Chapter 10). CFA modifies EFA in that the user specifies a priori which items should load on which factors. Although at first glance this appears to be a limitation, demanding that the user have more information (or more sophisticated hunches) before he or she begins is, in fact, a major benefit, for two reasons. First, it yields better evidence that the composition of the scale matches one's assumptions, compared with having to rely on after-the-fact pleading that the results are sufficiently congruent. Second, it allows the user to compare the properties of the scale across populations or versions.

SEM both incorporates CFA and extends path analysis by allowing the user to examine the relationships among latent – that is, unseen but hypothesized – variables. Each latent variable has two or more associated measured variables. Thus, each latent variable is a small CFA in its own right, testing the mini-hypothesis that the measured variables are, in fact, the measurable manifestations of the latent one. This also provides an added benefit in that the correlations among the measured variables are an indication of their reliability, which SEM can correct for. Consequently, the relationships among the latent variables reflect their true correlations, uncontaminated by measurement error.

ACKNOWLEDGMENT

The author would like to thank Dr. Chittaranjan Andrade for his very helpful comments on this and the previous paper in the series.

REFERENCES

Antony, M.M. (2001). Assessment of anxiety and the anxiety disorders: An overview. In M.M. Antony, S.M. Orsillo, & L. Roemer (Eds.), *Practitioner's guide to empirically based measures of anxiety* (pp. 9–17). New York: Kluver Academic/Plenum. http://dx.doi.org/10.1007/0-306-47628-2_2

Furukawa, T.A., Streiner, D.L., Azuma, H., Higuchi, T., Kamijima, K., Kanba, S., ..., & Miura, S. (2005, Oct). Cross-cultural equivalence in depression assessment: Japan-Europe-North American study. *Acta Psychiatrica Scandinavica, 112*(4), 279–285. http://dx.doi.org/10.1111/j.1600-0447.2005.00587.x Medline:16156835

Klein, R.B. (2011). *Principles and practice of structural equation modeling.* (3rd ed.). NY: Guilford.

Meehl, P. (1990). Why summaries of research on psychological theories are often uninterpretable. *Psychological Reports, 66,* 195–244.

Norman, G.R., & Streiner, D.L. (2008). *Biostatistics: The bare essentials.* (3rd ed.). Shelton, CT: PMPH USA.

Streiner, D.L. (1994, Apr). Figuring out factors: The use and misuse of factor analysis. *Canadian Journal of Psychiatry, 39*(3), 135–140. Medline:8033017

Streiner, D.L. (2005, Feb). Finding our way: An introduction to path analysis. *Canadian Journal of Psychiatry, 50*(2) , 115–122. Medline:15807228

Streiner, D.L., & Norman, G.R. (2008). *Health measurement scales: A practical guide to their development and use.* (4th ed.). Oxford: Oxford University Press.

TO READ FURTHER

Byrne, B.M. (2006). *Structural equation modeling with AMOS: Basic concepts, applications, and programming.* (2nd ed.). Mahwah, NJ: Lawrence Erlbaum & Associates.

Klein, R.B. (2011). *Principles and practice of structural equation modeling.* (3rd ed.). NY: Guilford.

Norman, G.R., & Streiner, D.L. (2008). *Biostatistics: The bare essentials.* (3rd ed.). Shelton, CT: PMPH USA.

18 Unicorns Do Exist: A Tutorial on "Proving" the Null Hypothesis

DAVID L. STREINER, PH.D.

Canadian Journal of Psychiatry, 2003, *48*, 756–761

In Philosophy 101, we learned that, if Person A posits the existence of some phenomenon, it is incumbent on Person A to prove its existence rather than it's being Person B's job to disprove it. For example, if I assert that there are pink unicorns with purple polka dots hiding deep in the forest, I cannot simply say, "Well, prove that they don't exist." For the scientific world to accept my claim, I have to bring one back, dead or alive. Is it ever legitimate to violate this injunction and try to prove the non-existence of something? In this paper, we'll take a look at trying to prove that something does not exist. In particular, we will examine the steps necessary to show that two treatments are equivalent – that, in essence, a difference between them does not exist. Let's start off, though, by looking at "normal" science.

In most instances, we design studies to show statistical significance. That is, we want to prove that one treatment is more effective or has fewer side effects than another, or we want to demonstrate that a relation exists between two variables, such as a history of sexual or physical abuse and the probability of having a psychiatric diagnosis (e.g., MacMillan et al., 1999). We begin by positing a *null hypothesis* that there is no difference between the groups or that there is no correlation between the variables, and then we do everything in our power to disprove it. If fortune deigns to smile upon us, and the statistical test has a p level less than or equal to 0.05, we conclude that we can reject the null hypothesis and therefore accept the alternative – that the treatments do differ or that the variables are correlated. The technical name for this is *null-hypothesis significance testing* (NHST). In NHST, if p is greater than

0.05, we do not say that we can accept (or prove) the null hypothesis; rather, we use the convoluted locution that we "have failed to disprove the null."

The reason for this, as I have said, harkens back to David Hume and the philosophy of science, which asserts that we cannot prove the non-existence of something (unless, of course, it violates one of the laws of nature, such as the notions of perpetual motion machines, travel that is faster than light, or politicians who tell the truth). To use our original example, no one has ever seen such a unicorn (at least while sober), but we cannot prove that it does not exist. Although it is highly unlikely, a unicorn may walk out of the forest tomorrow, much as the coelacanth was discovered in 1938, after it was thought to have been extinct for millions of years. Using an example closer to home, six randomized controlled studies failed to find that ASA had any beneficial effect in preventing reinfarctions. However, Canner's (1983) meta-analysis demonstrated that ASA reduced mortality by 10%, and it is now inconceivable that post-myocardial infarction patients would not be told to take it. The six studies didn't prove that the null hypothesis is true – that there is no difference between ASA and placebo – they simply failed to reject it; that is, all six suffered from a Type II error in failing to reject the null hypothesis when, in fact, it is false. There is a qualitative difference between "highly unlikely" and "impossible" that can never be breached, no matter how many studies have negative outcomes. Therefore, a negative result often means that we should just try harder next time.

The only problem with this philosophical purity is that, as noted, there are times when we do want to demonstrate a lack of difference. This occurs most often in evaluating "me too" drugs – drugs that are supposedly as good as existing ones but that may be cheaper or have fewer side effects. Here, the first task is to show that they are no less effective – in other words, to "prove" the null hypothesis of no difference. Similar situations exist when an outpatient program is compared with an inpatient one, or time-limited therapy is compared with therapy without a limit on the number of sessions, or a lower dosage of a drug is compared with a higher dosage (e.g., Bollini, Pampallona, Tibaldi, Kupelnick, & Munizza, 1999). In all these cases, it would be sufficient to show that the less expensive or less invasive therapies are not worse than the alternatives; it is not necessary to prove superiority in terms of outcome for them to be accepted as replacements. As we'll see, showing superiority versus non-inferiority or equivalence does not simply demonstrate opposite sides of the same coin.

The Statistical Theory

How do we reconcile the competing demands of wanting to prove equivalence on the one hand with the difficulty, if not impossibility, of proving the null hypothesis on the other? First, we have to correct a common misperception about the null hypothesis (H_0). In almost all situations, the null hypothesis is written as

$$H_0 : \mu_1 = \mu_2 \text{ or } H_0 : \pi_1 = \pi_2 \qquad [1]$$

when we are comparing means (μs) or proportions (πs); that is, the means or proportions of the two groups are the same, versus the alternative hypothesis (H_A),

$$H_A : \mu_1 \neq \mu_2 \text{ or } H_A : \pi_1 \neq \pi_2 \qquad [2]$$

that the two means or proportions are different. The mistake is to think that the null hypothesis always has to mean "no difference." In fact, the null hypothesis is the hypothesis to be nullified, or disproven. Cohen (1994) refers to the hypothesis of no difference by the delightful name, "nil hypothesis." In most cases, the null and the nil hypotheses are the same; however, this needn't necessarily be the case, and we will use this distinction in testing for equivalence.

A second point is that not all differences are created equal, and there are some we can safely ignore. Because of sampling error, there will always be a difference between groups, no matter how similar they maybe. Further, if we simply increase the sample size sufficiently, we will always be able to show that this difference is statistically significant. For example, let's assume that School A has a mean IQ score of 100, School B has a mean IQ score of 103, and the standard deviation is the usual 15 points. Most people would agree that this 3-point difference is clinically trivial. However, if we draw a sample of 400 students from each school, we will probably find that this difference is statistically significant. With larger sample sizes, we can find statistical significance with even smaller differences.

These two points – that the null hypothesis doesn't always mean no difference and that some differences may be statistically significant but clinically trivial – form the basis of testing for equivalence. First, rather than saying that the two means (or proportions, or whatever parameter we're interested in) have to be identical, we establish an *equivalence interval* within which we would say that the groups are "close enough." For instance, let's assume that, for sociophobic patients, Treatment A results in a mean score of 10 on a scale of social comfort (that is, $M_1 = 10$), where a higher score reflects greater comfort. How much lower can the score be with a different therapy (Treatment B) for us to say that the difference between the groups (which we call delta, or δ) is clinically unimportant – 1 point lower? 2 points? 3 points? This is not a statistical question, but rather is a clinical one, based on our knowledge of the condition, the scale, and the intervention. If the new treatment is significantly faster, cheaper, or – if it's a drug – has a better side-effect profile, we may be willing to accept a lower score (that is, somewhat poorer adjustment) than if the new therapy does not offer these advantages. As Kendall, Marrs-Garcia, Nath, and Sheldrick (1999) point out, though, there's a trade-off in the choice of this interval. The smaller its value, the more similar the treatments must be, but the harder it is to demonstrate equivalence statistically. Conversely, it is easier to show equivalence with wider intervals, but then we have to accept bigger differences between the two groups and still say they're not different.

There are two approaches to equivalence testing. The two-tailed approach tries to show that the two means or proportions are similar; that is, that one is neither much larger nor much smaller than the other. The one-tailed method is far more common and tests whether the second mean or proportion is different in only one direction. This is also referred to as *non-inferiority testing*, because it is often used to see whether a new therapy isn't any worse than usual treatment. We don't care whether it's better – in fact, we'd be ecstatic – we merely want to ensure that it's not significantly worse. The two-tailed method is certainly important and is often used in bio-availability studies, where the aim is to show that a new compound neither raises nor lowers some biological marker outside of a given range. However, on a practical level, it is much more likely that we would be interested in showing that the new treatment is not worse than the standard (non-inferiority testing), so we will restrict ourselves to that situation.

The first step is to use our clinical judgment to define the equivalence interval, which we designate δ. Using the previous example, assume that we'd accept a difference of 20% at most, which translates into $\delta = 2$ points. That means that the mean for the new treatment (M_2) cannot be less than 8 if it is to be deemed non-inferior.

Now, let's bring the first point into play and redefine the null hypothesis. Instead of the usual nil hypothesis of no difference, we say that the null hypothesis is

$$H_0 : \mu_1 - \mu_2 > \delta \qquad [3]$$

(or, in English, the first mean is more than δ points greater than the second), and the alternative hypothesis is

$$H_A : \mu_1 - \mu_2 \leq \delta \qquad [4]$$

(that is, the difference between the means is less than δ, which also covers the possibility that μ_2 is larger than μ_1). Note that if $\delta = 0$, these are simply the null and alternative hypotheses for a one-sided t-test.

This means that, if we can reject the null hypothesis, we are left by default with the alternative hypothesis that the difference between the means (or proportions) being smaller than is probably correct. The test for this looks very similar to the usual one, with the exception of δ in the numerator:

$$t(d) = \frac{(M_1 - M_2) - \delta}{S_{M_1 - M_2}}, \qquad [5]$$

where $S_{M_1 - M_2}$ is the standard error of the difference:

$$S_{M_1 - M_2} = \sqrt{\left[\frac{(n_1 - 1)s_1^2 + (n_2 - 1)s_2^2}{n_1 + n_2 - 2} \right] \times \left[\frac{1}{n_1} + \frac{1}{n_2} \right]}, \qquad [6]$$

and where $df = (n_1 + n_2 - 2)$, the n is the sample size in each group, and the s is the standard deviation. If we are dealing with proportions rather than means, then we simply replace M_1 with p_1 and M_2 with p_2 in Equation [5] (the proportions in each group), and use Equation [7] for the standard error:

$$S_{P_1 - P_2} = \sqrt{\frac{p_1(1 - p_1)}{n_1} + \frac{p_2(1 - p_2)}{n_2}}. \qquad [7]$$

Fig. 18.1 Hypothetical results of a new and a standard therapy

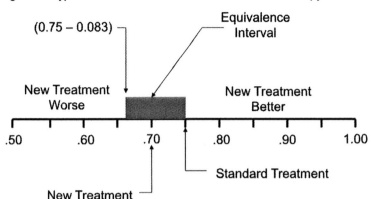

An Example

Let's work through an example. Assume that we specified ahead of time that we would consider two treatments for sociophobia equivalent if the new one worked for at least 85% as many patients as did the usual therapy. What we actually find is that, with 20 patients per group, 75% improve on the standard therapy, A (that is, $p_A = 0.75$), and 70% improve with the new treatment, B ($p_B = 0.70$). Since 15% of 0.75 is 0.083, we set δ to be 0.083. Thus, the null hypothesis is

$$H_0 : p_A - p_B > 0.083, \qquad [8]$$

and the alternative hypothesis is

$$H_A : p_A - p_B \leq 0.083. \qquad [9]$$

Spelled out, the null hypothesis is that the proportion of successful patients in the standard therapy group is more than 0.083 better than the proportion of successful patients in the new treatment group; the alternative hypothesis is that the difference in proportions is less than or equal to 0.083. This is shown in Figure 18.1.

Using Equation [7], we find that the standard error of the difference between these two proportions is 0.141 and, therefore,

$$t(38) = \frac{(0.75 - 0.70) - 0.083}{0.141} = 0.234. \qquad [10]$$

Since this is smaller than the critical value of 1.645 that we would need to reject a one-tailed hypothesis at the 0.05 level, we cannot reject the null hypothesis, and we have to conclude that the two treatments are not equivalent.

Sample Size and Power

In the example we just worked through, it would seem at first glance that the two treatments should have come out as equivalent. We said that we would accept a 15% difference from the effectiveness of the standard treatment or roughly 0.083 less effectiveness than that demonstrated for Treatment A: 0.75. The success rate for Treatment B, 0.70, seems to be this much less; in fact, the difference is only one subject per group (that is, 15/20 for A versus 14/20 for B). Why do these results seem to be counterintuitive?

Simply examining raw differences overlooks two important points. First, we cannot look only at the difference between the two groups. As is always the case, the means or proportions that emerge from a study are sample estimates of the true population parameters. Because of this, they deviate from the real values to some degree. The amount of this deviation is related to the variability in what is being measured (for example, the standard deviation) and the sample size, and these have to be taken into account when we test to see whether the difference is statistically significant.

The second point is that, in testing for equivalence, we reverse the usual meanings of the null and alternative hypotheses. This means that we have to alter both our interpretations of Type I and Type II errors and what we mean by power. In both NHST and equivalence testing, a Type I error occurs when we conclude that the null hypothesis is false when, in fact, it is true; a Type II error occurs when we erroneously conclude that the null hypothesis is true when it is not. Power is the ability to reject the null hypothesis when it is false.

In non-inferiority testing, though, the null hypothesis is that the standard treatment is better than the new one. This means that

1. A Type I error occurs when we say that the two treatments are equivalent, when in fact the standard treatment is better.

2. A Type II error occurs when we conclude that the standard treatment is better, when, in fact, the treatments are equivalent.
3. Power is the probability of accepting that the groups are equivalent when, in fact, they are equivalent (Hatch, 1996).

The issue, then, is the power of the test. As we would expect, with only 20 subjects per group, the power of the tests we just ran is low. The reality is that equivalence testing is at times less powerful than testing for a difference. That is, we would need more subjects to test when a given difference is within the equivalence interval than when we test to see whether the two groups differ.

To determine why this is so, let's take a look at the equations to calculate sample size (Rogers, Howard, & Vessey, 1993). For the equivalence of two means, the equation is

$$n = \frac{2(z_\alpha + z_{\beta/2})^2 s^2}{[(M_1 - M_2) - \delta]^2},$$ [11]

and for the equivalence of two proportions, it is

$$n = \frac{(z_\alpha + z_{\beta/2})^2 [p_1(1 - p_1) + p_2(1 - p_2)]}{[(p_1 - p_2) - \delta]^2}.$$ [12]

(If we are testing whether the two means or proportions are identical, then the denominator becomes simply δ^2.) These are very similar to the usual equations for sample size determination (Streiner, 1990; see Chapter 4) with two differences, one that has a small effect on the sample and one that has a potentially large effect. The difference with the small effect is that we now want to minimize the Type II error rather than the Type I error, as in NHST. Consequently, the values of α and β are reversed, in that we set β at 0.05 and α at 0.10 or 0.20. The difference that has a potentially large effect is the δ in the denominator.

If we use Equation [12] to figure out the required sample size for the example (setting $\alpha = 0.20$, $\beta = 0.05$, and therefore power = 0.95), we will find it to be 2255 subjects per group! Conversely, with only 20 subjects per group, the power of the test to detect a difference of 0.083 between these proportions is less than 30%.

The sample size to test for equivalences is not always larger than that for testing for differences; again, it depends on the value of δ. Table 18.1 gives the sample sizes needed to test for non-inferiority for various

Table 18.1 Sample size per group for one-tailed equivalence testing on proportions

p_s	p_e	δ				$p_s > p_e$
		0.10	0.15	0.20	0.25	
	0.90	117	54	31	21	–
	0.85	545	140	64	37	540
0.90	0.80		625	159	72	157
	0.75			691	175	79
	0.70				745	49
	0.80	200	89	51	33	–
	0.75	860	216	96	54	862
0.80	0.70		914	229	102	231
	0.65			956	238	109
	0.60				984	64
	0.70	260	116	65	42	–
	0.65	1080	270	120	67	1084
0.70	0.60		1109	276	122	281
	0.55			1126	280	128
	0.50				1130	74
	0.60	296	132	74	47	–
	0.55	1203	300	133	74	1208
0.60	0.50		1207	300	133	305
	0.45			1199	298	136
	0.40				1178	77
	0.50	309	137	77	49	–
	0.45	1288	306	135	76	1233
0.50	0.40		1207	300	133	305
	0.35			1174	292	134
	0.30				1130	74
	0.40	296	132	74	47	–
	0.35	1154	288	128	71	1159
0.40	0.30		1109	276	122	281
	0.25			1053	262	120
	0.20				984	64
	0.30	260	116	65	42	–
	0.25	982	246	109	62	986
0.30	0.20		914	229	102	231
	0.15			835	209	95
	0.10				745	49

Notes: p_s = proportion in standard group; p_e = proportion in experimental group; $\alpha = 0.20$, $\beta = 0.05$ for equivalence testing; $\alpha = 0.05$, $\beta = 0.20$ for $p_s > p_e$.

combinations of proportions in the standard treatment group, p_s, and the experimental group, p_e, where $\alpha = 0.20$ and $\beta = 0.05$. For comparison, the last column is the sample size required for the traditional NHST that $p_s > p_e$. When $\delta = 2$ $(p_s - p_e)$, the sample sizes are about equal for both types of tests. When $\delta < 2$ $(p_s - p_e)$, the sample size for equivalence testing is larger than for difference testing. When $\delta > 2$ $(p_s - p_e)$, it is smaller. Note that, when δ is larger than 2 $(p_s - p_e)$, the change in sample size is relatively small. However, when δ is smaller than 2 $(p_s - p_e)$, the sample size increases rapidly and exponentially. The same relation holds for testing the non-inferiority of means, with M_s and M_e replacing p_s and p_e.

Summary

At times, despite all philosophical injunctions to the contrary, we have to prove that there are no unicorns. The solution, as we've seen, is to reverse the meanings of the null and alternative hypotheses and try to show that the null hypothesis of a difference can be rejected. This leaves us, by elimination, with the alternative: there is no difference (or at least, the difference is small enough for us to ignore). The issue is that the closer the groups must be to be considered equivalent, the larger the sample size required. This is entirely analogous to the situation for the traditional NHST: larger sample sizes are needed to detect smaller differences between groups. In both cases, sample size is like magnification with a microscope: the smaller the object that's being observed, the more magnification we need.

ACKNOWLEDGMENTS

I am deeply grateful to Drs. Malcolm Binns and Elizabeth Lin for their careful reading of an earlier draft and for their many helpful comments.

REFERENCES

Bollini, P., Pampallona, S., Tibaldi, G., Kupelnick, B., & Munizza, C. (1999, Apr). Effectiveness of antidepressants. Meta-analysis of dose-effect relationships in randomised clinical trials. *British Journal of Psychiatry*, 174(4), 297–303. http://dx.doi.org/10.1192/bjp.174.4.297 Medline:10533547

Canner, P.L. (1983, May). Aspirin in coronary heart disease. Comparison of six clinical trials. *Israel Journal of Medical Sciences*, 19(5), 413–423. Medline:6345461

Cohen, J. (1994). The earth is round ($p < .05$). *American Psychologist, 49*(12), 997–1003. http://dx.doi.org/10.1037/0003-066X.49.12.997

Hatch, J.P. (1996, Jun). Using statistical equivalence testing in clinical biofeedback research. *Biofeedback and Self-Regulation, 21*(2), 105–119. http://dx.doi.org/10.1007/BF02284690 Medline:8805961

Kendall, P.C., Marrs-Garcia, A., Nath, S.R., & Sheldrick, R.C. (1999, Jun). Normative comparisons for the evaluation of clinical significance. *Journal of Consulting and Clinical Psychology, 67*(3), 285–299. http://dx.doi.org/10.1037/0022-006X.67.3.285 Medline:10369049

MacMillan, H.L., Boyle, M.H., Wong, M.Y., Duku, E.K., Fleming, J.E., & Walsh, C.A. (1999, Oct 5). Slapping and spanking in childhood and its association with lifetime prevalence of psychiatric disorders in a general population sample. *Canadian Medical Association Journal, 161*(7), 805–809. Medline:10530296

Rogers, J.L., Howard, K.I., & Vessey, J.T. (1993, May). Using significance tests to evaluate equivalence between two experimental groups. *Psychological Bulletin, 113*(3), 553–565. http://dx.doi.org/10.1037/0033-2909.113.3.553 Medline:8316613

Streiner, D.L. (1990, Oct). Sample size and power in psychiatric research. *Canadian Journal of Psychiatry, 35*(7), 616–620. Medline:2268843

TO READ FURTHER

Hatch, J.P. (1996, Jun). Using statistical equivalence testing in clinical biofeedback research. *Biofeedback and Self-Regulation, 21*(2), 105–119. http://dx.doi.org/10.1007/BF02284690 Medline:8805961

Rogers, J.L., Howard, K.I., & Vessey, J.T. (1993, May). Using significance tests to evaluate equivalence between two experimental groups. *Psychological Bulletin, 113*(3), 553–565. http://dx.doi.org/10.1037/0033-2909.113.3.553 Medline:8316613

PART THREE

Research Methods

19 Reconcilable Differences: The Marriage of Qualitative and Quantitative Methods

PAULA N. GOERING, PH.D., AND
DAVID L. STREINER, PH.D.

Canadian Journal of Psychiatry, 1996, 41, 491–497

In the previous chapters in this book, we've focused on various aspects of research, as the term is now commonly used in psychiatry. That is, when most psychiatrists say "research" (if they say it at all), they generally mean some form of quantitative study, involving a large number of subjects, perhaps with random assignment to different groups, using objective outcome measures, and analysed with inferential statistics. Indeed, the earlier chapters (and most of the forthcoming ones) address these different components of quantitative methodology. This chapter is unique in two ways: it focuses on qualitative research techniques, and it is authored by two people (one of whom actually knows what she's talking about). What we hope to do is introduce you to qualitative research and explore how it can be integrated with more traditional, quantitative methods so that studies benefit from the strengths of each approach.

In reality, a qualitative approach to gathering data is not new to psychiatry or to other branches of medicine, but is actually closer to its roots. After all, Freud's theories were derived from what we would now call in-depth interviews and life histories; Adolph Meyer used and taught a detailed life history approach; and many of our current diagnoses were derived from careful, systematic studies of a small number of cases (Lief, 1948). The tradition survives in the superb case descriptions of neurological patients by Oliver Sacks (1995). As we will see, though, there are important differences between interviews carried out within a qualitative research tradition and those done for clinical purposes, although the latter may lead to researchable questions. In this chapter, we will discuss (1) what qualitative methods are, (2) how they differ from "clinical practice," (3) why qualitative methods are useful, and (4) how they can complement quantitative approaches. Be forewarned (or reassured), though, that we will not delve too deeply into the differences among the various theoretical traditions in which qualitative methods are often embedded, nor will we go into much detail about the technical aspects of data analysis. For those who want to explore these topics in greater depth, we would recommend the work of Denzin and Lincoln (2000) and Pope, Ziebland, and Mays (2000).

Qualitative Research Methods Philosophy

Before we introduce the unique data collection, study design, and quality control techniques associated with qualitative research, some of the underlying assumptions that distinguish this type of research need to be understood. Various names are given to the basic paradigm, wherein the term "naturalistic" is often used by its practitioners in opposition to the traditional "rationalist" position (the latter is sometimes labelled "positivist," which is meant to be a derogatory term when used by "postmodernists"). Guba and Lincoln (1985) discuss the beliefs about the nature of reality and ways of knowing that differentiate these two paradigms. They stress that what is at issue is not the nature of self-evident truth, but rather the fit between the philosophy of science and the phenomenon that is under study. They do not advocate abandoning experimental methods when dealing with genetic and biological processes, but do argue that social and behavioural phenomena are best understood within a different framework.

The nature of reality within the naturalistic framework is less tangible and predictable than the rationalistic version. Rather than seeing human behaviour as a conglomerate of independent variables and processes that can be taken apart, examined, and eventually reassembled to get the total picture, emphasis is placed upon multiple, interacting realities that can be studied only as a whole. The focus is on subjectivity, that is, meaning and interpretation as constructions that exist in the minds of people. Echoing the early Gestalt psychologists, the assumption is that the sum of human experience is greater than and different from its parts. Enquiry is more like filming an ever-changing and unending story, rather than cutting out and putting together a jigsaw puzzle. Each filming should increase understanding, but there is no one correct version, and more questions may be raised than answered.

Moreover, the relationship between the enquirer (a term that is used in preference to "researcher") and the respondent is viewed differently within the naturalistic paradigm. Rather than trying to maintain a discrete distance between the observer and the observed, mutual interaction is seen as both inevitable and as a valuable source of knowledge. Just as film-makers focus and shoot in response to both the action on the set and their own interests and sensitivities, so scientists are viewed as adaptable and responsive "instruments" who guide and shape the discovery process. The desired outcome of research for the rationalist is a set of context-free generalizations based on similarities among units. The naturalist is more interested in developing an adequate and complete picture – what is called a "thick description" of the situation under study. Differences in time and context are as important as similarities.

Critics of the ongoing and often contentious academic debates feel that the philosophical differences between these two types of science have been exaggerated and overemphasized (Reichardt & Rallis, 1994). Still, recognizing that basic concepts such as objectivity and subjectivity are viewed somewhat differently in each ideological camp should help those new to the territory make sense of the unusual features of the terrain. It should be noted that lumping all of the various qualitative theoretical traditions into one philosophical pot is a little like talking about psychiatry as if there were only one school of thought. In reality, there are numerous types of qualitative research traditions, ranging from phenomenology, with its focus upon the lived experience of individuals, to grounded theory, which searches to identify the core processes within a particular social scene (Miller & Crabtree, 1992). Among these distinctive traditions and theories, there are various research methods, which we will describe, although we will not be going into greater detail regarding the ways the theories dictate the methods.

Data Collection Techniques

Quantitative research encompasses a wide spectrum of techniques, from in vitro examination of nerve endings through brain imaging to community surveys of prevalence and to randomized, controlled clinical trials of new drugs and other types of therapy. Each of these procedures was developed to address questions that the others could not deal with. In an analogous way, there are a multitude of qualitative techniques available to the researcher. None is useful in all situations, but collectively the techniques are capable of addressing a wide range of problems. *Ethnography*, made famous by social and cultural anthropologists, is probably the most well-known qualitative method. Immersing oneself in the daily life of a culture over an extended period of time, developing relationships with key community members, and taking extensive field notes were techniques originally developed for the investigation of foreign societies. Now they are also used to explore exotic locales and cultures such as pool halls (Polsky, 1967) and operating theatres (Lingard, Garwood, & Poenaru, 2004). Life narratives, case studies, and archival analyses are other tools in the qualitative realm. In this section we will briefly describe group and individual interviews and participant observation: qualitative methods of data collection that are closer to clinical practice and thus more feasible and accessible for psychiatric researchers.

Focus Groups

The focus group is becoming an increasingly popular research technique used to discover such universal truths as which brand of toothpaste we prefer or which politician we least dislike. Despite these disreputable associations, focus groups actually are a very valuable tool in qualitative research (Frey & Fontana, 1991). A focus group session is a discussion in which a small number of people (somewhere in the neighbourhood of six to ten) talk about a topic proposed by the moderator or facilitator. This is one major way in which a focus group differs from a therapy group: it is the researcher who sets the agenda, rather than the participants, and he or she tries to keep the group focused on that topic, sometimes using a series of probes to assure coverage of key concepts. Otherwise, the session is fairly open; the members may make comments on what they feel or believe or on what someone else has said, and they may ask questions of other members.

Group interviews have some advantages over a series of individual ones. Obviously, they are more efficient, allowing the researcher to hear from multiple perspectives in one session. They may also provide the safety and comfort associated with being among others who have shared similar experiences, a critical issue if particularly sensitive or stigmatizing subjects are being discussed, such as sexual or physical abuse, the use of illicit drugs, or abortions. The free-flowing interaction within the group often stimulates new ideas and allows participants to reflect differently than they might if it were only their own experiences that were being described. Questions, feedback, and challenges from peers can stimulate a much broader and richer exploration of a subject than a one-on-one interaction between a single participant and a researcher.

In some situations, it is best to have a relatively homogeneous group of people who have shared common experiences or who reflect similar points of view. This is particularly true if the topic under discussion involves acts that are censured or proscribed (such as child or spousal abuse), that are potentially embarrassing (such as having been arrested), or that only some people experience (such as childbirth). In other cases (sibling rivalry, for example), a more heterogeneous composition, such as brothers and sisters of different birth orders, could result in a richer understanding of the topic. Problems of group dynamics that can plague therapy groups can also occur in focus groups: one member may attempt to dominate and steer the conversation, other members may be chary about voicing contrary views because of peer pressure, and the group may move off topic. It takes considerable skill to decide on the appropriate composition of a focus group and to manage the group dynamics so that the process is productive. A team of two researchers is ideal – one to run the group and the other to take detailed notes – and if the meeting is not being taped, two are mandatory. Otherwise, observation and recording will be completely inadequate.

In-Depth Interviews

As implied by the name, the advantage of long, one-on-one interviews is the intensive and intimate opportunity to hear in detail from one individual. Rather than the breadth of multiple, interacting perspectives gained through a focus group, a more complete picture of the subjective experience and context for a particular person is obtained in individual interviews. The style can range from the informal and unstructured interaction that typifies an ethnographic field interview to a more formal and semi-structured "long interview" that purposively covers a set of pre-selected subtopics (McCracken, 1988). When using more structured approaches, one has to be on guard against slipping into doing a quantitative, interviewer-administered questionnaire "incognito."

For example, if you find yourself asking a series of closed-ended questions that can easily be answered with "yes" or "no" or employing a few fixed categories, then you have lapsed back into the quantitative mode. The essential components of in-depth interviews are open-ended questions and a flexible process, so that the interviewees can tell their stories in their own words and unanticipated leads can be followed. Quality data collection is dependent on sensitive and unobtrusive listening that elicits private thoughts and feelings in a non-judgmental manner. In-depth interviews can take many hours and may involve a series of meetings or sessions in order to adequately cover the topic under discussion. The end result should be not only the verbatim recorded words of the respondent(s) but also the field notes of the interviewer's impressions, which supplement the transcript.

Participant Observation

Participant observation involves the researcher observing the phenomenon under study in the naturalistic situation and in "real time." The balance between participation and observation is variable, ranging from actively taking part in the group that is being observed; through being defined as a member of the group, but not being a participant in all of its activities; to being seen as an observer who is not part of the group. As in most research decisions, trade-offs are involved. The more the researcher is seen as an active member, the more the group members will trust him or her and be open about their thoughts and feelings. There are circumstances in which it is obvious that the researcher must remain an outsider, however, such as in observing groups of forensic patients or ballet students.

In all cases, though, the involvement with the group is intensive, extends over a period of time, and is marked by communication and interaction, rather than passive reception of knowledge. The purposes of this extended involvement are manifold. A primary goal is that the researcher will be able to understand the way the group members think and interpret their world, rather than being simply an observer of their behaviour. Further, as the researcher becomes less of a novelty and is seen more as a member, his or her presence will not distort the dynamics of the group or the behaviour of the individuals; that is, the problem of reactivity should be lessened, thus increasing the validity of the observations.

Research Design

Sampling strategies also take a different form in qualitative studies. Two of the hallmarks of quantitative research are random sampling and predetermination of sample size (Streiner, 1990; see Chapter 4). Subjects are chosen at random for a number of reasons: to meet the assumptions of statistical tests, to avoid bias, and to allow valid generalizations to the population from which the sample was drawn. The sample size is calculated beforehand in order for the statistics to have enough power to detect whether differences between groups or changes over time are "real" or are simply reflections of the vagaries of sampling. The logic behind sample selection in qualitative research is quite different. For the most part, qualitative research relies on *purposive sampling*, in which respondents are selected precisely because the investigator can learn the most from them. They may have information that others do not have, they may represent the full range or most extreme examples of the phenomenon, they may be the most articulate spokespersons, or they may have a unique perspective (Sandelowski, 1995).

Snowball Sampling

One of the hardest tasks in purposive sampling is finding and making contact with the subjects, whether they be community leaders, patients, or, as in one of our studies (Taylor et al., 1991), people who felt they had suffered ill effects from an environmental accident. It is likely, however, that one member of a group knows others in the same situation and so could suggest names and even make the initial contact, smoothing the way for the researcher. In this way, the first person may identify three other people, each of whom may know three or four other people, so that the sample "snowballs" in size. One consequence of this sampling strategy, intended or not, is that the researcher may end up with a relatively homogeneous group of people, all of whom have shared similar experiences.

Key Informants

Key informants are people who, because of their position or experience, have a greater knowledge of what is being investigated than the average person. Their authority can derive from an "inside" perspective or from an external appointment. In the community, for example, they may be religious or political leaders or may be seen as the "elder spokespersons." For example, a student of Paula Goering (PG), Tina Pranger (1999), used qualitative methods to study consumer involvement in mental health service planning and delivery. In addition to holding in-depth interviews with consumers (her primary sources), she conducted key informant interviews with administrators and care providers within the four organizations under study. These individuals could give an overview of the organizational context and had a perspective different from that of the consumers. They also provided an entry into the settings and served as "go-betweens," introducing the researcher to the participants and "legitimizing" the research.

Extreme Cases

Assume that we are interested in studying the factors that predispose some people to physically abuse their children. If we were to select parents randomly, we would likely find only a small proportion who are abusers. By contrast, we could deliberately choose people who have been convicted of abuse and whose histories can thereby bring these factors to light more sharply, especially if they are contrasted with people who, by one criterion or another, are regarded as excellent parents. As another example, if we were looking at the effectiveness of a psychosocial rehabilitation program, we might learn more in less time by interviewing in depth a few people who did very well and a few who did very poorly, rather than by looking at a larger number of people, most of whose progress was average.

Sample Size

When is enough, enough? In quantitative research, we determine sample size a priori based on the magnitude of the effect we are hoping to detect. A very different criterion is used in qualitative studies: we continue to enrol new people until we are not learning anything new from the next few subjects. In the jargon of the field, we *sample to informational redundancy* or *sample to saturation*. This doesn't mean that numbers aren't important. In qualitative research, just as in quantitative studies, we can have sample sizes that are too small or too large to achieve the desired aims. If our interest is in the range of people's experiences (for example, the different paths to homelessness), then obviously we'll need a relatively large number of subjects, and a single case study would be insufficient. Conversely, large sample sizes could prevent us from fully understanding how people experienced some event (for example, what led to the first psychiatric admission), since there wouldn't be enough time to allow in-depth, detailed analyses (MacLean et al. 2010; Sandelowski, 1995). What is deemed to be an adequate sample size in qualitative studies is usually smaller than what we see in quantitative research, and it is not unusual for 15 to 20 subjects to be sufficient to meet our aims.

Assuring Data Quality

As is apparent from the discussion so far, the main research "tools" used in qualitative research are the investigators themselves – their impressions, feelings, and interpretations of what they see and hear. Because of this subjective nature of the data, quantitative researchers are apt to dismiss them as unreliable (the data, that is, if not the researchers themselves) and unverifiable. Indeed, the allegations that Margaret Mead saw what she wanted to see and that the tales of guiltless premarital sex were "Just So" stories made up by the Samoans unfortunately reinforced this image (Freeman, 1983). The reality is quite different. Although the techniques used by qualitative researchers to ensure the reliability and validity of their findings are different from those used by quantitative investigators, they do, in fact, exist, and they are as rigorous (Kirk & Miller, 1986).

A primary method to enhance the quality of the data is called *triangulation*, a technique that is familiar to coastal sailors and enthusiasts of World War II spy movies. You remember the scene: the OSS or SOE agent is sitting in an attic somewhere in Germany, hunched over his transmitter, while outside the Gestapo are riding around in a truck with a circular antenna on top. They pick up the direction of the radio, and draw a line on a map. Then they drive to another site, locate the radio again, and draw another line. The spot the lines intersect is where our unsuspecting hero is holed up. In qualitative research, the phenomenon being investigated is found not from different radio locations, but by using different techniques, observers, times, and places.

For example, in our studies of the psychosocial impact of environmental hazards (Taylor et al., 1991), we used a number of qualitative techniques: focus groups, key informants, and in-depth interviews. Next, the transcripts from these interviews were coded for themes by two researchers working independently. Last, our confidence in our conclusions was increased when the same themes emerged in different locales, which were faced with a variety of situations perceived as hazardous, such as landfill sites, solid-waste incinerators, and industrial accidents. As we'll discuss later, triangulation can also be achieved by combining qualitative and quantitative methods.

Comparison with Clinical Practice

There are clear similarities between psychiatric clinical practice and these qualitative research data collection methods. With appropriate training (Goering & Strauss, 1987), the interviewing skills of an expert clinician can be used to great advantage in this type of research where the "use of self as an instrument" is intrinsic. The differences lie in the purpose and the conduct of the research interviews – which are initiated by the researcher, not the client – in that they seek to understand rather than to solve problems or to provide assistance. Interpretation and advice are not offered, and the expert on the subject under discussion is the interviewee, not the interviewer.

There are also major differences in how the data are recorded, analysed, and reported following a group or individual interview, an aspect of qualitative research that is often underestimated by those who are not familiar with the careful and systematic process of repeated examination and coding that is involved. Irrespective of the actual data collection method used, the interview is almost always recorded and transcribed verbatim, and this record is supplemented by "field notes," which provide a context for the interview, as well as the researcher's comments about other aspects of the interaction that may not be apparent from simply reading the transcript. The transcript is then carefully scrutinized and coded for themes (a process that is now made easier by software programs specifically designed for that purpose) in an iterative process of sifting and categorizing to arrive at summary descriptions and conclusions. There is also continual attention to "quality control" in the research process (Sandelowski, 1986), such as having two or more coders working independently and documenting decisions made at each step of the coding process, so others can follow the inductive line of reasoning and be able to discriminate between good and bad scholarship.

Combining Qualitative and Quantitative Methods

Whether qualitative and quantitative methods can, or should, be combined has been the subject of heated debate. The purists in both the quantitative and the qualitative camps who argue against such a union stress that the two paradigms are based on completely different philosophical assumptions and values (e.g., Powers, 1987). To them, the thought of combining methods is tantamount to miscegenation, akin to a marriage between an anglophone and a francophone: people who communicate in different languages and to achieve different aims and thus are doomed to continual fighting if forced to live together. Those who argue for a combination see the methods as different tools, suited for different tasks but both potentially necessary in order to do a good job. The latter viewpoint has recently gained in popularity, particularly in the more pragmatic fields of program evaluation and policy research (Reichardt & Rallis, 1994), where triangulation has become trendy and much has been written about its value (although much less has been said about how to actually accomplish it). Even some people who espouse combining both techniques in one study don't see it as an equal marriage, however, believing that qualitative methods are appropriate only as an initial, hypothesis-generating stage and that a quantitative study must later be used to confirm or refute these hypotheses. What we hope to accomplish in this section is to show how the two techniques can be equal partners in the marriage, each helping the other at every step of the research endeavour: using the qualitative study prior to designing a quantitative one; running the two techniques simultaneously so that each can inform the other as the study progresses; and, where the qualitative study is done afterwards, helping to explain the findings of the quantitative investigation.

Quality before Quantity

The aim of many studies is to gain a better understanding in an area where there has already been much research done. The new project may involve modifying an existing therapy or applying it to a somewhat different group of subjects. We generally know beforehand what the important outcomes of a study will be and how we should measure them. When we're venturing into a new area, though, we often do not have these landmarks; we may not know what the key dependent, or even the independent, variables may be. Qualitative techniques can very profitably be used in such situations to demarcate areas of potential importance. For example, a former student of David Streiner (DS), Tuanchai Inthusoma, used qualitative techniques for this purpose in a study in Thailand. One aim of the World Health Organization's Expanded Program for Immunization is to achieve an 80% immunization rate in children. However, among children in Thailand's Klong Toey slums, where the investigator worked, the immunization rate for measles was far below this target. Some "trialists" were eager for her to do a randomized, controlled trial to determine if various interventions could increase compliance, such as educating mothers about the possible dangers of measles or how to recognize the disease. It became clear, though, that it would be a waste of time and effort to do such a study before there was a better understanding of people's perceptions of what measles meant to them and what barriers prevented them from having their children immunized (Serquina-Ramiro et al., 2001).

Inthusoma used a combination of focus groups with mothers from the slum area and in-depth interviews with both mothers and community leaders in her investigation. A number of factors quickly became apparent. First, any educational program designed to increase the mothers' ability to recognize measles or to see it as dangerous would be superfluous, as their knowledge was not deficient in either area. Second, the women relied on traditional Thai remedies – mainly different forms of cereals – to treat measles. Third, there was a belief that all children have measles as a normal part of growing up, as well as a prevailing feeling that normal patterns should not be interfered with. Thus, the problem was not ignorance of the need to treat measles per se, but rather a different belief system regarding what the proper treatment was and its purpose (they used cereals to ameliorate symptoms, rather than to attempt prevention). The interviews also revealed that the mothers' main source of information about etiology, treatment, and prognosis came from their mothers and mothers-in-law, not the formal health system. Consequently, the educational intervention had to be tailored to take these beliefs into account and the message targeted as much to the generation of grandparents as to the biological parents. Had she not known of this ahead of time, Inthusoma might have given a non-helpful message to the wrong people. The use of qualitative methods to check assumptions and refine research questions is valuable across and within cultures.

Another sequential use of qualitative followed by quantitative methods is during the development of measurement scales. Focus groups and in-depth interviewing of key informants can identify the domains that should be covered and can provide feedback about the appropriateness, face, and content validity of the individual questions. This approach is becoming very common in the burgeoning field of quality of life (QOL) measures. As one example, another student of DS, Gabriel Ronen, developed a QOL scale for children with epilepsy to be answered by the children themselves, rather than the more usual (but probably less accurate) method of asking the parents about the children (Ronen, Streiner, & Rosenbaum, 2003). He ran a series of focus groups with epileptic children and elicited a number of factors about which parents were unaware, such as the feeling of many children that they had to shield their parents from knowing the full impact of the epilepsy, since they felt that the grownups would overreact. Another example concerns the measurement of satisfaction with psychiatric care. Colleagues of PG, who have tested innovative methods for obtaining client satisfaction (Clark, Scott, & Krupa, 1993), used focus groups to generate the attributes of care that are important from the client's perspective as a first step in the development of a scale. They found, as have others using similar methods (Elbeck & Fecteau, 1990; Everett & Boydell, 1994), that interpersonal relationships with staff are of utmost importance and are not adequately represented in most standardized scales.

Quality and Quantity Together

Qualitative methods can be used in the same study with quantitative methods in order to extend and complement findings. PG is one of a team of investigators who conducted a study in Toronto of mental illness and pathways into homelessness (Tolomiczenko & Goering, 2000). A classical epidemiological design that includes a large number of subjects representative of the population of homeless was required in order to assess the distribution of mental illness and the factors that are associated with homelessness within subgroups. Questions of "how many" and "how much" can be answered with such an approach, but the question of "how" required a different method. In-depth interviews with a smaller subset of the larger sample, supplemented by collateral interviews with significant others (family, providers, friends) described in much greater detail and complexity the process by which individuals start using shelters or living in the street. The combination of a survey and long interviews allowed for revisiting familiar categories concerning diagnosis and social factors on a broad scale while exploring new territory about process and context in a more intensive fashion. Both types of information together provided a better basis for planning strategies for prevention.

Quantity before Quality

Finally, the interpretation and communication of quantitative findings can draw upon qualitative methods for valuable insights and helpful illustrations. In our work with environmental contaminants (Taylor et al., 1991), we found that there was a high degree of distress in communities that were potential sites for solid-waste storage facilities (the new euphemism for garbage dumps), but in communities that already housed such facilities or after the dump was operating, the level of stress was much lower and well within normal limits. The questions that arose after the quantitative study tried to pinpoint the cause of this phenomenon. Do the most distressed people move out of the neighbourhood? Do people adapt to a threatening situation? Was their initial assessment of the situation overly pessimistic? Do they change their evaluation of risk? The study found that all of these factors were present to varying degrees (Elliott et al., 1997). This is a situation where the quantitative study yielded hard data, but their meaning was unclear, so a qualitative study after the fact was necessary.

Practical Issues

In order to conduct studies that combine both methods, it is necessary to have access to a wide range of expertise and skills. This often means using a team approach and asking qualitative and quantitative experts to collaborate – a recipe for disaster (or at a minimum, confusion and dissention) unless the researchers from both traditions have a high degree of mutual respect and openness to learning. The ability to abandon technical jargon and speak plain English, a rare commodity within both methodological camps, is also critical when communicating across boundaries. Careful consideration must be given to design and operational issues. How and when will the two types of data be linked? In a fully integrated study, the team will meet and discuss assumptions and findings through all phases so that the results of each can inform the other. If triangulation is the aim, conclusions will be formed in a more separate fashion and then compared to assess the degree to which the multiple sources confirm or contradict each other. The latter is always a possibility, and it should not be assumed that quantitative findings always have greater authority. Erroneous assumptions, invalid measures, insufficient power, and other limitations may result in the quantitative findings being less valid than the qualitative ones (Estroff & Zimmer, 1994). The reporting of results also requires forethought. Journals tend to prefer one type of method over another, and page limits and style requirements are not always conducive to reports that include both types of methods. Despite these potential problems and demanding decisions, there are many rewards to be gained from combined studies, and efforts to reconcile methodological differences can lead to creative and synergistic research.

ACKNOWLEDGMENTS

The authors gratefully acknowledge the many helpful comments from Drs. Kathy Boydell, Cathy Charles, Deborah Cook, Janet Durbin, and Mita Giacomini.

REFERENCES

Clark, C., Scott, E., & Krupa, T. (1993, Oct). Involving clients in programme evaluation and research: A new methodology for occupational therapy. *Canadian Journal of Occupational Therapy, 60*(4), 192–199. Medline:10129021

Denzin, N.K., & Lincoln, Y.S. (Eds.). (2000). *Handbook of qualitative research.* (2nd ed.). Thousand Oaks, CA: Sage.

Elbeck, M., & Fecteau, G. (1990, Sep). Improving the validity of measures of patient satisfaction with psychiatric care and treatment. *Hospital & Community Psychiatry, 41*(9), 998–1001. Medline:2210711

Elliott, S.J., Taylor, S.M., Hampson, C., Dunn, J., Eyles, J., Walter, S., & Streiner, D.L. (1997). 'It's not because you like it any better...': Residents' reappraisal of a landfill site. *Journal of Environmental Psychology, 17*(3), 229–241. http://dx.doi.org/10.1006/jevp.1997.0055

Estroff, S.E., & Zimmer, C.M. (1994). Social networks, social support, and violence among persons with severe, persistent mental illness. In J. Mohahan & H.J. Steadman (Eds.), *Violence and mental disorder: Developments in risk assessment* (pp. 259–295). Chicago, IL: University of Chicago Press.

Everett, B., & Boydell, K.M. (1994, Jan). A methodology for including consumers' opinions in mental health evaluation research. *Hospital & Community Psychiatry, 45*(1), 76–78. Medline:8125469

Freeman, D. (1983). *Margaret Mead and Samoa: The making and unmaking of an anthropological myth.* Cambridge, MA: Harvard University Press.

Frey, J.H., & Fontana, A. (1991). The group interview in social research. *Social Science Journal, 28*(2), 175–187. http://dx.doi.org/10.1016/0362-3319(91)90003-M

Goering, P.N., & Strauss, J.S. (1987, Jul). Teaching clinical research: What clinicians need to know. *American Journal of Orthopsychiatry, 57*(3), 418–423. http://dx.doi.org/10.1111/j.1939-0025.1987.tb03551.x Medline:3618740

Guba, E.G., & Lincoln, Y.S. (1985). Epistemological and methodological bases of naturalistic inquiry. In Y.S. Lincoln & E.G. Guba (Eds.), *Naturalistic inquiry* (pp. 73–84). Beverly Hills, CA: Sage.

Kirk, J., & Miller, M.L. (1986). *Reliability and validity in qualitative research.* Newbury Park, CA: Sage.

Lief, A. (1948). *The commonsense psychiatry of Dr. Adolf Meyer.* New York: McGraw-Hill.

Lingard, L., Garwood, S., & Poenaru, D. (2004, Jul). Tensions influencing operating room team function: Does institutional context make a difference? *Medical Education, 38*(7), 691–699. http://dx.doi.org/10.1111/j.1365-2929.2004.01844.x Medline:15200393

MacLean, L., Estable, A., Meyer, M., Kothari, A., Edwards, N., & Riley, B. (2010). Drowsing over data: When less is more. In D.L. Streiner & S. Sidani (Eds.), *When research goes off the rails: Why it happens and what you can do about it* (pp. 283–289). New York: Guilford.

McCracken, G. (1988). *The long interview.* Newbury Park, CA: Sage.

Miller, W.L., & Crabtree, B.F. (1992). Primary care research: A multimethod typology and qualitative road map. In B.F. Crabtree & W.L. Miller (Eds.), *Doing qualitative research* (pp. 3–20). Newbury Park, CA: Sage.

Polsky, N. (1967). *Hustlers, beats, and others.* Chicago, IL: Aldine.

Pope, C., Ziebland, S., & Mays, N. (2000, Jan 8). Qualitative research in health care. Analysing qualitative data. *British Medical Journal, 320*(7227), 114–116. http://dx.doi.org/10.1136/bmj.320.7227.114 Medline:10625273

Powers, B.A. (1987, Mar-Apr). Taking sides: A response to Goodwin and Goodwin. [Commentary]. *Nursing Research, 36*(2), 122–126. Medline:3644258

Pranger, B. (1999). *Mental health consumer involvement in service level decision-making: Rhetoric and reality.* Unpublished doctoral thesis, University of Toronto.

Reichardt, C.S., & Rallis, S.F. (1994). *The qualitative-quantitative debate, new perspectives: New directions for program evaluation.* San Francisco, CA: Jossey-Bass.

Ronen, G.M., Streiner, D.L., Rosenbaum, P., & Canadian Pediatric Epilepsy Network. (2003). Health-related quality of life in children with epilepsy: Development and validation of self-report and parent proxy measures. *Epilepsia, 44*(4), 598–612. http://dx.doi.org/10.1046/j.1528-1157.2003.46302.x Medline:12681011

Sacks, O. (1995). *An anthropologist on Mars.* New York: Knopf.

Sandelowski, M. (1986, Apr). The problem of rigor in qualitative research. *ANS. Advances in Nursing Science, 8*(3), 27–37. Medline:3083765

Sandelowski, M. (1995, Apr). Sample size in qualitative research. *Research in Nursing & Health, 18*(2), 179–183. http://dx.doi.org/10.1002/nur.4770180211 Medline:7899572

Serquina-Ramiro, L., Kasniyah, N., Inthusoma, T., Higginbotham, N., Streiner, D.L., Nichter, M., & Freeman, S. (2001, Dec). Measles immunization acceptance in Southeast Asia: Past patterns and future challenges. *Southeast Asian Journal of Tropical Medicine and Public Health, 32*(4), 791–804. Medline:12041556

Streiner, D.L. (1990, Oct). Sample size and power in psychiatric research. *Canadian Journal of Psychiatry, 35*(7), 616–620. Medline:2268843

Taylor, S.M., Elliott, S., Eyles, J., Frank, J., Haight, M., Streiner, D.L., …, & Willms, D. (1991). Psychosocial impacts in populations exposed to solid waste facilities. *Social Science & Medicine, 33*(4), 441–447. http://dx.doi.org/10.1016/0277-9536(91)90326-8 Medline:1948158

Tolomiczenko, G., & Goering, P. (2000). The process and politics of community-based research with people recently homeless. *Psychiatric Rehabilitation Journal, 24,* 46–51.

TO READ FURTHER

Crabtree, B.F. & Miller, W.L. (Eds.). (1992). *Doing qualitative research.* Newbury Park, CA: Sage.

Denzin, N.K., & Lincoln, Y.S. (Eds.). (2000). *Handbook of qualitative research.* (2nd ed.). Thousand Oaks, CA: Sage.

Kirk, J., & Miller, M.L. (1986). *Reliability and validity in qualitative research.* Newbury Park, CA: Sage.

20 Thinking Small: Research Designs Appropriate for Clinical Practice

DAVID L. STREINER, PH.D.

Canadian Journal of Psychiatry, 1998, 43, 737–741

Open almost any textbook on research methods or evaluation, and you will see descriptions of procedures such as randomized controlled trials, case control methods, and non-equivalent control group designs, which are appropriate for looking at groups of patients to evaluate the efficacy or effectiveness of some intervention. This may lead the reader to conclude that the only way to study whether or not a treatment works is to have a large number of patients who can be studied. While it is true that large studies are needed to determine whether a therapy works in general for certain types of disorders, there are many evaluation techniques that can be used by individual clinicians to see if a treatment is effective for a specific in- or outpatient in their practices. In this chapter, we will look at a few of these designs.

First, let's discuss why, if a therapy has been shown to work in a large trial, the therapist should be concerned about its effectiveness at the individual level. There are three primary reasons: group versus individual effects; efficacy versus effectiveness; and the translation of "manualized" procedures into clinical practice.

Rationale

Group versus Individual Effects

Whenever we analyse a study to see if an intervention has worked, we compare the groups in relation to some summary statistic; for example, is the mean score on a depression inventory lower in the

Fig. 20.1 Hypothetical results of a study showing an effective treatment

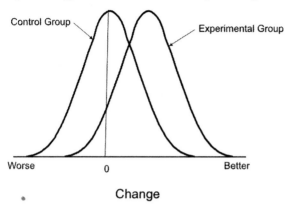

Change

group that received the newer treatment than in the group that had traditional therapy, or did a smaller proportion of patients relapse in one condition compared with another? Even if the results are in the desired direction, it does not mean that all patients benefited equally. It is quite possible and even expected that, while the majority of patients improved, some did not, and others may even have become worse. This follows from the fact that within each group, there is always a *distribution* of change scores. In Figure 20.1, for example, the mean change score of the experimental group is larger than that of the control group. However, it is obvious that some people in the control condition improved more than some people in the treatment arm and that some people in the experimental group were the same as or worse than when they started treatment. Thus, there is no guarantee that a therapy that works in general for the majority of people would be effective for a specific patient.

Efficacy versus Effectiveness

When we read an article describing the results of a study, we often find that the "Subjects" section has a long list of inclusion and exclusion criteria: patients are enrolled in the study only if they fulfil all of the criteria for the disorder being studied, fall within a certain age range, do not have any co-morbid disorders (especially brain damage or substance abuse problems), have not been on any other medication for one or two months, and so forth. Some studies even have a run-in period during which adherence to the treatment regimen is carefully monitored so that potentially non-compliant patients can be eliminated before they drop out and jeopardize the results. The reason for the many inclusion and exclusion criteria lies in the nature of all statistical tests that look at differences between or among groups. Whether we are talking about a *t*-test, an ANOVA, or something more sophisticated, they all boil down to a simple ratio of the variability *between* the groups divided by the variability *within* the groups. (Statisticians earn their keep by figuring out how to calculate these two indices of variability, which differs from one situation to the next.) So, to make the results statistically significant, we can make the difference between the groups as large as possible, the variability within the groups as small as possible, or both. There is often little we can do to increase the differences between the groups; that is determined by how good the drug or other intervention really is. However, we can reduce the within-group variability by making the subjects as homogeneous as possible, hence the rigid inclusion and exclusion criteria. The outcome of such a study tells us about the *efficacy* of the intervention; that is, can it work under ideal circumstances?

When treating patients in our offices or in hospital, we don't have the luxury of excluding people who do not quite fit the *Diagnostic and Statistical Manual of Mental Disorders* (DSM-IV) criteria, have something else wrong with them, or may be less than perfectly compliant with the treatment regimen; in other words, we are operating within the real world, filled (some might say unfortunately) with real patients. Thus, we are more interested in the *effectiveness* of the treatment: does it work within the constraints of actual practice? A certain drug, for example, may be extremely efficacious but have disturbing side effects. Patients may be willing to continue to take the medication while they are in a study, because they are being closely monitored by a research nurse and know that the study will end in a month or so. With no one to remind (or nag) them to take the drug, and after being on it for six months or so, compliance will begin to decline. This is a constant problem with any treatment that must be used for long periods, whether the therapy is for a psychological problem, hypertension, hyperlipidemia, or something else. Consequently, an efficacious therapy may not be at all effective. For more about the difference between efficacy and effectiveness trials, see Streiner (2002; see Chapter 21).

"Manualized" Versus Actual Therapy

Once a study is completed and it demonstrates that the treatment works, we need to know exactly what that therapy was: what exactly was done, by whom, and for how long. For that reason, treatment in a research context very often follows a strict protocol. For example, drug trials may stipulate that the patient receive a specific dose, to be increased by fixed amounts at regular intervals or if certain criteria are met. Similarly, therapists (providing cognitive-behavioural or interpersonal therapy, for instance) receive training and then must follow a manual, indicating what should and should not be said or done (Luborsky & DeRubeis, 1984). Often, the sessions are recorded and later evaluated by someone from the research team as a further check that the therapy provided conformed to the manual.

While this process ensures that we know exactly what was done in the study, it differs markedly from actual practice. We may start using a new type of therapy after reading some articles or attending a workshop, without the training and supervision provided to the research therapists; alterations in drug level would be made when the patient's condition changed, not when the calendar did; and we may "contaminate" treatment by bringing in elements of a different mode of therapy if the situation warrants it. Hence, the therapy we provide may differ in ways – some relatively trivial and others more substantial – from the therapy performed in the study.

What all of this means is that we cannot assume that, because a study showed that a given therapy works, it will be successful with the particular patient we have in treatment right now. In fact, Weisz, Donenberg, Han, and Weiss (1995) found that studies under highly controlled conditions showed considerably larger gains in the experimental groups than studies that were carried out in more naturalistic situations. The consequence is that we should look on each patient as a mini-experiment, a study with a sample size of 1. In the remainder of this article, we will discuss a few of the methods appropriate for "$N = 1$" studies.

Study Designs

Before-After Design

Perhaps the simplest design to envision is one in which a patient is measured on some attribute before therapy starts and again when therapy is near the end. The attribute can be measured using a questionnaire completed by the patient or someone in the patient's family, a behavioural test that taps the patient's ability to perform some task (for example, venture from the house, approach a feared animal, or start a conversation with a stranger), or anything else that reflects the person's difficulty. A technique this straightforward must have problems associated with it, and the before-after design has enough to fill volumes (and it has; Collins & Horn, 1991).

The first issue does not pertain only to before-after designs, although it is particularly problematic in this type of study, and that is the nature of the measure itself. First, it should be reliable and valid (Streiner, 1993; see Chapter 22). Second, the therapist should avoid the temptation to complete the measure him- or herself, as is required by, for example, the Hamilton Depression Rating Scale (HDRS; Hamilton, 1960). It is easy to see why this temptation exists: it is seemingly more objective than the patient's evaluation; it prevents "impression management" (Paulhus, 1984); and, after all, who is in a better position to rate the patient's condition than the therapist? The answer is just about everybody else in the world! There is far too much distortion caused by seeing what we want and expect to see, rather than what is really there (Rosenthal, 1966). In one meta-analysis, Greenberg and his colleagues showed that, across a number of studies, therapists reported about twice the improvement on tricyclic antidepressants (TCAs) than did the patients themselves (Greenberg, Bornstein, Greenberg, & Fisher, 1992). By the same token, relying exclusively on patient self-report is problematic. "Impression management" refers to the tendency of people to consciously or unconsciously give answers that reinforce a particular picture that they want to portray. For example, at the start of therapy, patients may overstate the magnitude and perhaps exaggerate the nature of their difficulties to ensure that they will receive help. Later, when they want to terminate, because either they feel they have improved sufficiently or they are just tired of attending therapy, they may minimize their problems. This "hello-goodbye" effect (Streiner & Norman, 2008) results in a dramatic improvement in test scores, even without any change in the patient's condition. So, how do we get an accurate report? The answer is to rely on objective indices as much as possible: indicators of behaviour that are observable, countable, and reproducible. (Sources of scales are given in Appendix B of Streiner & Norman, 2008, and criteria for evaluating scales in Streiner, 1993; see Chapter 22).

The second problem goes by many names: baseline effects, floor and ceiling effects, the law of initial values, and others. What they all refer to is that the changes in the measures we use, be they questionnaires or behavioural indices, rarely have the same meaning at the lower and upper levels. For example, if at the start of therapy, a compulsive patient spends 16 hours a day washing his hands, there is relatively little room to get worse (he *does* have to sleep, after all), but a lot of room for improvement. After some therapy, he may be down to washing "only" 4 hours daily. At this point, there is less room for improvement, but more scope to get worse. By the same token, while the *amount* of change is constant, the *rate* of change is not. A reduction of 4 hours, from 16 to 12 hours a day, represents a 25% improvement. Then, a further reduction of 4 hours daily is a 33% improvement, and the same decrease, from 8 to 4 hours daily, is a 50% change. Which description is correct: that there is a constant change of 4 hours daily each month or so, or that there is a steady decrease in the percentage of time spent hand washing? The answer is "both and neither." This somewhat less-than-helpful reply indicates that both indices yield useful information – there is a constant *amount* of change, and an increasing *rate* of change. The bottom line is that even this simple design can have problems with the interpretation of results.

A third issue is "how much change is significant?" Unfortunately, "significance" can have two meanings: "statistically unlikely to have arisen by chance" and "clinically meaningful." Simply subtracting the post-therapy score from the pre-therapy score on some test is not a sufficient measure. All tests have measurement error associated with them (Streiner & Norman, 2008); differences may arise because test scores differ from one occasion to the next, even without any clinical change having taken place. If a standardized test is used before and after treatment, then the best (Christensen & Mendoza, 1986) formula to determine if the change is statistically significant is

$$SC = \frac{X_{\text{Post}} - X_{\text{Pre}}}{\sqrt{2(SEM)^2}}, \qquad [1]$$

where SC = significant change, X_{Post} = post-therapy score, X_{Pre} = pre-therapy score, and SEM = standard error of the mean (Streiner & Norman, 2008). If SC exceeds 1.96, then the change was unlikely to have happened by chance.

But was the change clinically important? There are no formulae to answer this question. (Whether this is good or bad depends on your views about statistics and statisticians.) One recommendation (Jacobson, Follette, & Revenstorf, 1984) that appears sensible is to say that the patient has improved if three criteria are met: (1) the pre-therapy score is in the dysfunctional range, (2) the post-therapy score is within the range of scores of the normal population, and (3) the change is statistically significant.

Even when these three criteria are met, all we can be sure of is that change occurred *during the course* of therapy; we cannot be positive that it occurred *because* of therapy, much as we would like to believe that we were responsible (but only if the change is for the better). The reason is that therapy does not take place in a vacuum. The person is usually embedded within a rich social context including family, friends, the work setting, and leisure activities. Alterations in any of these may take place without our knowledge and affect the person's psychological state, positively or negatively. We want our mini-study to rule out, as much as possible, competing hypotheses about the cause of the change. The three designs we will discuss next – reversal studies, interrupted time series, and multiple baselines – do this better than the before-after design.

Reversal Studies

A more powerful design under some circumstances than the before-after method is called a *reversal study*, a *withdrawal study*, or an *A-B-A design* (Barlow, Nock, & Hersen, 2009), which was first used clinically to evaluate behaviour modification programs. The first A is a measure of the level of some behaviour (for example, socializing, trichotillomania, head banging) prior to the start of therapy. The B measures the level of the same behaviour once therapy is instituted, and the second A is the level of the behaviour when therapy has stopped. Of course, programs can be repeated and measured a number of times, resulting in A-B-A-B or A-B-A-B-A designs; or a different form of therapy can be introduced, resulting in an A-B-A-C-A design; and so on. The more times a reversal occurs involving a concomitant change in behaviour, the more confident we can be that the change is due to the presence or absence of the therapy, not to other causes, such as the natural history of the disorder.

The reversal study is powerful under some circumstances. There are two major restrictions in using this design. The first is that the behaviour is being influenced by the treatment and the intervention does not result

Fig. 20.2 Results from an A-B-A-B-A design

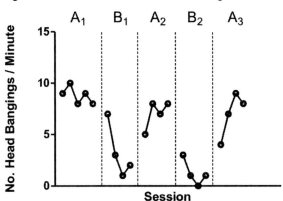

in long-term change. So, this design is very powerful when we are look-ing at the effects of short-acting drugs or operant conditioning programs (for example, token economies). It should not be used if the interven-tion is supposed to produce permanent change in behaviour (although it has been used to look at educational programs, which probably reflects a somewhat cynical view of the lasting effects of education or the train-ability of students). Since a permanent change is expected, if the patient reverts to baseline levels when therapy is stopped, then he or she would likely be entitled to a refund (with interest). The second limitation is ethi-cal: if therapy results in a decrease in a dangerous behaviour, such as head banging, then it may be unethical to withdraw it (Barlow et al., 2009).

Traditionally, the results of reversal designs are not analysed statisti-cally (heretical as that may sound). Rather, the behaviour is plotted on a graph, and a decision is made about whether the change from one condition to another is clinically important, as shown in Figure 20.2. The problem is that one person's clinical importance is another's barely noticeable change. It is probably safer (albeit more humbling) to rely on statistical tests designed for this type of study, in particular, what are called *randomization tests* (Edgington, 1996; May & Hunter, 1993).

Interrupted Time Series

Many interventions do not meet the major criteria for reversal trials, because either the treatment takes a while to begin or to stop working (as is the case with many psychotropic medications) or the results are

Fig. 20.3 An interrupted time series

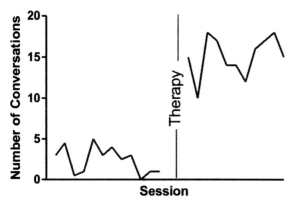

not (or at least should not be) reversible when the treatment is withheld. When this is the case, it is sometimes possible to use another design, an *interrupted time series* (Cook & Campbell, 1979). As an example, imagine that we want to evaluate the effectiveness of a program that is aimed at increasing a patient's comfort level in talking to people. We begin by asking the patient to record the number of people she talked to each day. Only after she has done this for a few weeks would we begin the treatment, and she would then record her behaviour for a few weeks after treatment had ended. What we hope to find is shown in Figure 20.3: a low socialization rate before therapy, followed by a break in the line (the effect of the therapy), and culminating in a consistently higher rate of social activities. The reason for delaying therapy for a while and asking the patient to record her behaviour for a few weeks after therapy has ended is to enable us to obtain good estimates of the pre- and post-therapy levels. Most of the phenomena we are interested in (for example, socialization, depressive symptoms, outbursts of anger, weight) fluctuate from one day to the next because of a host of factors outside our control. If we have only a few values before and after treatment (as we do with before-after designs), we are less sure that these are accurate reflections of the actual state of affairs. How many measurement points are needed? Ideally, we should have about 30 during each interval, that is, daily recordings for a month. This would allow us to analyse the data statistically using a technique called time-series analysis (Norman & Streiner, 2003). However, much as in reversal designs, many people use fewer data points and rely on "eyeball" tests of clinical change.

Multiple Baselines

In the previous two designs, we attempted to rule out competing hypotheses regarding the cause of change by testing a number of times if the therapy results in behavioural change (reversal studies) or measuring the behaviour over a long enough period to ensure that it was stable (interrupted time series). Multiple-baseline techniques use a third approach: assessing a number of different behaviours or traits at the same time, but intervening to modify only one at a time. For example, if the patient was experiencing difficulties with both shyness and driving, we would have the person monitor both behaviours, using a diary, questionnaire, or some other method. Therapy would initially target one area, and monitoring would continue for both. Once the first problem had been resolved, the therapy could focus on the second area.

The rationale behind the multiple-baseline technique is that, if factors other than therapy are influencing recovery, then they would likely affect a number of problem areas. If the change is due to the treatment, then its effects should be more focused on the particular difficulty, and the levels of the other behaviours should not change. The more areas measured simultaneously (up to the maximum number feasible, which is about four), the more confident we are that the change was a result of the therapy. What we have to ensure is that we do not choose behaviours that are related to one another. For example, if we were to measure how far a person is able to venture from home as one target behaviour and depressive symptoms as another, then it is possible that reducing the phobia might lift the depression to some degree. This may lead us to conclude erroneously that the change was due to other factors rather than to the therapy having had an effect in two areas.

Conclusion

It would be naïve of us to believe that we will be equally effective with all the patients we see. They differ with respect to the severity of their problems, the presence or absence of other conditions that affect the outcome, and other aspects of their lives. In turn, we work better with some patients than others, and the only people who are always consistent are those who are uniformly bad. Consequently, we should view each case as a small study of quality assurance, to ensure that we are having an effect (a positive one, ideally) on the patient. This chapter has outlined a few of the designs that are feasible for clinicians to use with individual cases. For those who want to read further, the classic texts in the area are those by Barlow et al. (2009) and Cook and Campbell (1979).

REFERENCES

Barlow, D.H., Nock, M.K., & Hersen, M. (2009). *Single case experimental designs: Strategies for studying behavior change*. (3rd ed.). New York: Pearson.

Christensen, L., & Mendoza, J.L. (1986). A method of assessing change in a single subject: An alteration of the RC index. *Behavior Therapy, 17*(3), 305–308. http://dx.doi.org/10.1016/S0005-7894(86)80060-0

Collins, L.M. & Horn, J.L. (Eds.). (1991). *Best methods for the analysis of change*. Washington, DC: American Psychological Association.

Cook, T.D., & Campbell, D.T. (1979). *Quasi-experimentation: Design and analysis issues for field settings*. Boston: Houghton-Mifflin.

Edgington, E.S. (1996, Jul). Randomized single-subject experimental designs. *Behaviour Research and Therapy, 34*(7), 567–574. http://dx.doi.org/10.1016/0005-7967(96)00012-5 Medline:8826764

Greenberg, R.P., Bornstein, R.F., Greenberg, M.D., & Fisher, S. (1992, Oct). A meta-analysis of antidepressant outcome under "blinder" conditions. *Journal of Consulting and Clinical Psychology, 60*(5), 664–669, discussion 670–677. http://dx.doi.org/10.1037/0022-006X.60.5.664 Medline:1401382

Hamilton, M. (1960, Feb). A rating scale for depression. *Journal of Neurology, Neurosurgery, and Psychiatry, 23*(1), 56–62. http://dx.doi.org/10.1136/jnnp.23.1.56 Medline:14399272

Jacobson, N.S., Follette, W.C., & Revenstorf, D. (1984). Psychotherapy outcome research: Methods for reporting variability and evaluating clinical significance. *Behavior Therapy, 15*(4), 336–352. http://dx.doi.org/10.1016/S0005-7894(84)80002-7

Luborsky, L., & DeRubeis, R. (1984). The use of psychotherapy treatment manuals: A small revolution in psychotherapy research style. *Clinical Psychology Review, 4*(1), 5–14. http://dx.doi.org/10.1016/0272-7358(84)90034-5

May, R.B., & Hunter, M.A. (1993). Some advantages of permutation tests. *Canadian Psychology, 34*(4), 401–407. http://dx.doi.org/10.1037/h0078862

Norman, G.R., & Streiner, D.L. (2003). *PDQ statistics*. (3rd ed.). Shelton, CT: PMPH USA.

Paulhus, D.L. (1984). Two-component models of socially desirable responding. *Journal of Personality and Social Psychology, 46*(3), 598–609. http://dx.doi.org/10.1037/0022-3514.46.3.598

Rosenthal, R. (1966). *Experimenter effects in behavioral research*. New York: Appleton-Century-Crofts.

Streiner, D.L. (1993, Mar). A checklist for evaluating the usefulness of rating scales. *Canadian Journal of Psychiatry, 38*(2), 140–148. Medline:8467441

Streiner, D.L. (2002). The two "Es" of research: Efficacy and effectiveness trials. *Canadian Journal of Psychiatry, 47*, 552–556.

Streiner, D.L., & Norman, G.R. (2008). *Health measurement scales: A practical guide to their development and use.* (4th ed.). Oxford: Oxford University Press.

Weisz, J.R., Donenberg, G.R., Han, S.S., & Weiss, B. (1995, Oct). Bridging the gap between laboratory and clinic in child and adolescent psychotherapy. *Journal of Consulting and Clinical Psychology, 63*(5), 688–701. http://dx.doi.org/10.1037/0022-006X.63.5.688 Medline:7593861

TO READ FURTHER

Barlow, D.H., Nock, M.K., & Hersen, M. (2009). *Single case experimental designs: Strategies for studying behavior change.* (3rd ed.). New York: Pearson.

Cook, T.D., & Campbell, D.T. (1979). *Quasi-experimentation: Design and analysis issues for field settings.* Boston: Houghton-Mifflin.

Edgington, E.S. (1996, Jul). Randomized single-subject experimental designs. *Behaviour Research and Therapy, 34*(7), 567–574. http://dx.doi.org/10.1016/0005-7967(96)00012-5 Medline:8826764

21 The Two "E's" of Research: Efficacy and Effectiveness Trials

DAVID L. STREINER, PH.D.

Canadian Journal of Psychiatry, 2002, 47, 552–556

It is fairly well accepted now that the best evidence for demonstrating that an intervention works comes from the results of a randomized controlled trial (RCT), in which eligible patients are randomly assigned to either a new therapy or to a comparison group. However, there are RCTs, and then there are RCTs. In other words, not all RCTs are the same. In this chapter, we will discuss the differences between RCTs designed to demonstrate the *effectiveness* of treatment and those that look at the *efficacy* of an intervention. Thus, it's first necessary to discuss the difference between efficacy and effectiveness.

Efficacy is concerned with the question, *Can* a treatment work under ideal circumstances? Conversely, effectiveness addresses the question, *Does* it work in the real world? Studies that focus on efficacy do everything possible to maximize the chances of showing an effect. The rationale is that if the treatment cannot be shown to work under the best conditions, there isn't a ghost of a chance that it will be effective in actual practice. On the other hand, effectiveness studies emphasize the applicability of the treatment and therefore try harder to duplicate the situations that clinicians will encounter in their practices. The two study types are referred to in terms that describe their differing aims and designs. They are sometimes distinguished as explanatory and pragmatic trials (Hotopf, Churchill, & Lewis, 1999; Schwartz & Lellouch, 1967); at other times they are called explanatory and management trials (Sackett & Gent, 1979). "Pragmatic" and "management" capture the flavour of the question "do things work in the real world?" However, "explanatory" is a bit misleading, because the emphasis in the study is more on "can" than on "why." So, I'll continue to use the terms "efficacy" and "effectiveness" in this chapter.

No matter what they're called, though, the difference between the two types has implications for who is selected to be in the study, how the intervention is delivered, how dropouts and people who receive the "wrong" treatment are handled, and how the results are analysed. In actuality, efficacy and effectiveness studies are the extremes of a continuum, and most studies fall somewhere in between. However, it is important for the reader of trials to be aware of these implications, because they affect (or should affect) how the results are interpreted: do you change your clinical practice today in light of the findings, or do you wait until more convincing evidence is in?

To illustrate the difference, I will focus on the treatment of a disorder that Geoff Norman and I discovered several years ago: photonumerophobia, or the fear that one's fear of numbers will come to light (Norman & Streiner, 2008; Streiner, 1998b; see Chapter 7). Unfortunately, this malady has not yet been recognized by DSM or ICD. Nevertheless, after teaching statistics to medical students, nurses, and grad students for more than four decades, we believe it is obvious that this is a widely prevalent and disabling condition, but one that is now amenable to treatment. The therapy we propose is teaching statistics using the essays in this "Research Methods in Psychiatry" (RMP) series. To test whether it works, we'll have a comparison group of people treated with another set of readings (the Other condition). The outcome will be the number of people who are not phobic at the end of the semester.

Subject Selection

Most parametric statistical tests, such as the t-test and the analysis of variance (ANOVA), compare how large the difference between the groups is in relation to the variability within groups. That is, they assume that differences among people within the same group is "error" (a better term would perhaps be "unexplained variability") and that the between-group variability must be larger than the within-group variance to show that something is going on. Therefore, when designing a study, we maximize the chances that we'll find a statistically significant result if we (1) make the difference between the groups as large as possible and (2) make the variability within the groups as small as possible. We have relatively little control over the first factor because it's a function primarily of how well the intervention works (although we'll soon see how we can exert that small degree of control). However, we can affect the within-group variability by making the groups as homogeneous as possible in terms of age, sex (to the degree allowed by the granting agencies), other treatments received within a certain time frame, and, most important, by ensuring the strictness of the diagnostic criteria and the absence of co-morbid disorders. This is why the "subjects" section of efficacy studies begins with a long list of inclusion and exclusion criteria: the criteria exist not only to ensure that the people in the trial actually have the disorder of interest but also to make the groups homogeneous and thus reduce the within-group variability.

Some efficacy studies go even further than making the groups homogeneous: they try to exclude those who may be "placebo responders" and to enrol only those patients who will be most compliant and most responsive to the intervention. For example, some studies use a single-blind run-in phase (e.g., Quitkin et al., 1998), during which all eligible patients are placed on a placebo. Those who show an improvement are eliminated from the study because they would inflate the change seen in the comparison group and thus reduce the between-group difference. Another tactic is to use an enriched sample of patients who have previously been shown to respond to the intervention (Calabrese, Rapport, Shelton, & Kimmel, 2001). A third approach, used in the Veterans Administration hypertension study, had patients take a riboflavin-labelled placebo (Veterans Administration, 1970). This allowed the investigators to determine which subjects would comply with taking medications and to reject the others.

The drawback of this approach is that the participants in the study become less and less like the patients encountered in actual practice. The practising clinician does not have the researcher's luxury of saying, "I can't treat your schizophrenia, because DSM-IV says you must have had your symptoms for six months, and yours have persisted for only five months," or "You also suffer from an anxiety disorder, so out you go." It is also difficult to test whether the patient will be compliant; in any case, the therapist must try to treat the patient even if there are concerns in this regard.

So, if we were designing an efficacy trial of RMP versus Other, we would apply very tight criteria for photonumerophobia and exclude all people who do not meet all of them. We would also reject from the study people who might have other psychological or medical disorders that could lessen the magnitude of the treatment effect or who were receiving some other form of therapy for their problem that would make it difficult to determine what the "active ingredient" was. Conversely, an effectiveness trial would include all people who present with this complaint: all would be accepted for therapy, irrespective of age, comorbidities, or other concurrent therapies. The sample size might have to be increased to compensate for these confounding conditions, but the results would be more generalizable to clinical practice.

The Intervention

I mentioned earlier that the main determinant of the difference between the groups is the effectiveness of the intervention itself and that we have little control over this. In fact, while we cannot enhance the true effect of the treatment, there are many ways to make it perform less well. Needless to say, efficacy studies try very hard to avoid these pitfalls, using various techniques. From the provider's perspective, these techniques include having therapists attend training sessions so that they can learn to perform the therapy systematically (Elkin, Parloff, Hadley, & Autry, 1985), using treatment manuals that detail what should and should not be done during the sessions (Luborsky & DeRubeis, 1984), tape-recording the sessions so that they can later be checked for adherence to the treatment protocol (Sensky et al., 2000), having fixed dosing regimens or algorithms in drug trials (Philipp, Kohnen, Hiller, Linde, and Berner, 1999), or having a fixed number of therapy sessions (Scott et al., 2000). Some surgical trials even go so far as to drop surgeons or centres that have high perioperative mortality or infection rates (Gasecki, Eliasziw, Ferguson, Hachinski, & Barnett, 1995). On the receiving side of the intervention, efficacy studies often have research nurses or assistants call the patients to remind them to take their medication, to reschedule missed appointments, and, sometimes, just to check on the patients between visits.

The advantages of these strategies are obvious. The therapy is delivered either by highly skilled and well-trained people or by advanced students who receive continual supervision and feedback from more senior clinicians. The intervention itself often follows the recommendations of best-practice guidelines, which are (or at least should be) based on the results of earlier clinical trials. When medications are used, a frequent requirement is ongoing monitoring of blood levels to ensure that the medications are within therapeutic levels. Follow-up and reminder calls maximize adherence to the therapy, and these contacts themselves may have some therapeutic effect.

Wouldn't life (or at least work) be wonderful if we all had these resources! The sad reality is that the extra staff and lab work are rarely available or affordable outside large, externally funded RCTs. Further, despite what we read in letters of recommendation, not everybody is in the top 5% of the profession: believe it or not, one-half of the therapists in this world are below average (Streiner, 2000; see Chapter 1). Even excellent therapists, though, rarely have the luxury of attending week- or month-long training courses after they finish residency or a fellowship. More often, they learn of new techniques through lectures, readings, or, at best, a one-day pre-conference workshop that does not have any provision for continuing supervision. The consequence is that therapy in real life is rarely delivered as effectively or uniformly as it is in controlled efficacy trials. Donoghue and Hylan (2001), for example, summarize the results of many surveys showing that in primary- and secondary-care settings, tricyclic antidepressants are frequently prescribed in dosages lower – often 50% lower – than those found to be efficacious in RCTs.

Effectiveness trials are closer to the end of the continuum that reflects therapy as it is actually given. For example, they impose fewer restrictions on how the treatment is delivered and monitor patient compliance less. Even so, it is rare to see a random selection of clinicians in effectiveness studies: they tend to be drawn from people in academia, often in tertiary-care teaching hospitals. It is also becoming increasingly more common for studies of both efficacy and effectiveness to use manualized therapy or drug algorithms (McMain et al., 2009), which is likely more usual in studies than in routine clinical practice. This means that, although there is probably still a difference between the way therapy is delivered in effectiveness trials and in real life, these studies tend to be more realistic than are efficacy studies.

Who Gets Counted

Let's assume we have gone through all the steps of finding 100 patients with phobia, allocating them to the two groups at random, and carrying out the intervention. At the end of the study, when we start looking at the data, we find that ten subjects in the Other group have actually stumbled across the RMP series on their own and have read all the articles. In the RMP group, two subjects committed suicide before the classes began, seven dropped out before writing the final exam, and three withdrew before the study began, claiming that their phobia was cured. Do we count these people? If so, to which group do we assign the results? That is, are the results of the subjects in the Other group who read the RMP articles attributed to RMP or to Other? The answer is, as one would expect from a statistician-psychologist, "It all depends."

The first thing it depends on is how many people we've lost. Ideally, we've taken measures to keep this number as small as possible, in which case it really won't matter much how we count their results, because it won't appreciably change the outcome. However, if despite our best efforts we've lost more than roughly 10% to 15% of the subjects, then we have to consider whether we are conducting an efficacy trial or an effectiveness one. If we are asking the question, "Can the intervention work?" (that is, if we are testing its efficacy), then we are in a bit of a bind. We can argue, on the one hand, that it doesn't make sense to blame the RMP intervention for the deaths of the two subjects if they were never exposed to RMP. Nor does it make sense to credit RMP with curing the three who got better before starting the trial. The ten in the Other group who actually read the RMP articles are a bit more troublesome, in that they were likely exposed to both conditions; however, we can again argue that the best course of action would be to drop them from the analyses, along with the seven subjects who withdrew. On the other hand (and there's always an other hand), the more subjects we drop from the analyses, the greater the possibility that we're biasing the results by deviating from random assignment. There's no easy solution to this conundrum. For therapies in which it is difficult to disentangle the beneficial effects from the side effects (for example, drug therapies), "can the intervention work?" and "does the intervention work?" may boil down to the same thing – so we should count people who dropped out. With other types of interventions, such as the talking therapies, it may be possible to alter those aspects that lead to dropping out without affecting the therapy itself (for example, by extending clinic hours or even bringing the therapy to the patient). In these situations, there may be a big difference between can and does, so it makes more sense not to count people who have dropped out.

The picture is entirely different for an effectiveness trial, in that the bind disappears – we have to count everybody. In real life, if patients become desperate and commit suicide before the treatment has had a chance to work, then that is the fault of the treatment and how it is delivered. One cannot ignore the fact that receiving therapy often involves being on a waiting list for a period of time or that the drug may not start to work for two or three weeks. Similarly, patients may discontinue a treatment because of adverse side effects, which can be anything from blurry vision caused by reading 28 essays, to the inconvenience of coming to class for an entire semester, to time lost from work. Finally, patients assigned to one treatment mode may deliberately or accidentally receive the other intervention. These are the realities of life and some of the reasons why the results of effectiveness trials are always equal to or worse, but never better, than those of efficacy studies. This last observation has been documented by Weisz, Donenberg, Han, and Weiss in a meta-analysis of child psychotherapy trials (1995). In well-controlled studies that were closer to the efficacy end of the continuum, the children in the experimental conditions scored 0.75 SD (standard deviation) above those in the control conditions. Translated into English, this means that 77% of the children who received the interventions did better than the average child who was a control subject. However, in studies that were carried out in regular clinic settings (that is, closer to the effectiveness end of the continuum), this difference virtually disappeared.

Analysis

The differences in the study objectives also affect the approach to the statistical analyses. Effectiveness trials must count all the patients in the group to which they were originally assigned. This is referred to as an "intention-to-treat" (ITT) analysis. As we have discussed, dropouts can jeopardize the results of effectiveness studies because we cannot assume that those who discontinued are a random subset of all the subjects (Streiner, 2002; see Chapter 8). Rather, they are more probably those who benefited the most or the least. Various statistical techniques have been developed – such as the Last Observation Carried Forward (LOCF), multiple imputation, or growth curve analysis – that allow subjects who miss appointments or who drop out entirely to be included in the analyses (Streiner, 2002).

These procedures are not required to the same degree in efficacy studies, because we are interested only in those patients who received the full course of treatment. As a consequence, we are not interested in those who discontinued early, for whatever reason, or those who were contaminated by receiving some or all of the wrong treatment. Here, imputation is used to fill in the blanks when some demographic data are missing, or if the patient skipped some appointments in the middle of the test. We would not impute data if a subject dropped out entirely.

Conclusions

Cook and Campbell (1979) differentiate between the internal validity of a study and its external validity. The former refers to the design aspects of the investigation – how well it was carried out, the degree to which various biases were avoided, and whether it had minimal dropouts. *Internal validity* affects the degree to which we can conclude that the outcome resulted from the intervention or from other factors, such as the groups' differing on key variables or differential dropouts from the various conditions. Of equal, if not greater, concern for clinicians is the study's *external validity*, which affects our ability to generalize the results of the trial to the conditions that obtain in real life. Very often, there is a trade-off between these two types of validity: tightening up admission criteria increases internal validity at the expense of external validity, as does increasing the control over what happens during the session. "To minimize potential sources of error, we have to sacrifice verisimilitude. Conversely, the more we try to mirror the reality of the therapeutic encounter, the greater the chances are that factors outside of our control (and perhaps of our knowledge) may be responsible for the results" (Streiner, 1998a, p. 117).

So, which should come first, effectiveness studies or efficacy studies? The answer is very definite: for the clinician, the most useful information comes from effectiveness studies. From this perspective, it would be wise to start with an effectiveness trial because it, and it alone, tells whether the intervention will work in real life. However, there's a risk associated with this approach. It is quite possible that the intervention can work, but there may have been problems in the treatment delivery – in patient selection criteria, in therapist training, in non-adherence due to side effects or the requirements of the study itself, or in other factors that led to finding no difference between the groups. This Type II error – concluding that there is no significant effect when, in fact, there is one – may prematurely cut off further research in the area. Had there been significant findings from a previous efficacy study, though, researchers would be more inclined to start investigating the reasons for the effectiveness study's failure, focusing on the way the therapy was delivered, rather than dismissing the treatment as ineffective.

No single study can answer all questions, and investigators must decide where they want to be on the efficacy-effectiveness spectrum. Consequently, to know more about the usefulness of an intervention, we require a series of studies, spanning the continuum from one end to the other.

REFERENCES

Calabrese, J.R., Rapport, D.J., Shelton, M.D., & Kimmel, S.E. (2001, Jun).
Evolving methodologies in bipolar disorder maintenance research. *British Journal of Psychiatry, 178*(Suppl 41), S157–S163. http://dx.doi.org/10.1192/bjp.178.41.s157 Medline:11388956

Cook, T.D., & Campbell, D.T. (1979). *Quasi-experimentation: Design and analysis issues for field settings.* Boston, MA: Houghton Mifflin.

Donoghue, J., & Hylan, T.R. (2001, Sep). Antidepressant use in clinical practice: Efficacy v. effectiveness. *British Journal of Psychiatry, 179*(Suppl 42), S9–S17. http://dx.doi.org/10.1192/bjp.179.42.s9 Medline:11532821

Elkin, I., Parloff, M.B., Hadley, S.W., & Autry, J.H. (1985, Mar). NIMH treatment of depression collaborative research program: Background and research plan. *Archives of General Psychiatry, 42*(3), 305–316. http://dx.doi.org/10.1001/archpsyc.1985.01790260103013 Medline:2983631

Gasecki, A.P., Eliasziw, M., Ferguson, G.G., Hachinski, V., Barnett, H.J., & North American Symptomatic Carotid Endarterectomy Trial (NASCET) Group. (1995, Nov). Long-term prognosis and effect of endarterectomy in patients with symptomatic severe carotid stenosis and contralateral carotid stenosis or occlusion: Results from NASCET. *Journal of Neurosurgery, 83*(5), 778–782. http://dx.doi.org/10.3171/jns.1995.83.5.0778 Medline:7472542

Hotopf, M., Churchill, R., & Lewis, G. (1999, Sep). Pragmatic randomised controlled trials in psychiatry. *British Journal of Psychiatry, 175*(3), 217–223. http://dx.doi.org/10.1192/bjp.175.3.217 Medline:10645321

Luborsky, L., & DeRubeis, R.J. (1984). The use of psychotherapy treatment manuals: A small revolution in psychotherapy research style. *Clinical Psychology Review, 4*(1), 5–14. http://dx.doi.org/10.1016/0272-7358(84)90034-5

McMain, S.F., Links, P.S., Gnam, W.H., Guimond, T., Cardish, R.J., Korman, L., & Streiner, D.L. (2009, Dec). A randomized trial of dialectical behavior therapy versus general psychiatric management for borderline personality disorder. *American Journal of Psychiatry, 166*(12), 1365–1374. http://dx.doi.org/10.1176/appi.ajp.2009.09010039 Medline:19755574

Norman, G.R., & Streiner, D.L. (2008). *Biostatistics: The bare essentials.* (3rd ed.). Shelton, CT: PMPH USA.

Philipp, M., Kohnen, R., Hiller, K.O., Linde, K., & Berner, M. (1999, Dec 11). Hypericum extract versus imipramine or placebo in patients with moderate depression: Randomised multicentre study of treatment for eight weeks. *BMJ (Clinical Research Ed.), 319*(7224), 1534–1538. http://dx.doi.org/10.1136/bmj.319.7224.1534 Medline:10591711

Quitkin, F.M., McGrath, P.J., Stewart, J.W., Ocepek-Welikson, K., Taylor, B.P., Nunes, E., ..., & Klein, D.F. (1998, Sep). Placebo run-in period in studies of depressive disorders. Clinical, heuristic and research implications. *British Journal of Psychiatry, 173*(3), 242–248. http://dx.doi.org/10.1192/bjp.173.3.242 Medline:9926101

Sackett, D.L., & Gent, M. (1979, Dec 27). Controversy in counting and attributing events in clinical trials. *New England Journal of Medicine, 301*(26), 1410–1412. http://dx.doi.org/10.1056/NEJM197912273012602 Medline:514321

Schwartz, D., & Lellouch, J. (1967, Aug). Explanatory and pragmatic attitudes in therapeutical trials. *Journal of Chronic Diseases, 20*(8), 637–648. http://dx.doi.org/10.1016/0021-9681(67)90041-0 Medline:4860352

Scott, J., Teasdale, J.D., Paykel, E.S., Johnson, A.L., Abbott, R., Hayhurst, H., ..., & Garland, A. (2000, Nov). Effects of cognitive therapy on psychological symptoms and social functioning in residual depression. *British Journal of Psychiatry, 177*(5), 440–446. http://dx.doi.org/10.1192/bjp.177.5.440 Medline:11059998

Sensky, T., Turkington, D., Kingdon, D., Scott, J.L., Scott, J., Siddle, R., ..., & Barnes, T.R. (2000, Feb). A randomized controlled trial of cognitive-behavioral therapy for persistent symptoms in schizophrenia resistant to medication. *Archives of General Psychiatry, 57*(2), 165–172. http://dx.doi.org/10.1001/archpsyc.57.2.165 Medline:10665619

Streiner, D.L. (1998a). Evaluating what we do. In S. Cullari S (Ed.), *Foundations of clinical psychology* (pp. 112–137). Boston, MA: Allyn and Bacon.

Streiner, D.L. (1998b, May). Risky business: Making sense of estimates of risk. *Canadian Journal of Psychiatry, 43*(4), 411–415. Medline:9598280

Streiner, D.L. (2000, Nov). Do you see what I mean? Indices of central tendency. *Canadian Journal of Psychiatry, 45*(9), 833–836. Medline:11143834

Streiner, D.L. (2002). The case of the missing data: Methods of dealing with drop-outs and other vagaries of research. *Canadian Journal of Psychiatry, 47,* 68–75.

Veterans Administration Cooperative Study Group on Antihypertensive Agents. (1970, Aug 17). Effects of treatment on morbidity in hypertension. II. Results in patients with diastolic blood pressure averaging 90 through 114 mm Hg. *Journal of the American Medical Association, 213*(7), 1143–1152. http://dx.doi.org/10.1001/jama.1970.03170330025003 Medline:4914579

Weisz, J.R., Donenberg, G.R., Han, S.S., & Weiss, B. (1995, Oct). Bridging the gap between laboratory and clinic in child and adolescent psychotherapy. *Journal of Consulting and Clinical Psychology, 63*(5), 688–701. http://dx.doi.org/10.1037/0022-006X.63.5.688 Medline:7593861

TO READ FURTHER

Donoghue, J., & Hylan, T.R. (2001, Sep). Antidepressant use in clinical practice: Efficacy v. effectiveness. *British Journal of Psychiatry, 179*(Suppl 42), S9–S17. http://dx.doi.org/10.1192/bjp.179.42.s9 Medline:11532821

Fritz, J.M., & Cleland, J.A. (2003, Apr). Effectiveness versus efficacy: More than a debate over language. *Journal of Orthopaedic and Sports Physical Therapy, 33*(4), 163–165. Medline:12723672

PART FOUR

Measurement

22 A Checklist for Evaluating the Usefulness of Rating Scales

DAVID L. STREINER, PH.D.

Canadian Journal of Psychiatry, 1993, *38*, 140–148

Rating scales are ubiquitous in psychiatry. They are used to measure symptoms which are found in most disorders, such as depressed mood (Beck, Steer & Brown, 1996; Hamilton, 1980), anxiety (Spielberger, Gorsuch, Lushene, Vagg, & Jacobs, 1983), or positive and negative symptoms of schizophrenia (Kay, Fiszbein, & Opler, 1987), to determine the presence of some trait, such as self-esteem (Herzberger, Chan, & Katz, 1984); or for a variety of other purposes. In many studies, a scale is used as the only criterion to rate the effectiveness of an intervention (e.g., Lambourn & Gill, 1978; Olmsted et al., 1991). Consequently, we must have some confidence that the scale measures what it purports to and that it does so with a minimum of error. In this chapter, we will examine some of the characteristics of scales and give some criteria which can be used to evaluate their utility. The intended audience are people who want to be better able to evaluate articles which have used rating scales and those who intend to use existing scales in their research. This paper is not meant to be a primer in how to construct scales; those who are interested in doing so would be better served by reading one of the more complete texts (e.g., Anastasi & Urbina, 1997; Nunnally & Bernstein, 1994; Streiner & Norman, 2008).

It may be useful to begin by differentiating the term "scale" from other, similar terms such as index, inventory, test, or schedule. Some authors have tried to distinguish a *scale* from an *index* on the basis of the tool's measurement properties; one yields a score which is on an ordinal scale (the intervals between the numbers cannot be assumed to reflect equal increments in the trait being measured), and the other produces a score on an interval scale (that is, the intervals represent equal increases in the trait). Unfortunately, people can't agree on which term is which. Others say a scale is made up of questions which are correlated, whereas an index is closer to a checklist of separate items (Streiner, 2003a). By this definition, the Apgar scale (Apgar, 1953) is really an index, and the International Index of Erectile Function (Rosen et al., 1997) is actually a scale. So much for that differentiation.

Yet a third term, *inventory*, can also be used as a synonym, although most people use it to refer to an instrument which consists of a number of different independent scales, such as the Minnesota Multiphasic Personality Inventory-2 (MMPI-2; Butcher, Dahlstrom, Graham, Tellegen, & Kaemmer, 1989) or the Millon Clinical Multiaxial Inventory-III (Millon, Millon, & Davis, 1994). A *test* used to refer to an instrument which a person could pass or fail, such as the final exams ("achievement tests" in more formal parlance) we struggled through in school, or the admission tests we took to get into graduate or professional school. However, there are exceptions to this usage: the Test of Attentional and Interpersonal Style (Nideffer, 1976), for instance, would more accurately be called an inventory.

What all of these instruments have in common, despite their differences in terminology, is that they are attempting to measure the amount of some attribute, be it anxiety, depression, or knowledge of cardiac functioning. A schedule, such as the Diagnostic Interview Schedule (DIS; Robins, Helzer, Croughan, & Ratcliff, 1981) or the Schedule for Affective Disorders and Schizophrenia (SADS; Spitzer & Endicott, 1982), is more like a checklist, which counts the number of signs or symptoms present. This is then used to arrive at a diagnosis, based on a certain number of items being endorsed or the pattern of endorsement of specific items. Rarely do schedules yield a number which can be manipulated statistically.

In this chapter, we will focus on scales, since the methods used to develop and validate them differ from those used in the development of schedules. The chapter itself will centre around a checklist, which can be used when assessing a scale's potential utility (see Table 22.1).

The Items

Where They Come From

Scales, unlike the goddess Athena, rarely spring full-grown from their creators' heads. Rather, there is usually a process of gathering potentially useful items from various sources and then winnowing out those which do not meet certain criteria. Items may come from existing scales,

Table 22.1 A checklist for evaluating scales

Items
Where did they come from?
- Previous scales
- Clinical observation
- Expert opinion
- Patients' reports
- Research findings
- Theory

Were they assessed for
- Endorsement frequency?
- Restrictions in range?
- Comprehension?
- Lack of ambiguity?
- Lack of value-laden or offensive content?

Reliability
- Was the scale checked for internal consistency?
- Does it have good test-retest reliability?
- Does it have good inter-rater agreement (if appropriate)?
- On what groups were the reliabilities estimated?
- How was reliability calculated?

Validity
- Does the scale have face validity? Should it?
- Is there evidence of content validity?
- Has it been evaluated for criterion validity (if possible)?
- What studies have been done to assess construct validity?
- With what groups has the scale been validated?

Utility
- Can the scale be completed in a reasonable amount of time?
- How much training is needed to learn how to administer it?
- Is it easy to score?

---

clinical observation, expert opinion, patients' reports of their subjective experiences, research findings, and theory. There are advantages and disadvantages associated with each of these sources. The user should be aware of where the scale's items came from and the possible biases which may therefore have been introduced.

Existing Scales

It is sometimes said that borrowing from one source is plagiarism, but taking from two or more is research; the same principle holds true in scale development. Older scales may be deemed inadequate because they do not adequately cover all aspects of an area. However, their items are frequently quite useful and may have gone through their own process of weeding out bad ones. Moreover, if one were trying to tap depressive mood, for example, it would be difficult to ask about appetite loss in a way that hasn't been used before. Consequently, items from earlier scales often appear on more recent ones. However, there is the danger that their terminology may have become outdated in the interim. Until it was modified in 1987, the MMPI contained such quaint terms as "deportment," "cutting up," and "drop the handkerchief." Endorsement of these items revealed more about a person's age than his or her behaviour.

Clinical Observation

The impetus for developing a new scale, either in an area where previous scales exist or in virginal territories, is clinical observation – seeing phenomena which aren't tapped by existing tools. The major problem with this is that the person developing the scale may have "seen" phenomena which aren't apparent to other people. Unfortunately, psychiatry's history is replete with such spurious observations (McDonald, 1958). If a scale is based on these unreplicated findings, a later user of the instrument may expend considerable effort executing a study, only to find out in the end that the dependent measure is of little clinical use.

Expert Opinion

A step up from the clinical wisdom of one person is the collective wisdom of a panel of experts. The obvious advantage is that a range of opinions can be expressed, so that the scale is less the result of one idiosyncratic way of thinking or limited by one person's clinical experience. However, there is always the danger that the "panel of experts" was chosen because all of its members are known to the senior author of the scale, and all share his or her viewpoint and biases regarding the domain to be measured. In this case, there is probably more of an illusion of a breadth of opinions, rather than the reality of it. Consequently, just because the items were contributed by a panel, do not automatically assume that they reflect a broader spectrum of ideas.

Patients' Reports

Clinicians may see the behavioural manifestations of a disorder, but only the patient is able to report on the subjective elements. Quite often, it is these aspects which differentiate one disorder from another, or which provide the best clues about severity. Some scales though, such as the Hamilton Rating Scale for Depression (Hamilton, 1980), are based on a phenomenological approach to psychiatry, so there is a decreased emphasis on the patient's subjective state. If the patient's experience is important to you, for example, you may wish to look for a different scale of dysphoria. However, this could be determined only if the scale's author reported this orientation in the original paper.

Research Findings

Empirical research provides another fruitful source of potential items (for example, many of the items on scales which differentiate "process" from "reactive" schizophrenics were based on empirical findings), such as the increased probability of the involvement of alcohol among reactive schizophrenics (Ullmann & Giovannoni, 1964). However, just because one paper reported a finding is no guarantee that it will be replicated (McDonald, 1958).

Theory

Most scales used in psychiatry reflect some theoretical approach, although this may not be stated explicitly in the paper describing the scale's development, or even acknowledged by the scale's author. However, the wide disparity in content among various scales of social support is a manifestation of the authors' theories of that concept: for example, whether social support does or does not involve elements of reciprocity, or if the key ingredients are the number of people in the network, or the frequency of contacts, or both (Thoits, 1982; Wallston, Alagna, DeVillis, & DeVillis, 1983). Unless the scale's developer was explicit about the belief system underlying the instrument's development, it may be necessary for the user to compare the items on the scale with the beliefs about what the scale should cover, using the "content validity matrix" described below under "Validity."

Assessment of the Items

Developing a pool of items is a necessary first step in scale construction. However, it is extremely unlikely that each of the items will perform as intended. Some will not be understood or will be misinterpreted by respondents, and others may not discriminate between people who have the trait and those who do not. Consequently, it is necessary to cut out bad items if they do not meet certain criteria, some of which include the following.

Endorsement Frequency. If one item on a depression scale read, "I have cried at least once in my life," it is obvious that the vast majority of people would answer "yes." If we don't even bother to ask the question, but simply assume the answer to be yes, no information would be lost. In fact, we would probably have less measurement error by not asking the question, since the response would not be contaminated by random responding, lying, illiteracy, or anything else which might affect the true answer. The moral of the story is that if some items are answered in one direction or another more than 90% or 95% of the time, they may be even worse than useless.

Restriction in Range. A similar problem may exist with questions which allow a range of answers, such as a 7-point scale to rate student performance which goes from "much below average" to "much above average." Often, people avoid the extreme categories (the "end aversion bias"), thus turning it into a 5-point scale. Moreover, no supervisor has ever seen a student who was below average, which thereby forces the responses into the two remaining boxes – those above the mid-point, but not including the end. It is obvious that this item's ability to discriminate among students is limited.

A test developer should have checked for items which suffer from a high (or low) endorsement frequency or which show only a restricted range of answers. These questions contribute nothing to a scale except noise and should have been weeded out.

Comprehension. Unfortunately, health care professionals spend many years unlearning the mother tongue and replacing it with a language called jargon or medicalese. People talk about "mood"; professionals speak of "affect." Respondents to a scale either may not know these technical terms or may misinterpret them. Many lay people think the continuum of anxiety is calm, tense, and hypertensive. Hypertension is an emotional state, rather than a fancy term for high blood pressure. Furthermore, the reading ability of many people with a high school diploma is closer to a grade 6 than a grade 12 level. So, the fact that you or your colleague can understand the items is no guarantee that the average respondent can. What this means is that the scale should have been pretested on the target group to determine if the terms are comprehensible. If there is no assurance that this was done, the potential test user should take this step.

Lack of Ambiguity. A "no" response to the statement "I like my mother," does not necessarily mean that he or she hates mom. Rather, it may simply reflect the fact that the subject's mother is dead, and the person did not feel free to interpret the statement in the past tense. Similarly, if a questionnaire to assess knowledge of side effects asks whether or not they were explained by the physician, the person may have difficulty answering if the nurse did all the explaining; yes, the side effects were described, but no, not by the doctor.

Items like these are ambiguous, in that it is not always clear to the subject how she or he should answer; nor is the investigator always clear about what the answer denotes. Like problems in comprehension, items should have been pretested on people similar to the intended users to eliminate such ambiguities, or this must be done by the scale's user.

Value Laden or Offensive Content. How would you expect a patient to respond to the item, "I often bother my doctor with trivial complaints"? Nobody wants to admit bothering his or her physician, especially if the complaints are trivial. These terms, as well as a host of others, lead the respondent to answer the tenor of the question as much as the content. Words which signal to the respondent which answers are desirable and which are not introduce a definite bias into the questionnaire and should not appear in items.

The original version of the MMPI (Hathaway & McKinley, 1951) contained a number of items tapping religious beliefs. Although this could be justified on psychometric grounds, in that many patients exhibit an increase in religiosity just prior to a psychotic break, the items were sometimes seen as an unwarranted intrusion into personal affairs and made an easy target for those opposed to the use of personality testing. The revised version (Butcher et al., 1989) dropped these offending items, which increased the acceptance of the test.

The potential user of questionnaires should scan the scales (or preferably have a lay person do so) to determine if any items appear leading, value laden, or offensive.

Reliability

Reliability means that "measurements of individuals on different occasions, or by different observers, or by similar or parallel tests, produce the same or similar results" (Streiner & Norman, 2008). If the person has not changed, then two different measurements should yield similar scores on the scale. If this has not been demonstrated, then the potential user of the test should stop right there and relegate it to the wastepaper basket. An article which introduces a new scale and does not report its reliability is hiding something and should be read with a healthy dose of scepticism.

One point that cannot be emphasized strongly enough is that reliability (and, as we'll see, validity) is not a fixed property of a test. It depends on three factors: the scale itself, the group to which it was administered, and the circumstances under which it was given. A scale that shows good reliability under one set of conditions may not be reliable with different people (for example, those from other cultures or with different diagnoses) or given in a different context (a research versus a clinical setting). You cannot assume that the scale's reported reliability will be the same when these factors have changed.

There are a number of different indices of reliability, each of which reflects a different attribute of the test. Not all are necessary for any one scale; an instrument that is self-administered, for example, does not have to demonstrate inter-rater reliability. In this section, we will go through some of the more common forms of reliability and how they should be measured.

Internal Consistency

If a scale is measuring a single attribute, such as self-esteem or anxiety, then all of the items should be tapping it to varying degrees. So, if a person states on one item that he or she is tense, the person should also endorse other items which ask about nervousness, being on edge, and so on. To the extent that items on the scale are not answered in a consistent manner, the instrument is either measuring a number of different things or the subjects are responding in an inconsistent manner, perhaps because the items are badly worded.

Since the early 1950s, the most widely used measure of a scale's internal consistency is Cronbach's α (alpha), also referred to as coefficient α (Cronbach, 1951). Alpha, like all coefficients of reliability, can range between 0.00 and 1.00. Scales with coefficients under 0.70 should usually be avoided. However, α usually increases with the number of items in the scale, so 20-item tests often have values in the 0.80s, even if they have poor internal consistency (Cortina, 1993), and other indices should be used (Streiner, 2003b). A high value of α is necessary, but not sufficient, since it yields the most "optimistic" estimate of scale's reliability, that is, one that is higher than the other indices discussed below.

Test-Retest Reliability

A scale should be stable over time, assuming that nothing has changed in the interim. If a patient completes a depression inventory today and again next week, then the results should reflect an equivalent degree of dysphoria (again assuming the person hasn't gotten any better or worse). If the score is different in the absence of change, then it is impossible to know which number is an accurate reflection of the person's status.

The acceptable value of the test-retest reliability coefficient depends on two factors: the interval between the two administrations and the hypothesized stability of the trait being measured. Unless the test is very long, the retest should not have occurred less than two weeks after the first testing. Otherwise, the person may have been recalling his or her previous answers and repeated these, rather than responding to the questions themselves. (We assume that the person can't remember responses to 100 or so items, so longer tests can have a shorter retest interval). The interval should not have been so long that whatever was being measured may have changed. Within these limits, test-retest reliabilities in the 0.60s are marginal, those in the 0.70s are acceptable, and anything over 0.80 would be considered high for research purposes. If the scale is to be used to make decisions about an individual, the reliability should be over 0.90 (Nunnally & Bernstein, 1994).

Inter-Rater Reliability

Some indices, such as the Hamilton Rating Scale for Depression (Hamilton, 1980), are completed by a rater rather than by the patient. The issue here is that two or more observers, independently evaluating the same person, should come up with similar scores. Like test-retest reliability, a lack of agreement usually means that none of the results can be trusted.

Acceptable values for inter-rater reliability are similar to those for test-retest reliability. However, if each rater must interview the patient independently in order to complete the scale (as opposed to the raters assessing the patient simultaneously through a one-way mirror or based on previous observations), then somewhat lower reliability values are expected. The reason is that there are now two sources of error instead of one: the raters are different, and the patients may have changed in the interim or altered their responses for the different evaluators. Even so, the inter-rater reliability should never drop below 0.60, and ideally should be at least in the low 0.80s.

A note of caution is in order for the person who wants to use an observer-based scale. Just because the article reported a high inter-rater reliability does not mean that you will necessarily achieve the same level. Most of these scales require some degree of observer training; if the training is inadequate or inaccurate, then the reliability will suffer accordingly. By the same token, if you do a better job of training than the original authors, inter-rater reliability may actually increase.

Choice of Sample

The reliability of an instrument depends on its ability to discriminate among people. Paradoxical as it may sound, if all of the subjects get the same score on the scale, then its reliability is zero, since it is not discriminating at all. The implication of this is that if a reliability study for an anxiety scale used a mixed bag of people, ranging from mountain climbers and sky divers to agoraphobics and obsessive compulsives, then the reliability estimate will be quite high. However, if the scale is intended to be used only among patients suffering from anxiety disorders, then it will have much greater difficulty discriminating among these people, who have a more restricted range of anxiety, and the reliability will drop. Conversely, an estimate based on a sample of patients in an anxiety disorders clinic will underestimate the scale's reliability when it is used in a general outpatient clinic.

There are two conclusions to be drawn. First, when evaluating an article reporting reliability, we need to ensure its sample is similar to the people it will be used with. Second, if the sample is different, it may be necessary to conduct your own reliability study. However, if the test's standard deviations are known for the original sample and the new sample, it is possible to estimate how much the reliability will change (Streiner & Norman, 2008).

Fig. 22.1 Line 1 shows perfect association and agreement;
line 2 shows perfect association and no agreement

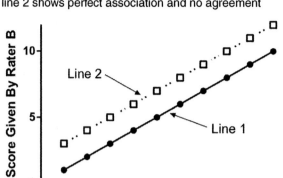

How Was Reliability Calculated?

The most common way to calculate a reliability coefficient is to calculate a Pearson correlation coefficient between the two scores: the
test and retest scores, or those based on the two observers (Norman
& Streiner, 2003). Although it is the most widely used index, it is not
necessarily the best for two reasons. First, it cannot readily handle the
situation where there are more than two observers. The only way it
can do so is by correlating rater A versus rater B, A versus C, and B
versus C. Unfortunately, this violates one of the basic assumptions of
the correlation, that all of the tests are independent. Obviously, they are
not, since each rater's data enter into the calculations twice. Second,
Pearson correlation is sensitive to differences in association, but not in
agreement; Figure 22.1 helps to distinguish between these terms. In the
situation shown by line 1, there is perfect agreement and perfect association between the two raters; whenever rater A assigned a score of 3
to a subject, so did rater B, and similarly for all other ratings. In line 2,
there is a systematic bias. Rater B's scores are always two points higher
than rater A's, so that whenever A gave a 2, B gave a 4. In this case, the
association is perfect (a high score from A is associated with a high one
from B, and similarly for low scores), but the agreement is zero; they
never give the same score to a subject. Pearson's r in both of these cases
is identical: 1.00. The same problem appears in a test-retest situation; if

the scores on readministration are systematically higher or lower than at Time 1, Pearson's r would not pick it up. This doesn't mean that the test is unreliable; since people are rank ordered exactly the same both times, the test still conveys useful information.

Since the Pearson correlation coefficient is insensitive to systematic biases between observers or administration times, it is somewhat optimistic. It would be preferable if authors reported an intra-class correlation (ICC), which is identical to Pearson's r if no bias is present, but lower than r when there is any bias (Streiner & Norman, 2008).

Validity

Now that we know that the test is measuring something reliably, the next question is "what exactly is it measuring?" Validity addresses what conclusions can legitimately be drawn about people who attain various scores on the scale; for instance, if the test purports to measure social support, are we safe in saying that people who score higher on it actually have more social support? Like reliability, there are a number of ways of assessing this, each telling something different about the scale, not all of which are appropriate for any given instrument. But there is one major difference between determining reliability and assessing validity.

In the former case, it is often sufficient for the test constructor to have done one study and arrive at a definitive answer. Validity is an ongoing process and there is rarely a time we can say "enough." The reason is that we can always learn more about the types of conclusions we can draw, and this varies with the sample, the situation, time, and a host of other factors.

There are two points that should be emphasized before we delve into the ways we establish validity. The first is that the definition of validity has changed over the past few decades. If you read older books on the topic (or more recent works by people who haven't kept up with the field), you'll see validity defined as telling us what the scale "really" measures. Thus, the focus was on the test. Nowadays, as we saw a couple of paragraphs ago, validity is concerned with the conclusions we can make about a person's *score* on a test. This isn't just semantics. Instead, it reinforces the second point, that validity (like reliability) is not a fixed property of the test. A given score may tell us one thing about a person from one group, assessed in a specific situation, but it may mean something entirely different (or nothing) about a person from another group tested in a different situation.

Traditionally, psychometricians have talked about the "three Cs" of validity – content, criterion, and construct validity. Although this tradition has given way to a more global conception of validity testing (Streiner & Norman, 2008), it is still easier to begin thinking about validity within the context of these three terms. To this "holy trinity" is added one other term: face validity. But bear in mind that there aren't different "types" of validity: everything is an attempt to demonstrate construct validity (which we'll define below). So, we'll talk about content *validation* (that is, a method) rather than content *validity* (that is, a "type" of validity).

Face Validation

Face validation addresses a very simple, qualitative question: do the items appear, on the face of it, to be measuring what the scale says it measures? The presence of face validation does not improve the psychometric properties of the index, nor does its lack detract from it. Rather, it is more a matter of acceptability from the respondent's point of view. That is, the person may be more willing to complete a depression inventory if the items seem to be asking about affect than if they seem irrelevant. An item such as "My shirt collar seems looser now" may be excellent from a psychometric point of view, since a "yes" response may reflect appetite and weight loss; however, if the respondent feels that the items are silly and unrelated to his or her problems, they may be answered randomly or not at all. There may be times where the test user wishes to avoid face validity. If there is concern that the person may deliberately falsify his or her responses by faking bad or faking good in order to achieve some aim (for example, to ensure hospitalization or to get discharged), then it may be wise to avoid scales which have high face validity.

Content Validation

In order to be sure that a scale which purports to measure family functioning is, in fact, tapping this area, the items should at a minimum meet two criteria: all relevant areas of family functioning are assessed (content coverage), and the items shouldn't be tapping topics that are unrelated (content relevance). Like face validation, this is a judgment call by the test developer and user and is usually not reduced to a single number.

Table 22.2 A content validation matrix

	Domain			
Item	Communication	Role definition	...	Autonomy
1	✓			
2				✓
3		✓		
.				
.				
.				
20	✓			

The best way to check the content validation of a scale is to construct a matrix, such as the one in Table 22.2. Each column represents a domain deemed to be important, and each row is an item. In a scale of family functioning, for example, the domains could be "communication," "role definition," "autonomy," and so forth. To evaluate the utility of an existing scale, these domains should be determined by the user of the test, rather than simply be a reflection of the developer's ideas.

A check mark is placed under the domain tapped by the item. Each item should have a check mark under one (and preferably, only one) domain; otherwise, its relevance for the test is questionable. At the same time, each domain should have at least a few check marks under it; all else being equal, the more items in a domain, the more reliably it's assessed (Streiner & Norman, 2008). Naturally, this technique can be used only with items which are face valid; otherwise, it would be difficult to determine the correct domains they tap.

Criterion Validation

A test which is supposed to tap an attribute such as suicidal potential should correlate with other, accepted measures of the same trait. If both the scale being evaluated and the "gold standard" test were administered at the same time, this is called concurrent criterion validation. In some circumstances, the criterion may occur only sometime in the future; the new test is evaluated by how well it predicts what the criterion score will be.

Although the distinction between these two types of validation appears relatively minor, consisting of when the criterion is measured, the difference is actually quite substantial. If a gold standard exists which can be given at the same time as the new test, then the question should arise, "Why develop a new measure at all?" The only reason (except for wanting to immortalize one's name as a test) is that the new measure is better – cheaper, faster, less invasive, or easier to use. In this case, the two tests should correlate quite strongly, 0.80 or above. If the new scale is supposed to be more valid than the old one, then concurrent validation is necessary, but by no means sufficient. In this case, the two measures should not correlate too highly; if the correlation between the new and gold standard tests is 0.70 or over, then the two are tapping very much the same thing and there is little room for the new test to be any better than the original. If the correlation is too low (below 0.30 or so), then the measures are not related at all, meaning that the new scale is measuring something entirely different from the gold standard. In this case, the test developer is looking for a correlation somewhere between 0.30 and 0.70.

If the test developer used predictive validation, this implies that the behaviour or attribute being measured will occur only sometime after the test is completed by the person, and there is no comparable measure which can be given at the same time. This type of validation is used most often in school admission tests, where the criterion is whether or not the person will graduate three or four years later, and diagnostic tests, where the criterion is whether or not the person later develops a disorder or certain results show up on biopsy or autopsy. In the latter case, the correlation should be quite high, at least 0.70 if the test is used for research purposes and 0.85 or higher if clinical decisions are made on the basis of the test results.

Construct Validity

In much of medicine and the social sciences, the usual state of affairs is that either no other test exists which taps the same attribute, or the existing ones are inadequate for one reason or another. Consequently, criterion validation is either impossible to establish or insufficient. Moreover, the trait that is being studied is what is referred to in psychology as a "hypothetical construct" (Cronbach & Meehl, 1955) or a "construct" for short. Unlike blood pressure or height, for example, which can be easily measured or seen, constructs such as anxiety and intelligence are abstract variables which cannot be directly observed. We do not see anxiety; we note a variety of symptoms, signs, and behaviours, such as sweatiness, tachycardia, impaired concentration, or avoidance of certain situations. What we then do is infer that all of these are caused by an underlying process which we call "anxiety." It is fair to say that most of the variables we deal with in psychiatry, such as "self-esteem," "repression," or "locus of control," are hypothetical constructs. This also pertains to many of the diagnoses used in medicine and psychiatry: we don't see schizophrenia or irritable bowel disease; rather, we see constellations of symptoms that usually occur together and are then attributed to the underlying disorder.

How would a person go about validating a new test in an area such as somatic preoccupation (SP)? No criterion exists other than clinical judgment, and that in itself is flawed, so the scale developer must use construct validity. A construct can be thought of as a "mini-theory," so the first step is to make some predictions based on the theory. These may include the following: people with a high degree of SP should see their family physicians more frequently than patients who have lower SP scores; high-SP people will have more over-the-counter medications in their homes than low-SP people; or scores for high-SP people should increase following the announcement of a flu epidemic. Each of these predictions can be tested, and every study with a positive outcome strengthens the construct and increases the validity of the scale.

It is obvious that a construct can lead to literally hundreds of hypotheses. Further, not all of them can be (or need to be) tested. As the reviewer of a scale, the first questions you have to ask for each study are (1) is the study a good test of the construct, and (2) did the measure perform as it should have? Then, based on all of the validity studies which have been done, the final question is (3) have enough studies been done so that the scale can be considered valid for the people you want to assess and within the context that you evaluate them (at least until contrary results come along)? The major point is that there is no single study which can establish construct validity; it must be shown over a number of studies, tapping various aspects of the hypothetical construct. Moreover, what the test developer considers to be sufficient proof of validity may not be the same as what the user of the scale deems necessary.

The Validation Sample

One of the major areas about which a test developer and a test user can disagree regarding the adequacy of a study is the choice of people on whom the scale was validated. Because of their ready availability, university students have served as a prime source of data. This is true even for scales which are meant to be used in clinical situations, such as the Social Avoidance and Distress Scale (Watson & Friend, 1969), or the Ego Identity Scale (Tan, Kendis, Fine, & Porac, 1977). The problems are twofold: university-trained students may not interpret the questions in the same way as the general population does; with few exceptions, not many will have the trait to the same degree as does the average person. Thus, they are rarely representative of the intended audience. And, to drive the point home yet again, since validity is an interaction among the test, the specific population, and the circumstances, "validity" with students in a classroom setting does not guarantee validity with patients in a clinical setting.

Another major shortcoming of some validation studies is that they show only that the test can discriminate between two extreme populations, such as hospitalized patients versus normal individuals. Tests are rarely needed to distinguish between these two groups; rather, they are used clinically where there is a large element of uncertainty, such as differentiating depression from early dementia. Consequently, while it is necessary to have a measure which discriminates between extreme groups (and indeed this is one form of construct validation), that is not sufficient; the test must be shown to work with the groups in which it will ultimately be used.

Even when the sample is appropriate, it is important to remember that different tests which tap an area may have been validated on different samples. For instance, both the Beck Depression Inventory-2 (BDI-2; Beck et al., 1996) and the Center for Epidemiologic Studies – Depression (CES-D; Radloff, 1977) are depression inventories. However, the former was validated on (and for) hospitalized psychiatric patients and the latter on community-dwelling normal individuals. The norms for the CES-D would be totally misleading if it were used with patients, while the BDI-2 would be inappropriate in studies of mood disturbances among newly diagnosed multiple sclerosis patients or with any other non-psychiatric group.

Just like the case with reliability, it is easy to make a scale look "valid" if the samples are chosen judiciously. However, if the members bear little resemblance to the groups with whom the test will ultimately be used, the "validity" is more apparent than real. The conclusion is that the user should ensure not only that appropriate validity testing was done, but that meaningful groups of subjects are used.

Utility

The last element a test user must think about is the utility of the measure. Even if it is highly reliable and valid for your purposes, it may not be feasible if it requires two weeks to train interviewers, takes three or four hours to administer and requires a $500 computer program to do the scoring.

Completion Time

There is no absolute criterion for deciding if a test takes too long to complete. The answer depends on the setting, the acuity of the disorder, and the context in which the test is given. People who have to take time off work to attend an outpatient clinic may feel burdened by a questionnaire which keeps them there an additional 10 minutes, while inpatients may welcome the break from routine offered by sitting in an office for the three hours required to complete the MMPI-2. Similarly, a patient in acute distress may find it difficult to sustain his or her attention long enough to complete a lengthy questionnaire. It is often the case in a research setting that a number of scales are given to the subjects. The issue then becomes the length of time that the entire battery takes and the additional time required to complete another scale.

As we mentioned earlier, it is usually the rule that longer tests are more reliable and often more valid than shorter ones. But, based on considerations of time, it may be necessary at times to sacrifice some degree of validity for brevity.

Training Time

An important issue in determining the utility of a test is the length of time necessary to master its use. Training may be required in two areas: learning how to administer the test and how to interpret the results. At one extreme, some scales simply are given to the subject and the total checked against norms to determine if the person's score falls above or below some criterion (e.g., Spielberger et al., 1983). At the other extreme, extensive training of an interviewer may needed for diagnostic schedules such as the SADS (Spitzer & Endicott, 1982), even if he or she is a mental health care professional, or the interpretation may require a solid background in psychopathology, as is the case with the MMPI-2 (Butcher et al., 1989) or the MCMI-III (Millon et al., 1994).

Tests which are completed by the patient have the advantage that no time is required to learn how to administer them. However, they require the person to be literate in English, motivated, and able to concentrate. Those which use an interviewer or a rater, such as the Hamilton Depression Rating Scale (Hamilton, 1980) do not have these problems, but often require training to reach an acceptable level of inter-rater reliability. In some cases, simply reading a manual may suffice, but the requisite training may be so intensive as to involve attendance at a workshop for three to five days (Robins et al., 1981; Spitzer & Endicott, 1982). Moreover, as we mentioned in the second section of this chapter, there is no guarantee that any two raters in a new setting will achieve the same inter-rater reliability which was reported by the test developer.

Learning how to interpret a test may again involve nothing more than memorizing what the cut-off point is between normal and abnormal. It usually requires a minimum of one year of supervision to master personality inventories like the MMPI-2. If the test is used solely for research purposes, this may not be an issue, since most often only group data are compared. However, the aspect of training time may be an important consideration if an instrument is to be used for clinical purposes.

The user of the test must determine how much time is necessary to learn how to use the test. This must then be weighed against the reported validity of the test, in comparison with scales which may not be as valid, but which do not require as much training.

Scoring

Scoring some scales may consist of simply adding up the number of endorsed items. Other inventories may need either a computer program or dozens of hand-scoring templates. This may be a critical component of its utility especially if the instrument is used with a large number of people.

In summary, scales are useful components of most research and clinical programs. However, there is considerable variability from one to another regarding their psychometric properties and usefulness. There are two very helpful sources of information about these properties: the *Mental Measurements Yearbook* (MMY; Spies, Carlson, & Geisinger, 2010) and *Test Critiques* (Keyser & Sweetland, 1994). Both books have new editions every few years (MMY now has 18 volumes; *Test Critiques* has 10), with reviews of copyrighted scales by experienced psychologists. Other books, (Corcoran & Fischer, 2006; Fischer & Corcoran, 2006; McDowell & Newell, 2006) are often more selective in the choice of tests listed, but can provide very useful information. The potential user of a test would do well to invest some time with these and other sources to determine if it meets the minimum standards of reliability and validity, and if it is practical to use in their situation.

REFERENCES

Anastasi, A., & Urbina, S. (1997). *Psychological testing.* (7th ed.). New York: Macmillan.

Apgar, V. (1953, Jul-Aug). A proposal for a new method of evaluation of the newborn infant. *Current Researches in Anesthesia & Analgesia, 32*(4), 260–267. Medline:13083014

Beck, A.T., Steer, R.A., & Brown, G.K. (1996). *Manual for the Beck Depression Inventory – II.* San Antonia, TX: Psychological Corporation.

Butcher, J.N., Dahlstrom, W.G., Graham, J.R., Tellegen, A., & Kaemmer, B. (1989). *Minnesota Multiphasic Personality Inventory (MMPI-2). Manual for administration and scoring.* Minneapolis, MN: University of Minnesota Press.

Corcoran, K., & Fischer, J. (2006). *Measures for clinical practice and research: Vol. 2. Adults.* (4th ed.). New York: Oxford University Press.

Cortina, J.M. (1993). What is coefficient alpha? An examination of theory and applications. *Journal of Applied Psychology, 78*(1), 98–104. http://dx.doi.org/10.1037/0021-9010.78.1.98

Cronbach, L.J. (1951). Coefficient alpha and the internal structure of tests. *Psychometrika, 16*(3), 297–334. http://dx.doi.org/10.1007/BF02310555

Cronbach, L.J., & Meehl, P.E. (1955, Jul). Construct validity in psychological tests. *Psychological Bulletin, 52*(4), 281–302. http://dx.doi.org/10.1037/h0040957 Medline:13245896

Fischer, J., & Corcoran, K. (2006). *Measures for clinical practice and research: Vol. 1. Couples, families, and children.* (4th ed.). New York: Oxford University Press.

Hamilton, M. (1980, Dec). Rating depressive patients. *Journal of Clinical Psychiatry, 41*(12 Pt 2), 21–24. Medline:7440521

Hathaway, S.R., & McKinley, J.C. (1951). *Manual for the Minnesota Multiphasic Personality Inventory. (rev.).* New York: Psychological Corporation.

Herzberger, S.D., Chan, E., & Katz, J. (1984, Jun). The development of an assertiveness self-report inventory. *Journal of Personality Assessment, 48*(3), 317–323. http://dx.doi.org/10.1207/s15327752jpa4803_16 Medline:16367532

Kay, S.R., Fiszbein, A., & Opler, L.A. (1987). The positive and negative syndrome scale (PANSS) for schizophrenia. *Schizophrenia Bulletin, 13*(2), 261–276. Medline:3616518

Keyser, D.J., & Sweetland, R.C. (1994). *Test critiques*. Kansas City, MO: Test Corporation of America.

Lambourn, J., & Gill, D. (1978, Dec). A controlled comparison of simulated and real ECT. *British Journal of Psychiatry*, 133(6), 514–519. http://dx.doi. org/10.1192/bjp.133.6.514 Medline:367479

McDonald, R.K. (1958, Sep). Problems in biologic research in schizophrenia. *Journal of Chronic Diseases*, 8(3), 366–371. http://dx.doi.org/10.1016/0021-9681(58)90202-9 Medline:13575509

McDowell, I., & Newell, C. (2006). *Measuring health: A guide to rating scales and questionnaires*. (3rd ed.). New York: Oxford University Press.

Millon, T., Millon, C., & Davis, R.D. (1994). *Manual for the Millon Multiaxial Clinical Inventory-III (MCMI-II)*. Minneapolis, MN: National Computer Systems.

Nideffer, R.M. (1976). Test of Attentional and Interpersonal Style. *Journal of Personality and Social Psychology*, 34(3), 394–404. http://dx.doi.org/10.1037/0022-3514.34.3.394

Norman, G.R., & Streiner, D.L. (2003). *PDQ statistics*. (3rd ed.). Shelton, CT: PMPH USA.

Nunnally, J.C., & Bernstein, I.H. (1994). *Psychometric theory*. (3rd ed.). New York: McGraw-Hill.

Olmsted, M.P., Davis, R., Garner, D.M., Eagle, M., Rockert, W., & Irvine, M.J. (1991). Efficacy of a brief group psychoeducational intervention for bulimia nervosa. *Behaviour Research and Therapy*, 29(1), 71–83. http://dx.doi. org/10.1016/S0005-7967(09)80009-0 Medline:2012591

Radloff, L.S. (1977). The CES-D scale: A self-report depression scale for research in the general population. *Applied Psychological Measurement*, 1(3), 385–401. http://dx.doi.org/10.1177/014662167700100306

Robins, L.N., Helzer, J.E., Croughan, J., & Ratcliff, K.S. (1981, Apr). National Institute of Mental Health Diagnostic Interview Schedule. Its history, characteristics, and validity. *Archives of General Psychiatry*, 38(4), 381–389. http://dx.doi.org/10.1001/archpsyc.1981.01780290015001 Medline:6260053

Rosen, R.C., Riley, A., Wagner, G., Osterloh, I.H., Kirkpatrick, J., & Mishra, A. (1997, Jun). The international index of erectile function (IIEF): A multidimensional scale for assessment of erectile dysfunction. *Urology*, 49(6), 822–830. http://dx.doi.org/10.1016/S0090-4295(97)00238-0 Medline:9187685

Spielberger, C.D., Gorsuch, R.L., Lushene, R.E., Vagg, P.R., & Jacobs, G.A. (1983). *Manual for the State-Trait Anxiety Inventory*. Palo Alto, CA: Consulting Psychologists Press.

Spies, R.A., Carlson, J.F., & Geisinger, K.F. (2010). *The 18th mental measurements yearbook*. Omaha, NE: University of Nebraska Press.

Spitzer, R., & Endicott, J. (1982). *Schedule for Affective Disorders and Schizophrenia (SADS)*. New York: New York State Psychiatric Institute.

Streiner, D.L. (2003a, Jun). Being inconsistent about consistency: When coefficient alpha does and doesn't matter. *Journal of Personality Assessment, 80*(3), 217–222. http://dx.doi.org/10.1207/S15327752JPA8003_01 Medline: 12763696

Streiner, D.L. (2003b, Feb). Starting at the beginning: An introduction to coefficient alpha and internal consistency. *Journal of Personality Assessment, 80*(1), 99–103. http://dx.doi.org/10.1207/S15327752JPA8001_18 Medline:12584072

Streiner, D.L., & Norman, G.R. (2008). *Health measurement scales: A practical guide to their development and use.* (4th ed.). Oxford: Oxford University Press.

Tan, A.L., Kendis, R.J., Fine, J.T., & Porac, J. (1977, Jun). A short measure of Eriksonian ego identity. *Journal of Personality Assessment, 41*(3), 279–284. http://dx.doi.org/10.1207/s15327752jpa4103_9 Medline:16367232

Thoits, P.A. (1982, Jun). Conceptual, methodological, and theoretical problems in studying social support as a buffer against life stress. *Journal of Health and Social Behavior, 23*(2), 145–159. http://dx.doi.org/10.2307/2136511 Medline: 7108180

Ullmann, L.P., & Giovannoni, J.M. (1964, Jan). The development of a self-report measure of the process-reactive continuum. *Journal of Nervous and Mental Disease, 138*(1), 38–42. http://dx.doi.org/10.1097/00005053-196401000-00005 Medline:14106322

Wallston, B.S., Alagna, S.W., DeVellis, B.M., & DeVellis, R.F. (1983). Social support and physical health. *Health Psychology, 2*(4), 367–391. http://dx.doi.org/10.1037/0278-6133.2.4.367

Watson, D., & Friend, R. (1969, Aug). Measurement of social-evaluative anxiety. *Journal of Consulting and Clinical Psychology, 33*(4), 448–457. http://dx.doi.org/10.1037/h0027806 Medline:5810590

TO READ FURTHER

Furr, R.M., & Bacharach, V.R. (2008). *Psychometrics: An introduction.* Thousand Oaks, CA: Sage.

Streiner, D.L., & Norman, G.R. (2008). *Health measurement scales: A practical guide to their development and use.* (4th ed.). Oxford: Oxford University Press.

23 Learning How to Differ: Agreement and Reliability Statistics

DAVID L. STREINER, PH.D.

Canadian Journal of Psychiatry, 1995, 40, 60–66

In psychiatry, as in other branches of medicine, diagnosis is as much an art as a science. Although each edition of the *Diagnostic and Statistical Manual* has set out increasingly more objective criteria for the various disorders, and while structured clinical interviews such as the CIDI (Kessler & Üstün, 2004) and the SADS (Spitzer & Endicott, 1982) have reduced the variation among diagnosticians in terms of what the patient is asked, differences among clinicians still remain. One interviewer may feel that the patient's report of rapid speech is a manifestation of mania, while another may judge it to be within the normal range of differences among people. Since so many of the diagnostic criteria rely on the judgment of the evaluator, it is not surprising that agreement is far from perfect. For example, Anthony et al. (1985) reported agreement rates between the DIS and clinical reappraisal ranging between −0.02 for panic disorder to a high of 0.35 for alcohol-use disorder.

These disagreements are not limited to the "soft" field of psychiatry. Even when purportedly objective diagnostic tests are used, physicians often differ among themselves in their interpretation. For instance, one study (Musch, Landis, Higgins, Gilson, & Jones,1984) looked at three radiologists examining films for the presence or absence of pneumoconiosis. When the analyses were restricted to X-rays that had satisfactory quality, the agreement among the raters ranged from 0.20 to only 0.40 (with poor-quality films, the highest agreement was 0.25). Thus, differences among clinicians, in both research and clinical settings, is and will remain a fact of life. This raises two issues: (1) how can we quantify the degree of agreement and disagreement; and (2) how can we best

Table 23.1 Representation of agreement and disagreement between two raters

		Rater 2	
		Present	Absent
Rater 1	Present	A	B
	Absent	C	D

Table 23.2 Presence or absence of dyskinesia assessed by two raters

		Rater 2		
		Present	Absent	
Rater 1	Present	17	18	35
	Absent	13	52	65
		30	70	100

resolve differences among the raters? In this chapter, we'll discuss various indices of agreement and different statistical strategies for arriving at a consensus opinion.

Assessing agreement is easiest when the decision is a binary one: a symptom, sign, or diagnosis is either present or not. If there are only two judges, the situation can be represented in a 2 × 2 table, as in Table 23.1. Cell A shows the number of cases in which both raters agree that the attribute is present, Cell D the number of times they agree that it is absent. The other two cells reflect disagreement between the judges: in Cell B, rater 1 believes it to be present and rater 2 feels it is absent; and Cell C indicates the number of times the opposite situation occurs.

The most direct index of agreement would seem to be relatively straightforward: simply add the number of times that the two raters agree with one another (A + D), divide by the total number of cases (N = A + B + C + D) and multiply by 100 in order to end up with a percentage. Let's assume that we did a study in which two raters looked for signs of tardive dyskinesia among 100 patients treated with neuroleptics, and we came up with the results shown in Table 23.2. In this case, the agreement rate would be [(17 + 52)/100] × 100, or 69%, which is fairly respectable. Should we conclude, therefore, that, based on these (fictitious) data, psychiatrists are reliable judges of the presence or absence of this symptom?

Those of you who have been reading previous essays in this series should know by now that, if it looks easy and straightforward, there must be a problem, and in fact there are many problems. The first challenge is a surfeit of methods that can be used to estimate agreement. Especially for 2 × 2 tables, there are at least 20 different indices (Fleiss, 1981; Grove, Andreasen, McDonald-Scott, Keller, & Shapiro, 1981; House, House, & Campbell, 1981; Kramer & Feinstein, 1981).

The index that we just calculated is an example of one class of agreement statistics, called percentage agreement. All such formulae are of the form:

$$\frac{\text{Agreements}}{\text{Agreements} + \text{Disagreements}} \times 100. \qquad [1]$$

They differ among themselves regarding what should be counted in the agreement and disagreement terms. What we have just calculated is called *Total* or *Raw* agreement: all observations (that is, all four cells) were included. A difficulty arises, though, when events occur at either a very high or a very low frequency. In these situations, the large number of cases in Cell A (for high-prevalence outcomes) or D (for low-prevalence ones) will produce high agreement rates, even if the number in the other cell (D or A, respectively) is zero. For example, imagine that two raters are charged with determining whether or not patients show signs of thought broadcasting. Let us make two assumptions: first, that it occurs only 5% of the time among the 100 patients in this study; second, that the raters never agree as to when it is present. In this case, the numbers in the four cells are A = 0, B = 5, C = 5, and D = 90. The raw agreement is therefore $[(0 + 90)/100] \times 100 = 90\%$, despite the fact that there is no concordance between the judges regarding the occurrence of this symptom.

One way around this problem is to look only at the cells in which an event occurred (or should have occurred) and to ignore Cell D, where both raters agree that it did not appear. (Of course, we can also do the reverse and ignore Cell A, if we want to measure the agreement of non-occurrence.) Now the problem is the converse of the previous one: the index is probably too conservative. In the example we just used, the occurrence agreement would be 0%, even though the judges were quite good in ruling it out. Other percentage agreement indices, which we will not go into here, try to find some balance between these two extremes. For those who are interested, many of the formulae are given in House et al. (1981).

The second difficulty in our original example, which is common to all of the percent agreement approaches, is that they do not take agreement

Table 23.3 The number of times the two raters will agree by chance

		Rater 2		
		Present	Absent	
Rater 1	Present	11	21	32
	Absent	22	45	67
		33	66	99

by chance into account. For once, a statistical term means just what you would expect;: agreement by chance refers to the fact that, even if the two judges had never seen the patients but simply said "present" or "absent" randomly, they would give the same label to a certain proportion of the subjects. What proportion would that be? If we look again at Table 23.2, we see that each psychiatrist sees dyskinesia in roughly one-third of the patients. This means that rater 1 will label about 33 of her patients as dyskinetic and 67 as symptom-free. Of these 33 patients, rater 2 will say that one-third (that is, 11) have dyskinesia and 22 do not; of the remaining 67, the rater will say that one-third (22) are dyskinetic and 45 are not. We can summarize this in Table 23.3 (the numbers don't add to 100 because of rounding error). Thus, just by chance, they will agree in (11 + 45) cases, or 56% of the time. Now, the 69% raw agreement does not look quite as impressive.

We can formalize the amount of agreement over and above chance in an equation called Cohen's kappa, or κ (Cohen, 1960), which is also referred to chance-corrected agreement. Kappa can be used if three conditions are met: (1) the patients (or whatever else we are rating) are independent of each other; (2) the raters make their judgments independently of one another; (3) the categories are mutually exclusive and collectively exhaustive (that is, a patient must fall into one and only one category). The equation can be written in two ways, depending on whether we use the actual number of cases, or the proportion of cases. When we use the raw data, the equation is

$$\kappa = \frac{n_o - n_e}{N - n_e},$$
[2]

where n_o is the observed number of cases of agreement, n_e is the number of cases of agreement expected by chance, and N is the total number of cases.

When we deal with the proportion of cases in each cell, the equation becomes

$$\kappa = \frac{p_o - p_e}{1 - p_e}, \qquad\qquad [3]$$

where p_o is the proportion observed; and p_e the proportion expected by chance.

The next step is to determine how many cases are expected by chance alone. To make our work a bit easier, we have to do this only for Cells A and D, since Cells B and C don't enter into the equation. For Cell A, we take the total number of cases in its row (17 + 18 in Table 23.2), multiply this figure by the total number of cases in its column (17 + 13), and divide by the total number of cases (100 in this example). The answer is 35 × 30/100, or 10.5. Similarly for Cell D, the row marginal is 65, the column marginal is 70, and the expected frequency is 65 × 70/100 = 45.5 (if you're interested in the rationale for this calculation, see the chapter on chi-squared in Norman & Streiner, 2008). We can now put these numbers into Equation [2], which results in

$$\kappa = \frac{69 - 56}{100 - 56} = 0.296. \qquad\qquad [4]$$

Thus, chance-corrected agreement is only 29.6%.

Kappa is one example of the second class of formulae, those that use a correction for chance agreement. As is the case with percent agreement statistics, the problem is an embarrassment of riches. Again, most of the formulae differ with respect to which events are counted and also in terms of how chance agreement is calculated. However, none has properties that would unequivocally recommend it over kappa.

The use of kappa to replace raw agreement has been of great benefit in terms of giving us a more accurate estimate of how well (or how poorly) we are performing as diagnosticians. However, there are three problems with kappa as it was originally proposed: (1) it could not deal with situations in which there may be more than two judges; (2) it could handle only binary, dichotomous outcomes; (3) its maximum value is not 1.0 in all situations, but is significantly less when the proportion of positive cases is very high or very low. We'll deal with each of these problems in turn.

The first problem, having more than two judges, has been dealt with by a relatively simple extension of the equation (Conger, 1980; Fleiss, 1971). The equations are somewhat too complex to describe here and, as we'll see, there are better ways than kappa of handling multiple raters, so we'll forgo any further discussion.

The second issue, when there are three or more categories, is a bit more complex at one level, but, as we'll see later, it will show us the way to greatly simplify our lives. Usually, when we have more than two categories, we are dealing with ordinal, rather than nominal, data; that is, the categories are usually in some sort of order, such as never/sometimes/always, or mild/moderate/severe, or poor/fair/satisfactory/excellent. We can, of course, make a table with the three or four categories as rows for rater 1 and as columns for rater 2, much as we did in Table 23.1. Agreement would then be the number of patients in the cells along the main diagonal, that is, for example, where both raters say "never," "sometimes," or "always." Similarly, we can determine the number of patients we would expect to be in those cells by chance and then calculate kappa.

Intuitive as this procedure may sound, there are two drawbacks to figuring out agreement in this way. First, as the number of categories or levels increases, the chance that the two judges will have precisely the same rating for a patient or student drops. This goes against everything we know from test construction: the more levels a scale has (within reason), the higher is the reliability (Streiner & Norman, 2008). Second, it does not differentiate among degrees of disagreement: a difference between the judges of one level is considered to be as much a disagreement as a difference between them of five levels.

The solution is to weight the amount of disagreement, so that a difference of many levels is penalized more than a difference of only a few levels (Cohen, 1968). The question then becomes: what weights should we use? In fact, we can use any weighting scheme we choose, such as 1 point for every level of disagreement, or 1 point if the judges are within two levels of each other and 5 points if they differ by more than two levels, and so on. If we use such an arbitrary system, though, we can manipulate the value of kappa to show low or high agreement with the same data, and two researchers can come up with very different answers regarding the reliability of the assessment. By convention (and for reasons we will outline shortly), most people use *quadratic weights*. This simply means that the disagreement is weighted by the square of the number of levels separating the judges. So, a disagreement of one level is given a weight of one, a disagreement of two levels is assigned

Table 23.4 Calculating weighted kappa

			Rater 2			
			None	Moderate	Severe	
	None	w_{ij}	0	1	4	
		Observed	15	10	5	30
		Expected	8.1	12.6	9.3	
Rater 1	Moderate	w_{ij}	1	0	1	
		Observed	8	17	12	37
		Expected	10.0	15.5	11.5	
	Severe	w_{ij}	4	1	0	
		Observed	4	15	14	33
		Expected	8.9	13.9	10.2	
			27	42	31	100

Notes: Numerator = 0 (15) + 1 (10) + 4 (5) + 1 (8) + 0 (17) + 1 (12) + 4 (4) + 1 (15) + 0 (14) = 81. Denominator = 0 (8.1) + 1 (12.6) + 4 (9.3) + 1 (10.0) + 0 (15.5) + 1 (11.5) + 4 (8.9) + 1 (13.9) + 0 (10.2) = 120.8.

$$\kappa_w = 1 - \frac{81.0}{120.8} = 0.33.$$

a weight of four, three levels a weight of nine, and so on. Whichever weight we use, the formula for weighted kappa (κ_w) is the same:

$$\kappa_w = 1 - \frac{\sum w_{ij} fo_{ij}}{\sum w_{ij} fe_{ij}}. \qquad [5]$$

This looks pretty formidable, but it means simply that, for the numerator, we multiply the weight for each cell by the observed frequency (f_o) and add them all; for the denominator, we do the same thing for the expected frequencies (f_e). If we are dealing with proportions, we substitute the observed and expected proportions (p_o and p_e) for f_o and f_e. We have worked through an example in Table 23.4 just to make things a bit more explicit. In each cell, the top number is the quadratic weight, the middle is the observed frequency, and the bottom is the expected frequency.

Although kappa looks at agreement, and weighted kappa at disagreement, the result is the same: an index of chance-corrected agreement.

The first major advantage of using the quadratic system of weights is that it transforms the ordinal data into a ratio scale by ordering the levels along a unidimensional continuum (Soeken & Prescott, 1986), which means that we can use more powerful parametric statistics with them.

The second advantage is that quadratic weighting of kappa can yield exactly the same result as another index of reliability that is far more flexible, the intraclass correlation (ICC; Fleiss & Cohen, 1973), which we will discuss shortly.

Before we turn to ICC, though, let us discuss the third potential shortcoming of kappa (and weighted kappa): the fact that in many instances, its maximum value is less than 1.0. Indeed, it can be 1.0 only when two conditions are met: (1) when all the off-diagonal cells (for example, cells B and C in Table 23.1) are empty; (2) as a consequence, when both raters have exactly the same number of cases in each category or level (in statistical parlance, when their marginal distributions are equal). The latter condition, though, is rare, since it would require both raters to agree perfectly on the number of cases and non-cases. In most situations, therefore, a kappa (or weighted kappa) of 0.80 is considered to be almost perfect agreement (Landis & Koch, 1977). When the marginal distributions are very discordant (for example, the split between cases and non-cases is 20% versus 80% in either direction, or more extreme), the maximum value of kappa falls close to 0.1 or 0.2 (Spitznagel & Helzer, 1985; Walter, 1984).

To overcome this problem, many other statistics have been proposed, such as Yule's Q and R (Yule, 1912), Van Eerdewegh's V (Spitznagel & Helzer, 1985), Finn's R (Finn, 1970), and Relative Improvement Over Chance (Copas & Loeber, 1990). However, none of them can deal with tables that are larger than 2 × 2 and they have not garnered widespread support.

Because of the relative ease of calculating κ_w, its use in medicine is now almost universal. However, when there are at least three raters for each subject, there are better ways to calculate agreement, based on maximum likelihood estimation (MLE) methods (Hui & Walter, 1980; Walter, 1984). The mathematics, though, are somewhat arcane and not as intuitively obvious as kappa to the non-statistician. Compounding the problem, calculation of MLEs requires a computer with special software. Consequently, its use in psychiatry is still somewhat limited (Miller, Streiner, & Parkinson, 1992; Streiner & Miller, 1990), although it will likely become more widespread as the programs become more available.

Continuous Outcomes

Evaluating agreement when the outcome is continuous is even more straightforward but not by the method most people would think of first. If we have two continuous measures, one from each rater, it may seem

Table 23.5 ANOVA summary table for inter-rater agreement

Source of variation	Sum of squares (SS)	df	Mean square (MS)	F
Students (S)	66	9	7.33	16.50
Raters (R)	5	1	5.00	11.25
Error (E)	4	9	0.44	
Total	75	29		

obvious that we should measure agreement by calculating a Pearson correlation (abbreviated as r) between them. As we pointed out in a previous chapter, though, association (what is measured by r) and agreement are not the same (Streiner, 1993; see Chapter 22). To recapitulate this point briefly, consider two situations. In the first, rater A assigns a grade between 1 and 4 to a series of residents. Rater B is more lenient and gives each resident a grade one mark higher, using points 2 through 5 on the scale. Thus, whenever rater A gives a 2, rater B gives a 3, and so on. Their agreement (that is, assigning the same mark to a resident) is zero, but association is perfect: those who rater A said were best were also rated best by rater B, and similarly for those judged as worst. In another situation, let's assume both raters give scores of 3 to all residents, meaning that their agreement is perfect. However, since the scale does not discriminate among residents, its reliability (and hence any association) is, by definition, zero (Streiner & Norman, 2008). Thus, we can have association without agreement and agreement without association.

Pearson's r, as we have said, measures association, but is blind to any systematic bias between raters. A better index is the one we mentioned previously, the intraclass correlation, which is sensitive to both agreement and association. If we continue with our example of two raters evaluating 10 residents, we would first analyse the results using an analysis of variance (ANOVA) and would come up with a summary table similar to Table 23.5.

The ICC for the reliability of the mean of the two judges in this situation is

$$\text{ICC} = \frac{\text{MS}_S - \text{MS}_E}{\text{MS}_S + (\text{MS}_R - \text{MS}_E)/n}, \qquad [6]$$

where n is the number of subjects, and the various MS terms are defined in the table. Substituting the numbers from Table 23.5, we get

$$\text{ICC} = \frac{7.33 - 0.44}{7.33 + (5.00 - 0.44)/10} = 0.885. \tag{7}$$

Let's take a closer look at the equation and see what it tells us. The numerator ($MS_S - MS_E$) reflects the variability among the residents (if you are interested in why the MS_E term is present, see a textbook such as Streiner & Norman, 2008). If all people get the same grade, then there is no among-resident variation and the numerator becomes zero. Hence, the reliability is zero or less, which reinforces what we said earlier: we can have perfect agreement and yet have zero reliability. The denominator consists of the variance among the residents plus the variance among the judges, as we would expect. That is, the more the judges vary among themselves, the lower will be the reliability. The n term means that estimates based on a large number of subjects will be more reliable than those based on a smaller number. Notice that there is no term in the equation reflecting the number of judges, k, because we assume here that we pool their ratings and use the mean of their scores for each subject. By the same token, the MS_R term is influenced by how much the raters differ from each other for each subject. So, if rater A assigns a 3 to Subject 1, and rater B assigns a 5 to her, their mean for that subject is 4. Since both raters differ from that average, the MS_R term increases, hence lowering the reliability. This shows how the ICC is affected by any systematic bias between the raters, while the Pearson correlation is not.

If we wanted to estimate the reliability of each of the judges acting alone, we would use a variant of the equation, which takes the differences among the raters into account:

$$\text{ICC} = \frac{MS_S - MS_E}{MS_S + (k-1)\,MS_E + k\,(MS_R - MS_E)/n}, \tag{8}$$

which comes out to 0.793. Again, this makes intuitive sense: the reliability of the average score for two raters is higher than the reliability of each judge individually.

What the difference between these two equations makes clear is that, although we talked about "the" ICC, there are, in fact, a number of different equations, depending on the situation. The equations presented here are used in the most common type of reliability study: the k raters are seen as a random sample of all possible judges and each evaluates all of the subjects. Different equations exist if the raters in the study are the only ones we are interested in (that is, we want to look at the reliability of raters in our setting and are not trying to generalize to other judges), or if different combinations of judges evaluate each subject. A fuller description of these other, less commonly used, variants is presented in a number of different articles and texts (Bartko, 1976; Lahey, Downey, & Saal, 1983; Shrout & Fleiss, 1979; Streiner & Norman, 2008).

People who took a course in introductory statistics (specifically the fewer who actually remember what they were taught) will know that techniques like ANOVA should be used only with interval and ratio data, that is, where there are equal intervals between successive points on the scale. By definition, categorical data do not meet this criterion, so how can we calculate ICCs on them? Easily – by ignoring this restriction and treating the ordinal categories as if they were interval. If we do this and plug the appropriate MS terms from the ANOVA table into the equation, we will end up with a number that, in most situations, is identical to weighted kappa using quadratic weights (Fleiss & Cohen, 1973).

The question then arises: why should we go through the bother of calculating an ICC, which requires a computer, rather than κ_w, which we can do by hand? The main reason is that ICCs are far more flexible and can handle situations that are difficult to deal with using κ_w. These include circumstances in which there are missing data, where different people evaluate different subjects, and where there are more than two raters (Streiner & Norman, 2008). There are three other reasons. First, ICCs provide a unifying framework, so that the same statistic is used for all types of data. Second, they are a subset of generalizability theory, which is an extremely powerful tool for examining the reliability of tests in a variety of circumstances (Streiner & Norman, 2008). Last, it may prevent some people from committing the abomination of taking interval data and dividing it into arbitrary categories in order to fit them into a manageable kappa table.

Resolving Differences

Given the fact that raters seldom agree to the degree we would like them to, the next issue is what to do about unacceptable levels of disagreement. There are two possible solutions (assuming that the raters are experienced and further training will not increase their reliability): (1) increase the number of raters, or (2) eliminate those who are least reliable.

One of the basic tenets of test theory is that, if errors are random, then increasing the number of observations will lead to more reliable results. This is the rationale for having many items on a scale. Over the long run, random errors will tend to cancel each other out, so the errors of those items that lead to an overestimate of the true score will be counterbalanced by errors in other items that lead to underestimates. The same explanation applies to the number of raters: the more there are, the greater the chances that their errors will cancel out.

How many raters are needed to achieve adequate reliability? Again, generalizability theory can provide an answer. If we do a reliability study using two or more evaluators, we can calculate a generalizability coefficient for raters. Then, we can do a series of Decision (or D) studies. The advantage is that these studies are done using only paper and pencil; it's not necessary to actually run more subjects. By using the coefficient that we found, we plug different numbers of raters into the equation, to determine how much the reliability is improved as the number of judges increases. Within the last few years, a free computer program called "G-String" is available to do all the nasty calculations for you (Streiner & Norman, 2008).

Needless to say, reality often rears its ugly head. The more raters there are, the more complicated any study becomes. Further, if the scale requires that the patients be interviewed, then there is a limit to how many times we can ask subjects to answer the same questions. If we are lucky, the subjects will follow Nancy Reagan's advice and "just say no"; if we are not so lucky, they will consent to more interviews, but they will give different answers to each rater, which will really create havoc with our reliability estimates. The object, then, is to select the best subset of raters and to select the best compromise in terms of balancing the number of raters against the added cost and complexity. For example, if there are three raters, this is done by calculating the inter-rater reliabilities among all possible pairs – rater A versus rater B, rater A versus rater C, and rater B versus rater C. If the average correlation among the raters is high, then adding raters will increase the overall reliability only slightly, and the best option would be to select the pair with the highest reliability and eliminate the least reliable one. If the average reliability is low, then even adding more raters or deleting poor ones would not help a dismal situation. When the average reliability is in the intermediate range, then the best solution would be to add more raters. For those faced with this situation, a very neat technique is given by Strahan (1980) for calculating the relative gain achieved by adding more raters.

Summary

Figuring out the agreement or reliability among raters is not as simple as it may first appear. Raw agreement for categorical variables is usually quite inadequate and has been replaced by chance-corrected agreement, usually in the form of Cohen's kappa. Weighted kappa is often used for ordinal variables, but, as we have seen, this can often be replaced by the intraclass correlation, which is a subset of generalizability theory. In the case of interval data, kappa is a poor choice, and Pearson's correlation coefficient is insensitive to systematic differences between the raters. A better technique is the ICC, which has the added advantage that it can be used when there are more than two raters, when judges evaluate different sets of subjects, and where there may be missing observations. Generalizability theory can also assist with decisions about adding more raters or evaluation times to improve levels of agreement.

REFERENCES

Anthony, J.C., Folstein, M., Romanoski, A.J., Von Korff, M.R., Nestadt, G.R., Chahal, R., …, & Gruenberg, E.M. (1985, Jul). Comparison of the lay Diagnostic Interview Schedule and a standardized psychiatric diagnosis. Experience in eastern Baltimore. *Archives of General Psychiatry, 42*(7), 667–675. http://dx.doi.org/10.1001/archpsyc.1985.01790300029004 Medline:4015308

Bartko, J.J. (1976). On various intraclass correlation reliability coefficients. *Psychological Bulletin, 83*(5), 762–765. http://dx.doi.org/10.1037/0033-2909.83.5.762

Cohen, J. (1960). A coefficient of agreement for nominal scales. *Educational and Psychological Measurement, 20*(1), 37–46. http://dx.doi.org/10.1177/001316446002000104

Cohen, J. (1968, Oct). Weighted kappa: Nominal scale agreement with provision for scaled disagreement or partial credit. *Psychological Bulletin, 70*(4), 213–220. http://dx.doi.org/10.1037/h0026256 Medline:19673146

Conger, A.T. (1980). Integration and generalization of kappa for multiple raters. *Psychological Bulletin, 88*(2), 322–328. http://dx.doi.org/10.1037/0033-2909.88.2.322

Copas, J.B., & Loeber, R. (1990). Relative improvement over chance (RIOC) for 2 x 2 tables. *British Journal of Mathematical and Statistical Psychology, 43*(2), 293–307. http://dx.doi.org/10.1111/j.2044-8317.1990.tb00942.x

Finn, R.H. (1970). A note on estimating the reliability of categorical data. *Educational and Psychological Measurement, 30*(1), 71–76. http://dx.doi.org/10.1177/001316447003000106

Fleiss, J.L. (1971). Measuring nominal scale agreement among many raters. *Psychological Bulletin, 76*(5), 378–382. http://dx.doi.org/10.1037/h0031619

Fleiss, J.L. (1981). *Statistical methods for rates and proportions.* (2nd ed.). New York, NY: Wiley.

Fleiss, J.L., & Cohen, J. (1973). The equivalence of weighted kappa and the intraclass correlation coefficient as measures of reliability. *Educational and Psychological Measurement, 33*(3), 613–619. http://dx.doi.org/10.1177/001316447303300309

Grove, W.M., Andreasen, N.C., McDonald-Scott, P., Keller, M.B., & Shapiro, R.W. (1981, Apr). Reliability studies of psychiatric diagnosis. Theory and practice. *Archives of General Psychiatry, 38*(4), 408–413. http://dx.doi.org/10.1001/archpsyc.1981.01780290042004 Medline:7212971

House, A.E., House, B.J., & Campbell, M.B. (1981). Measures of interobserver agreement: Calculation formulas and distribution effects. *Journal of Behavioral Assessment, 3*(1), 37–57. http://dx.doi.org/10.1007/BF01321350

Hui, S.L., & Walter, S.D. (1980, Mar). Estimating the error rates of diagnostic tests. *Biometrics, 36*(1), 167–171. http://dx.doi.org/10.2307/2530508 Medline:7370371

Kessler, R.C., & Üstün, T.B. (2004). The World Mental Health (WMH) Survey Initiative Version of the World Health Organization (WHO) Composite International Diagnostic Interview (CIDI). *International Journal of Methods in Psychiatric Research, 13*(2), 93–121. http://dx.doi.org/10.1002/mpr.168 Medline:15297906

Kramer, M.S., & Feinstein, A.R. (1981, Jan). Clinical biostatistics. LIV. The biostatistics of concordance. *Clinical Pharmacology and Therapeutics, 29*(1), 111–123. http://dx.doi.org/10.1038/clpt.1981.18 Medline:7460469

Lahey, M.A., Downey, R.G., & Saal, F.E. (1983). Intraclass correlations: There's more there than meets the eye. *Psychological Bulletin, 93*(3), 586–595. http://dx.doi.org/10.1037/0033-2909.93.3.586

Landis, J.R., & Koch, G.G. (1977). A one-way components of variance model for categorical data. *Biometrics, 33*(4), 671–679. http://dx.doi.org/10.2307/2529465

Miller, H.R., Streiner, D.L., & Parkinson, A. (1992, Aug). Maximum likelihood estimates of the ability of the MMPI and MCMI personality disorder scales and the SIDP to identify personality disorders. *Journal of Personality Assessment, 59*(1), 1–13. http://dx.doi.org/10.1207/s15327752jpa5901_1 Medline:1512671

Musch, D.C., Landis, J.R., Higgins, I.T.T., Gilson, J.C., & Jones, R.N. (1984, Jan–Mar). An application of kappa-type analyses to interobserver variation in classifying chest radiographs for pneumoconiosis. *Statistics in Medicine, 3*(1), 73–83. http://dx.doi.org/10.1002/sim.4780030109 Medline:6729290

Norman, G.R., & Streiner, D.L. (2008). *Biostatistics: The bare essentials.* (3rd ed.). Shelton, CT: PMPH USA.

Shrout, P.E., & Fleiss, J.L. (1979, Mar). Intraclass correlations: Uses in assessing rater reliability. *Psychological Bulletin, 86*(2), 420–428. http://dx.doi.org/10.1037/0033-2909.86.2.420 Medline:18839484

Soeken, K.L., & Prescott, P.A. (1986, Aug). Issues in the use of kappa to estimate reliability. *Medical Care, 24*(8), 733–741. http://dx.doi.org/10.1097/00005650-198608000-00008 Medline:3736144

Spitzer, R., & Endicott, J. (1982). *Schedule for Affective Disorders and Schizophrenia (SADS)*. New York: New York State Psychiatric Institute.

Spitznagel, E.L., & Helzer, J.E. (1985, Jul). A proposed solution to the base rate problem in the kappa statistic. *Archives of General Psychiatry, 42*(7), 725–728. http://dx.doi.org/10.1001/archpsyc.1985.01790300093012 Medline:4015315

Strahan, R.F. (1980). More on averaging judges ratings: Determining the most reliable composite. *Journal of Consulting and Clinical Psychology, 48*(5), 587–589. http://dx.doi.org/10.1037/0022-006X.48.5.587

Streiner, D.L. (1993, Mar). A checklist for evaluating the usefulness of rating scales. *Canadian Journal of Psychiatry, 38*(2), 140–148. Medline:8467441

Streiner, D.L., & Miller, H.R. (1990). Maximum likelihood estimates of the accuracy of four diagnostic techniques. *Educational and Psychological Measurement, 50*(3), 653–662. http://dx.doi.org/10.1177/0013164490503023

Streiner, D.L., & Norman, G.R. (2008). *Health measurement scales: A practical guide to their construction and use.* (4th ed.). Oxford: Oxford University Press.

Walter, S.D. (1984). Measuring the reliability of clinical data: The case for using three observers. *Revue d'Epidémiologie et de Santé Publique, 32*(3-4), 206–211. Medline:6522735

Yule, G.U. (1912). On the methods of measuring association between two attributes. *Journal of the Royal Statistical Society, 75*(6), 579–642. http://dx.doi.org/10.2307/2340126

TO READ FURTHER

Agresti, A. (1992). Modelling patterns of agreement and disagreement. *Statistical Methods in Medical Research, 1*(2), 201–218. http://dx.doi.org/10.1177/096228029200100205 Medline:1341658

Fleiss, J.L. (1981). *Statistical methods for rates and proportions.* (2nd ed.). New York, NY: Wiley.

Helzer, J.E., Robins, L.N., Taibleson, M., Woodruff, R.A., Jr., Reich, T., & Wish, E.D. (1977, Feb). Reliability of psychiatric diagnosis. I. A methodological review. *Archives of General Psychiatry, 34*(2), 129–133. http://dx.doi.org/10.1001/archpsyc.1977.01770140019001 Medline:320954

Streiner, D.L., & Norman, G.R. (2008). *Health measurement scales: A practical guide to their construction and use.* (4th ed.). Oxford: Oxford University Press.

24 What's under the ROC?
An Introduction to Receiver Operating
Characteristic Curves

DAVID L. STREINER, PH.D., AND JOHN CAIRNEY, PH.D.

Canadian Journal of Psychiatry, 2007, 52, 121–128

Those of you who have read this series of essays religiously know that, because of the tremendous loss of information incurred, you should never dichotomize continuous variables (Streiner, 2002; see Chapter 3). Never! Nohow! Ever! Under no circumstances! Except, of course, when it makes sense to do so. One very legitimate reason for dichotomizing is when a statistical test requires a linear relationship between variables (for example, multiple regression), but the actual relationship isn't linear. It then makes sense to trichotomize the predictor variable. A more common reason occurs when a dichotomous decision must be predicated on a continuous scale. For clinical or research purposes, it may be necessary to divide people into two groups – say, with or without depression – on the basis of an interview or a scale of depressive symptoms. This is done, for example, with the CES-D (Radloff, 1977), where the score can range from 0 to 60. Those who score 17 or more are deemed to suffer from depression; those with lower scores are classified as being without depression. The issue now becomes how we choose the cut-point that best divides the sample into these two groups.

For historical reasons, the method that's used is called ROC analysis. The name dates back to World War II and the merging of signal detection theory with the development of radar. When the gain of the radar set (comparable to the volume control on a radio) is at zero, no signal (in this case representing an enemy plane) is detected. Increasing the gain lets more signals in, but it also increases the amount of noise that is picked up and possibly misinterpreted as a true signal. At low levels of gain, the noise is very weak and unlikely to be falsely labelled, but at the same time, only very strong signals (very large or close planes, to continue the example) are detected and many true signals are missed. As the gain is turned up even further, weaker signals are picked up, but so is more noise (things that can seem like aircraft but are not, such as rain clouds or a flock of birds). At some point, further increases become counterproductive, in that the noise (false positives) begins to outweigh the signals (true positives).

If this terminology reminds you of the language we use in evaluating diagnostic tests, it's not a coincidence. Soon after the war, it was noted that ROC curves could be used in experimental psychology and psychophysics for studies of signal detection (Green & Swets, 1966). People then realized that signal detection theory is exactly what was being used in laboratory medicine and radiology (Goodenough, Rossmann, & Lusted, 1974; Swets, 1979), albeit most practitioners were unaware of the fact (much like Molière's M. Jourdain being unaware that he had been speaking prose for more than 40 years). The "signal" is a test finding indicative of the presence of some abnormality, and the "noise" consists of spurious images that could be misinterpreted as a true signal. The lowest level of "gain" would correspond to a judgment of "definitely, or almost definitely, normal" after, say, reading a computer axial tomography or radionuclide scan to detect a brain tumour (Swets et al., 1979). No false positives are made, but then again no abnormalities are detected either. A moderate level of gain would be a judgment of "abnormal," and the highest "definitely, or almost definitely, abnormal." Giving the last label to all suspect scans would most definitely catch nearly all of the tumours, but at the cost of subjecting many patients to unnecessary follow-up investigations or even surgery. Obviously, the radiologist wants to choose a subjective cut-point that, in his or her own mind, balances these two types of mistake.

Deriving the ROC Curve

To see how the choice of cut-point is made in signal detection theory, we'll return to that dread disorder we've discussed before, photonumerophobia (PNP), and the scale used to detect it (Streiner, 2006; see Chapter 17). We'll assume that the scale to measure PNP, the SPNP, is measured on a scale ranging from 1 (no phobia) to 10 (the highest degree of phobia). To do a study that will derive the ideal cut-point, we will administer the scale to, say, 50 individuals with phobia and 50

Fig. 24.1 Distributions of SPNP scores for individuals with and without phobia, with different cut scores

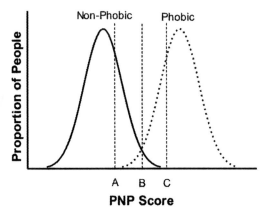

without phobia. We also need one other thing: an independent criterion of whether or not the person suffers from PNP. Although this is commonly referred to as the gold standard, we are often in a position where the quality of the standard, such as clinical judgment or chart diagnosis, is closer to tin or lead. However, in the absence of anything better, it must serve as the gold standard.

The rationale behind finding a cut-point is based on the assumption that we are dealing with two distributions of scores that are relatively normal: one from people who have PNP, as determined by the gold standard, and one from individuals who do not have the disorder (as shown in Figure 24.1). Notice that the curves overlap, as they almost always do in real life. Some individuals with phobia have SPNP scores that are lower than those of some individuals without phobia. That means that, no matter what we choose as the value of the cut-point, we're going to make some mistakes. If we use A on the graph as the dividing line, then we'll catch all of the individuals with phobia, but at the cost of erroneously labelling as phobic a large number of non-fearful individuals. Conversely, C doesn't result in any false negatives, but we'll miss a large number of those with phobia. Cut-point B is a compromise position: there will be both false positives and false negatives, but the total number of erroneously classified individuals is smallest at this point. Later, we'll discuss why B isn't always the best option, but first, let's see how to quantify the errors at each possible cut-point and turn those into an ROC curve.

Table 24.1 The number of people in each group receiving a given score

| SPNP score | Group | | Total |
	With phobia	Without phobia	
1	1	20	21
2	2	9	11
3	1	3	4
4	1	1	2
5	1	3	4
6	1	1	2
7	3	7	10
8	7	3	10
9	13	2	15
10	20	1	21
Total	50	50	100

Table 24.2 The number of individuals with and without phobia scoring above and below a cut-point of 5/6

| Cut-point | Group | | Total |
	With phobia	Without phobia	
6 or above	44 (A)	14 (B)	58
5 or below	6 (C)	36 (D)	42
Total	50	50	100

We begin by making a table, like Table 24.1, that shows the number of individuals in each group, as defined by the gold standard, who receive each score on the test. From this, we (or, more accurately and fortunately, the computer) derive a series of 2 × 2 tables. Because the scale has 10 points, we'll get nine tables: one for each cut-point. The first table is derived from the number of those who score 1 compared with those who score 2 or more; the second table gives the data for those who score 1 or 2 compared with those who score 3 or more; and so on, each table reflecting a progressively higher cut-point. In Table 24.2, we show the results for one of these tables, using a cut-point of 5/6. The letters in the table are used simply to identify the four cells; we'll use them a bit later.

From this table, we can derive the two indices that we need: the sensitivity and the specificity (Streiner, 2003) of the SPNP. Sensitivity refers

Table 24.3 Sensitivity and (1 – Specificity) for each
cut-point of the SPNP

Cut-point	Sensitivity	1 – Specificity
< 1	1.00	1.00
1 / 2	0.98	0.60
2 / 3	0.94	0.42
3 / 4	0.92	0.36
4 / 5	0.90	0.34
5 / 6	0.88	0.28
6 / 7	0.86	0.26
7 / 8	0.80	0.12
8 / 9	0.66	0.06
9 / 10	0.40	0.02
> 10	0.00	0.00

to the ability of the test to detect people who actually have the disorder. The formula is

$$\text{Sensitivity} = \frac{A}{A+C}. \qquad [1]$$

For a cut-point of 5/6, the sensitivity is therefore 44/50 = 0.88. The term "specificity" means that the test is specific to the disorder being assessed, and that it does not give a positive result because of other conditions. The formula is

$$\text{Specificity} = \frac{D}{B+D}, \qquad [2]$$

which in this case is 36/50 = 0.72.

This procedure is done for each of the nine tables, and we then list the sensitivity and (1 – specificity), as in Table 24.3. Note that we've added two extra rows to the table, one above the lowest point (a cut-point below 1) and one below the highest (a cut-point over 10). These are obviously impossible values, but we use them so that the curve that we draw will begin in the lower left corner and end at the upper right one. These pairs of values are plotted, with (1 – specificity) on the X-axis and the sensitivity on the Y-axis, yielding the curve in Figure 24.2. Note that the True Positive (TP) rate is synonymous with sensitivity, the True Negative (TN) rate is the same as specificity, and the False Positive

Fig. 24.2 The ROC curve based on the data in Table 24.3

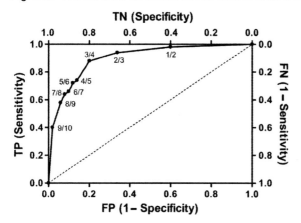

(FP) rate means the same as (1 – specificity); they're simply alternative terms for the same parameters. (To be totally accurate, although a bit pedantic, they are commonly called rates, but strictly speaking they are not: they are proportions, because a rate has time in the denominator; see Chapter 6.)

We've drawn the graph with two extra axes, one on top and one on the right side. These are not usually shown when the results of a study are presented, but we've included them to illustrate the relations among the parameters. As we can see, the sum of the TP rate and the FN rate is 1; when the TP rate increases, the FN rate decreases. Similarly, the TN and FP rates add to 1 and have the same reciprocal relationship to one another.

The lower left-hand corner of the curve is analogous to setting the gain to zero on the radar set: no spurious signals are misidentified (the FP rate is zero), but by the same token, no true signals are detected either (the TP rate is zero). Increasing the gain means moving up the curve: the TP rate increases, and so does the FP rate. Initially, the TP rate increases faster than the FP rate, until the curve is nearest to the upper left-hand corner. After this point, the TP rate continues to increase, but the FP rate starts to increase faster.

Before we begin to discuss some properties of the ROC, there are a couple of points to note about sensitivity and specificity. First, sensitivity depends only on those who have the disorder and specificity only on those who do not. Consequently, we can derive these estimates, and the ROC curve itself, without having to worry about whether the proportion of individuals in each group is representative of the prevalence in the population. Second, as we mentioned before, sensitivity and specificity are like the two ends of a seesaw: if one goes up, then the other goes down. Changing the cut-point favours one over the other, but we can't increase both without going back and improving the overall performance of the test.

Properties of the ROC Curve

As we'll see, there are a number of statistics that can be derived from the ROC, but as is often the case, it's best to begin by simply looking at the curve. The dotted line indicates the curve for a useless test; one that does not discriminate at all between individuals with and without phobia. A perfect test (which exists only in the dreams of test developers) would run straight up the Y-axis to the top and then horizontally to the right. The more the ROC curve deviates from the dotted line and tends towards the upper left-hand corner, the better the sensitivity and specificity of the test. Further, the cut-point that's closest to the corner is the one that minimizes the overall number of errors; in this case, it is 7/8.

The primary statistic we get from the ROC is the *area under the curve* (AUC). In this case, it is 0.899. This can be compared to the null hypothesis – that the test is useless – which has an AUC of 0.50; that is, half of the area in the graph falls below the dotted line, so that 0.399 is between the line and the ROC curve. The AUC can be interpreted in a very useful way. It is the probability that the test will yield a higher value for a randomly chosen individual with the disorder than for a randomly chosen person who does not have the disorder (Lasko, Bhagwat, Zou, & Ohno-Machado, 2005). That means that, in this example with an AUC of 0.899, if we take two individuals at random – one with and one without PNP – the probability is nearly 90% that the first person will have a higher score than the second. (For those who are more statistically inclined, it can be shown that value of the AUC is identical to the result from doing a Wilcoxon or Mann-Whitney U-test; Bamber, 1975; Hanley & McNeil, 1982.) A rough rule of thumb is that the accuracy of tests with AUCs between 0.50 and 0.70 is low; between 0.70 and 0.90, the accuracy is moderate; and it is high for AUCs over 0.90 (Fischer, Bachmann, & Jaeschke, 2003).

As is the case with any parameter, the AUC is an estimate, so that there is a standard error (SE) associated with it (0.031 for these data).

The SE can be used in two ways. First, the ratio of the AUC to the SE is a *t*-test that can be used to see if the AUC differs significantly from the null. Second, we can put a 95% confidence interval (CI) around the estimate of the AUC with the formula:

$$CI_{95} = AUC \pm 1.96 \times SE. \qquad [3]$$

One problem with the AUC is that there are many ways to estimate it. The issue is that, at a theoretical level, the ROC curve is a smooth, continuous function. However, we are trying to estimate it from a finite number of points, leading to the somewhat jagged shape seen in Figure 24.2. No single method of determining the AUC is ideal, because the choice depends on the number of points on the scale, the sample sizes of the two groups, and the degree of separation between the groups. A fuller, albeit somewhat mathematical and technical, explanation of the various methods is given by Lasko et al. (2005), who also list some of the free and commercially available software.

Comparing ROC Curves

At first glance, it may seem tempting to compare two tests or two versions of the same test by simply seeing which one has the larger AUC. However, like many things in life that are tempting, it's not necessarily the wisest thing to do. Simply comparing AUCs works only if the two ROC curves do not cross at any point, that is, that one curve is consistently higher than the other. However, Figure 24.3 shows two ROC curves with equivalent AUCs but having very different properties. Even if the AUCs aren't the same, but the lines cross, it's necessary to choose between them by using a finer-grained test, called the partial AUC, or pAUC (Lasko et al., 2005; Obuchowski, 2003). Rather than calculating the AUC over the entire range of the test, we focus our attention on that portion of curves that is of most interest to us when we are actually using the test, such as that between an FP rate of 0.2 to 0.4 or between sensitivities of 0.7 to 0.8. Calculating the pAUC can be difficult, but we can simplify the situation by looking at a specific FP rate rather than a range. Whichever test produces a higher curve at that specific rate is the more useful one. The problem with this simplification is that a small change in the chosen FP rate may change the conclusion if the curves cross in that general area. It's also worth noting that,

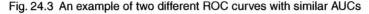

Fig. 24.3 An example of two different ROC curves with similar AUCs

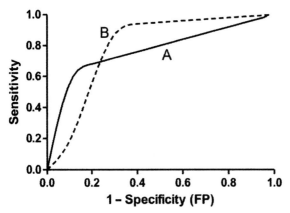

by using the pAUC, we may end up selecting the test that has a smaller AUC. The consequence is that we might opt for one test, based on its pAUC at a specific point, but we'd end up with the poorer test if it were used in a different situation, where we want a higher or lower FP rate (a point we'll discuss in the next section). This further reinforces the fact that validity is not a property of a test; rather, it depends on the use to which the test is put, and for a specific population (Streiner & Norman, 2008; see also Chapter 22). An example that compares two ROC curves, albeit non-crossing ones, is discussed by Cairney, Veldhuizen, Wade, Kurdyak, and Streiner (2007).

Choosing a Cut-Point

Using the cut-point that is nearest to the upper left-hand corner is equivalent to selecting B in Figure 24.1 as the dividing line between normal and abnormal. It's the point that will result in the lowest number of overall errors: FN + FP. In many instances, this is our goal, so it is the chosen cut-point . However, the assumption, either explicit or (more often) implicit, is that the cost of making an FP mistake is the same as making an FN one. "Cost" in this case doesn't mean just a financial burden. It also includes the consequences of missing a true case or erroneously labelling a person as abnormal. For example, in screening blood for hepatitis or HIV/AIDS, the cost of an FN must take into account the risk of infecting a blood recipient, whereas the cost of an FP is merely discarding a unit of blood that otherwise could have been used. Conversely, giving drugs to a child who has been erroneously diagnosed as having attention-deficit hyperactivity disorder exposes him to all of the risks of the medication in addition to the adverse consequences of labelling (Alderman, Charlson, & Melcher, 1981; Bergman & Stamm, 1967), whereas missing the diagnosis may simply delay the intervention until the next trip to a specialist.

Swets (1992) quantifies the relationship between the choice of cut-points with the formula:

$$S_{opt} = \frac{P(neg)}{P(pos)} \times \frac{(B_{TN} - C_{FP})}{(B_{TP} - C_{FN})},$$ [4]

where S_{opt} is the optimal slope of the ROC (more about this in a minute); $P(neg)$ is the is prior probability, or base rate, of a negative finding; $P(pos)$ that of a positive finding; and the Bs and Cs are the benefits and costs, respectively, of the various outcomes – True Negative, False Positive, and so on. If you remember high school geometry, you'll recall that a slope of 1 represents a line, tangent to the curve, going up at a 45° angle; that's just where the curve is nearest the upper left corner. Steeper slopes are further down the curve towards the lower left corner, reflecting more stringent criteria; and shallower slopes are nearer to the top of the curve, representing more lenient cut-points.

So, what does this formula tell us? First, let's keep a fixed set of costs and benefits; that is, we'll ignore what's to the right of the multiplication sign. Then, if the base rate of the disorder is low – that is, we're trying to diagnose a rare condition – $P(neg)$ is greater than $P(pos)$, so the slope is greater than 1. The less prevalent the condition, the more stringent our criterion must be. This reflects the old medical school adage that, if you hear the sound of footsteps, it's more likely to be a horse than a zebra (at least outside Africa). Conversely, for common disorders, we should use a more lenient criterion. Thus, if we were diagnosing PNP in a community survey, we would select a higher cut-point than if we were to use the SPNP in an anxiety disorders clinic. In the latter situation, a higher FP rate is more acceptable, because the number of negative cases is relatively small compared with a community sample.

Now let's keep the ratio of the prior probabilities constant and look at what the right-most part of the formula is telling us. When an intervention's effectiveness is less than ideal, and the cost of treating someone without the disorder is high, the cut-point should be set at a very stringent level. Conversely, when the benefit of treatment is high and the cost of missing a case is low, we set the cut-point much lower.

It's often difficult to quantify the various costs and benefits in units that can be plugged into the equation. One approach is to use relative rather than absolute values for the costs and benefits (Erdreich & Lee, 1981). For example, we could assume that a given disorder is so serious that the cost of an FN is five times that of a TP diagnosis. In this case, C_{FN} would be 5 and $B_{TP} = 1$. We would do the same with the cost of an FP diagnosis relative to the benefit of a TN. Even though these are rough approximations, we should still use the formula at a conceptual level, so that we keep in mind the trade-offs we make in selecting any given cut-point.

Sample Size

We need to figure out sample sizes for two situations: calculating the AUC for one ROC curve, and comparing two ROC curves. We can approach the sample size problem for one ROC curve in two different ways: by testing the hypothesis that the AUC is significantly different from the null hypothesis (that it is equal to 0.50), or by specifying the size of the SE. Let's start with the latter approach; because the former is very similar to testing the difference between two AUCs, we can deal with them together.

The rationale for determining the sample size by setting the magnitude of the SE is predicated on the fact that we are not testing a hypothesis; rather, we are estimating a parameter, the AUC. As is always the case in parameter estimation, sample size determines the SE and, by extension, the width of the CI. That means that we have to approach the problem backwards, by deciding ahead of time what should be the maximum size of the SE or width of the CI and then seeing, on the basis of our best guess of what the AUC will be, the sample size that we'll need to achieve this. The calculations can be quite tedious, but Hanley and McNeil (1982) give a nomogram for sample sizes of various AUCs and SEs.

Testing whether an AUC is significantly different from the null can be seen as being the same as determining if two AUCs differ from one another, the second test having an area of 0.50. However, when we test for the difference between two AUCs, we have to take one other factor into consideration: the correlation between the two tests. Again, the formulae are fairly formidable, but using a program for sample size

Table 24.4 Sample sizes for each group needed to test the differences between two AUCs, for a correlation between the tests of 0.6 (above the main diagonal) and 0.3 (below the diagonal)

AUC(2)	AUC(1)									
	0.50	0.55	0.60	0.65	0.70	0.75	0.80	0.85	0.90	0.95
0.50	–	404	104	48	28	18	13	9	7	6
0.55	700	–	414	107	49	28	18	12	9	7
0.60	176	700	–	428	110	50	28	17	12	9
0.65	78	175	700	–	440	111	49	28	18	12
0.70	44	78	175	695	–	445	108	49	28	18
0.75	28	44	78	173	680	–	431	110	48	27
0.80	20	28	44	76	168	646	–	421	103	45
0.85	14	19	28	43	74	159	585	–	367	89
0.90	11	14	19	27	41	69	142	486	–	269
0.95	8	11	14	18	25	37	61	115	339	–

calculation (Hintze, 2002), we generated Table 24.4, which gives the sizes for each group for an alpha of 0.5, a beta of 0.20, as well as two values of the correlation: 0.6 and 0.3. Like all sample size calculations, these should be looked on as rough approximations, not as additions to the Gospels.

Summary

From detecting enemy planes to assessing the efficiency of a diagnostic test, signal detection theory has produced many interesting applications (our personal preference is for non-military applications, but that's another story). Increasingly, ROC analysis is being adopted in psychiatry to evaluate the accuracy of field-based methods for identifying cases of disorder in population studies (e.g., Furukawa, Kessler, Slade, & Andrews, 2003; Kessler et al. 2002) and to screening for disorder in clinical settings (e.g., Nasr, Popli, & Wendt, 2005). Despite the attendant limitations we have identified, ROC analysis is a useful tool for what has always been a dilemma for clinical medicine (whether some clinicians choose to recognize it or not): the trade-off between being right or wrong and the costs of making mistakes in either direction. While these statistics cannot be substitutes for thinking (what we sometimes refer to as clinical judgment), they do provide a systematic approach for dealing with this problem.

REFERENCES

Alderman, M.H., Charlson, M.E., & Melcher, L.A. (1981). Labelling and absenteeism: The Massachusetts Mutual experience. *Clinical and Investigative Medicine. Médecine Clinique et Experimentale, 4*(3-4), 165–171. Medline:7337987

Bamber, D. (1975). The area above the ordinal dominance graph and the area below the receiver operating characteristic graph. *Journal of Mathematical Psychology, 12*(4), 387–415. http://dx.doi.org/10.1016/0022-2496(75)90001-2

Bergman, A.B., & Stamm, S.J. (1967, May 4). The morbidity of cardiac nondisease in schoolchildren. *New England Journal of Medicine, 276*(18), 1008–1013. http://dx.doi.org/10.1056/NEJM196705042761804 Medline:6022469

Cairney, J., Veldhuizen, S., Wade, T.J., Kurdyak, P., & Streiner, D.L. (2007). Evaluation of two measures of psychosocial distress as screeners for depression in the general population. *Canadian Journal of Psychiatry, 52*, 111–120.

Erdreich, L.S., & Lee, E.T. (1981, Nov). Use of relative operating characteristic analysis in epidemiology. A method for dealing with subjective judgment. *American Journal of Epidemiology, 114*(5), 649–662. Medline:7304595

Fischer, J.E., Bachmann, L.M., & Jaeschke, R. (2003, Jul). A readers' guide to the interpretation of diagnostic test properties: Clinical example of sepsis. *Intensive Care Medicine, 29*(7), 1043–1051. http://dx.doi.org/10.1007/s00134-003-1761-8 Medline:12734652

Furukawa, T.A., Kessler, R.C., Slade, T., & Andrews, G. (2003, Feb). The performance of the K6 and K10 screening scales for psychological distress in the Australian National Survey of Mental Health and Well-Being. *Psychological Medicine, 33*(2), 357–362. http://dx.doi.org/10.1017/S0033291702006700 Medline:12622315

Goodenough, D.J., Rossmann, K., & Lusted, L.B. (1974, Jan). Radiographic applications of receiver operating characteristic (ROC) curves. *Radiology, 110*(1), 89–95. Medline:4808546

Green, D.M., & Swets, J.A. (1966). *Signal detection theory and psychophysics.* New York: John Wiley & Sons.

Hanley, J.A., & McNeil, B.J. (1982, Apr). The meaning and use of the area under a receiver operating characteristic (ROC) curve. *Radiology, 143*(1), 29–36. Medline:7063747

Hintze, J.L. (2002). *PASS user's guide - II.* Kaysville, UT: NCSS.

Kessler, R.C., Andrews, G., Colpe, L.J., Hiripi, E., Mroczek, D.K., Normand, S.-L.T., . . ., & Zaslavsky, A.M. (2002, Aug). Short screening scales to monitor population prevalences and trends in non-specific psychological distress. *Psychological Medicine, 32*(6), 959–976. http://dx.doi.org/10.1017/S0033291702006074 Medline:12214795

Lasko, T.A., Bhagwat, J.G., Zou, K.H., & Ohno-Machado, L. (2005, Oct). The use of receiver operating characteristic curves in biomedical informatics. *Journal of Biomedical Informatics, 38*(5), 404–415. http://dx.doi.org/10.1016/j.jbi.2005.02.008 Medline:16198999

Nasr, S., Popli, A., & Wendt, B. (2005, Jun). Can the MiniSCID improve the detection of bipolarity in private practice? *Journal of Affective Disorders, 86*(2-3), 289–293. http://dx.doi.org/10.1016/j.jad.2005.01.008 Medline:15935249

Obuchowski, N.A. (2003, Oct). Receiver operating characteristic curves and their use in radiology. *Radiology, 229*(1), 3–8. http://dx.doi.org/10.1148/radiol.2291010898 Medline:14519861

Radloff, L.S. (1977). The CES-D scale: A self-report depression scale for research in the general population. *Applied Psychological Measurement, 1*(3), 385–401. http://dx.doi.org/10.1177/014662167700100306

Streiner, D.L. (2002, Apr). Breaking up is hard to do: The heartbreak of dichotomizing continuous data. *Canadian Journal of Psychiatry, 47*(3), 262–266. Medline:11987478

Streiner, D.L. (2003, Dec). Diagnosing tests: Using and misusing diagnostic and screening tests. *Journal of Personality Assessment, 81*(3), 209–219. http://dx.doi.org/10.1207/S15327752JPA8103_03 Medline:14638445

Streiner, D.L. (2006, Apr). Building a better model: An introduction to structural equation modelling. *Canadian Journal of Psychiatry, 51*(5), 317–324. Medline:16986821

Streiner, D.L., & Norman, G.R. (2008). *Health measurement scales: A practical guide to their development and use.* (4th ed.). Oxford: Oxford University Press.

Swets, J.A. (1979, Mar-Apr). ROC analysis applied to the evaluation of medical imaging techniques. *Investigative Radiology, 14*(2), 109–121. http://dx.doi.org/10.1097/00004424-197903000-00002 Medline:478799

Swets, J.A. (1992, Apr). The science of choosing the right decision threshold in high-stakes diagnostics. *American Psychologist, 47*(4), 522–532. http://dx.doi.org/10.1037/0003-066X.47.4.522 Medline:1595983

Swets, J.A., Pickett, R.M., Whitehead, S.F., Getty, D.J., Schnur, J.A., Swets, J.B., & Freeman, B.A. (1979, Aug 24). Assessment of diagnostic technologies. *Science, 205*(4408), 753–759. http://dx.doi.org/10.1126/science.462188 Medline:462188

25 Measure for Measure: New Developments in Measurement and Item Response Theory

DAVID L. STREINER, PH.D.

Canadian Journal of Psychiatry, 2010, 55, 180–186

If there is one theme that has permeated our culture over the past century, it is that bigger is better: hamburgers that surpass the mouth's ability to encompass them, SUVs that can easily transport Jumbo the elephant, and remote controls that require reading a 75-page manual just to find out how to turn the TV on. However, spurred on by health warnings, gas price increases, and baby boomers who have increasing difficulty in reading fine print, this trend may be reversing, replaced by the mantra, "small is beautiful." The same trend exists in creating scales to measure constructs such as anxiety, depression, pain, and coping. Previously, the longer the scale the better (at least from the test developer's standpoint, if not from the test-taker's), because longer scales were usually more reliable, and better reliability translates into better validity (Streiner & Norman, 2008). Over the past few decades, though, this "received wisdom" has been challenged by a new technique called *item response theory* (IRT), which promises shorter scales that are as, if not more, reliable than longer ones (Hambleton, 1996). In this chapter, we'll explore the basics of IRT and how it's revolutionizing the field of scale development.

Classical Test Theory

In order to understand how the rules have changed, it helps to know what the rules have been. In this case, they derive from what is called *classical test theory*, or CTT, which has ruled the game for the past 70 years or so. One reason for its dominance is that its assumptions are relatively weak, meaning that they apply in most situations (Hambleton & Swaminathan, 1985). The primary assumptions are that the amount of error associated with any particular item is unrelated to the true score (where the 'true score' is a hypothetical value, as if there were no measurement error), and that if we add up the error terms for all of the items, the sum will be, in the long run, equal to zero. In practical terms, these assumptions mean that the more items there are in a scale, the less random error will be associated with the total score. The reason is the same as why larger samples give more accurate estimates of the mean than do smaller ones; there's more opportunity for random errors to cancel each other out. The upshot is that we now have scales that are reliable and valid, but relatively long – for example, 21 items on the BDI (Beck, Steer, & Brown, 1996) and 57 items on the Depression scale of the MMPI-II (Butcher, Dahlstrom, Graham, Tellegen, & Kaemmer, 1989). These scales may not seem overly long, but when given in conjunction with other scales, they can add significantly to the test-taker's burden.

However, despite its obvious utility, there are some problems associated with CTT, in addition to its resulting in long scales. The first is *sample dependency*. This means that the psychometric properties of the scale are dependent on the sample in which the scale was tested. We have often raised the admonition that reliability and validity are not intrinsic characteristics of a measurement tool, but are an interaction between the scale and the sample (Streiner, 2007, see Chapter 28; Streiner, 1993, see Chapter 22; Streiner & Norman, 2008). Consequently, if the scale is to be used with a different population, it must be re-normed and the psychometric characteristics determined for that new group. Similarly, any change to the instrument, such as the removal or addition of items, requires a re-evaluation of the test's properties. Another implication of sample dependency is that there is a *circular dependency* between the scale's characteristics and those of the sample: how much of a trait people have depends on the test, and the norms of the test depend on how much of the trait the people in the sample have. We can't totally ignore sample characteristics in IRT; if everyone has either a lot or a little of the attribute we're measuring, nothing can compensate for the information we don't have at the other end of the scale. But, as long as the entire range of trait is sampled, then the distribution doesn't matter, as it does in CTT.

The second problem with CTT is the assumption of *item equivalence*: that all of the items contribute equally to the total score, or that the total score on a scale is simply the sum of the individual items. So, even if we think one item may be a better indicator of a trait than another, we can't easily build this belief into the scale. Adding the items to create a total score presents another difficulty: we have to assume that the items are measured on an interval scale (that is, the increase between, say, a score of 1 and a score of 2 means the same as the increase between 7 and 8), though they rarely, if ever, are. In CTT, we deal with this problem in a not particularly sophisticated manner – we cover our eyes and hope it will go away (which it never does).

A third problem involves the *standard error of measurement* (SEM; which, to make life confusing, is also the abbreviation for the standard error of the mean and structural equation modelling – but not in this paper). Very briefly, the SEM can be defined as how much people's scores would change on repeated administrations of the scale because of its unreliability. In CTT, we have one estimate of the SEM for the whole scale, irrespective of any individual's specific score. We know this isn't right – scores at the extremes usually have more error associated with them than scores in the middle of the range – but it's the best we can do. So, we'll all cover our eyes yet again and play "let's pretend."

Item Response Theory

The solution to these difficulties can be found in IRT. As is true with many developments, different people were working on the problem simultaneously, in this case Allan Birnbaum in the US (Birnbaum, 1968) and Georg Rasch in Denmark (Rasch, 1960). The two weak assumptions of CTT are replaced by two 'hard' assumptions in IRT: the scale is unidimensional (that is, it measures only one trait or attribute); and that, at any given level of the trait, the probability of endorsing one item is unrelated to the probability of endorsing any other item (a property called *local independence*). In actuality, it's unusual to encounter local dependence outside of achievement tests (i.e., those that assess how well a person knows a subject), so it's rarely an issue. Unlike the weak assumptions of CTT, the hard assumptions are more difficult to meet, but you violate them at your peril; if they're not met, the results of the IRT analysis are meaningless.

If a scale meets these two assumptions, then we can draw an *item characteristic curve* (ICC) for each item. Let's start simply and deal with items that are answered on a dichotomy, such as true/false or yes/no; later, we'll talk about items that allow more response alternatives.

Fig. 25.1 Two item characteristic curves differing in terms of difficulty level

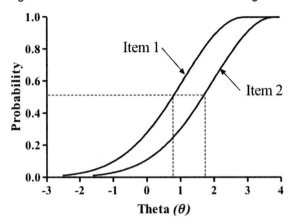

In Figure 25.1, the ICC shows the relationship between the amount of the trait (denoted by the Greek letter theta, θ) and the probability of endorsing the item. There are a few points to note about the ICC. First, θ is expressed very much like a standardized score; it has a mean of zero and a standard deviation of 1. If the trait that we're measuring is depression, then someone who is more depressed than average has a positive value of θ, and a negative score means that the person is less depressed than average. The second thing to note is the shape of the curve. The technical name for it is a *logistic function*; at the low end, increases in the trait result in only small increases in the probability of endorsing the item, and the same is true at the high end. In the middle, though, small increases in θ produce relatively large increases in the likelihood that a person will endorse the item. If we draw a horizontal line from the 50% probability mark to the ICCs and then drop a line down to the X-axis, we note a third property: the two items differ in terms of 'difficulty' (a term that's a holdover from IRT's origins in achievement testing). Item 2 is 'harder' than Item 1, because one needs more depression in order to endorse the item; that is, Item 2 taps more serious depression than does Item 1. Because the curves in Figure 25.1 differ from each other only in terms of difficulty, this is called the *one-parameter logistic model*, or 1PLM.

There are two other points to note about the ICCs in Figure 25.1. One is that when the trait has a value of around -3θ, the probability

Fig. 25.2 Two item characteristic curves differing
in terms of difficulty and discrimination

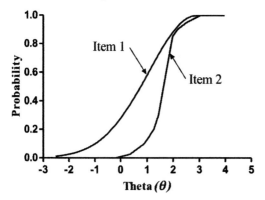

of endorsing the item is very close to zero. The second point is that the
curves are parallel; they don't differ from each other in terms of their
slope, reflecting the assumption in the 1PLM that all of the items discriminate equally. But neither of these points is an absolute requirement
of IRT. First, we can relax the requirement that the curves be parallel, as
in Figure 25.2. Since the curves can now differ in two respects – the difficulty and the slope – this is referred to as the *two-parameter logistic model*,
or 2PLM. The slopes reflect the discrimination ability of the item. Item 2
has a steeper slope than Item 1, indicating that it is a better discrimi-
nator, because the transition from not endorsing the item to endorsing
it is more acute. Thus, there is less ambiguity about the meaning of a
response: non-depressed people don't answer it and depressed people
do. Ideally, the curve would be perfectly vertical, but that's rarely seen.

The *three-parameter logistic model* (3PLM) does away with the requirement that the curve has to bottom out at a probability level of zero. This
is called the "guessing parameter," because it allows for the fact that, if a
person is unsure of an answer, he or she may guess at the right response.
Even though there may be some guessing (or random responding) that
takes place in mood and personality scales, the 3PLM is rarely used
apart from achievement testing. For the most part, mood and personality scales are constructed or modified using the 1PLM or 2PLM.

The ICCs that we've discussed so far apply to dichotomous items. In
fact, the original 1PLM, called the *Rasch model*, was developed for this
type of question, and it is a very useful technique. But, the real beauty

Fig. 25.3 Thresholds for a five-point Likert scale (SD = Strongly Disagree, D = Disagree, N = Neutral, A = Agree, SA = Strongly Agree)

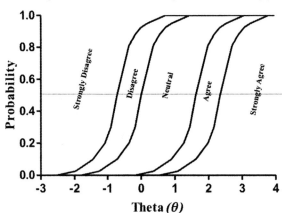

of IRT is in its application to items that are answered on a continuum, such as adjectival scales (for example, None, Somewhat, A Lot, A Great Deal) or Likert scales (for example, Strongly Disagree, Disagree, Neutral, Agree, Strongly Agree). (As an aside, do not pronounce his name "Like-urt"; it's "Lick-urt.") In CTT, we handle these items by continuing to play the game of "Let's pretend." In this case, the pretending is that the responses are equally spaced along the continuum, so that the amount that the trait increases as we move from Strongly Disagree to Disagree is the same as the increase between Disagree and Neutral (that is, that it is an interval scale). This allows us to blithely add up the responses to all of the items to arrive at a total score. With IRT, though, we can actually see if the response options are equally spaced and, even more important, whether all are useful.

In Figure 25.3, we've shown what looks like four ICCs from four dichotomous items. However, they are actually *threshold* curves for one item in a multi-item scale. They show where on the trait continuum there is a transition from answering with one response option to the next. For example, for values of θ less than −1, the most probable response is Strongly Disagree (SD); people whose θ levels are between −1 and −0.2 are most likely to answer Disagree. It can be seen from this diagram that the options aren't equally spaced along the trait continuum; the Strongly Disagree, Neutral, and Strongly Agree options seem to include more people than the Disagree and Agree ones. We get even more information

Fig. 25.4 Response curves for the item in Figure 25.3

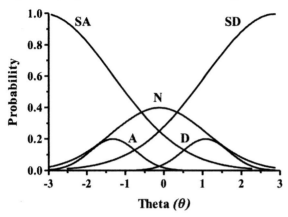

if we plot the *response curves* for this item, as in Figure 25.4. This figure shows the probability of giving each response for different values of θ. At any point along the X-axis, the sum of the probabilities is 1.0, because there is a 100% probability that the person will select one of the options. This figure tells us that the respondents aren't Canadian; they choose either the extreme options (Strongly Agree and Strongly Disagree) or the Neutral category, but not the wishy-washy Agree or Disagree. That means that we should either reduce the number of options to three or, if we want to maintain five choices, to be consistent with other items, we should combine Agree with Strongly Agree, and Disagree with Strongly Disagree when we score this item.

Another very useful bit of information we can derive with IRT is called *differential item functioning*, or DIF. Strictly speaking, if IRT is truly independent of the sample, then everyone should respond similarly to each item. However, there are times when the assumption breaks down, and the response depends not only on θ, but on some other dimension as well. For example, remember those math questions from school: "One train is travelling east at 50 km/hr. On the same track, another train is travelling west at 80 km/hr. If they start off 500 km from each other, how long will it be until they crash?" The ability to answer this question correctly depends on a person's ability in math (which is good), but is also a function of reading ability (which is bad, because it isn't what the test is supposed to measure). Within the context of IRT, DIF allows us to tell whether different groups respond to each item similarly or if there are differences in terms of difficulty or discriminating ability. This is very useful if we want to see if the items on the original and translated versions of a scale are performing equivalently. If a difference emerges, it may point to either problems in the translated item or cultural differences that affect how people respond to the content of the items (e.g., Azocar, Areán, Miranda, & Muñoz, 2001). We can also use DIF if we want to select items that are answered similarly by men and women or by other groups of people.

Finally, we can test the "fit" of each item. Fit statistics tell us two things: whether the items truly form a unidimensional scale and where on the θ scale each item belongs. Usually, before we do an IRT analysis, we factor analyse the items to test for unidimensionality. Ideally, what we will find is a very strong first factor, on which most of the items load (although no one quite knows what "a very strong first factor" actually means). Even so, there may still be items that really don't belong because they're not on the same dimension, and the fit statistic will flag them as a second check. Be careful, though: unidimensionality can be a slippery concept to pin down. Needless to say, if we're developing a scale to measure anxiety, for instance, we wouldn't want to include items that tap other constructs, such as demoralization or ego strength. But is anxiety itself uni- or multidimensional? As you're probably tired of hearing me say, "It all depends." What it depends on is how finely we want to measure it and for what purpose. If we were simply interested in screening people for the presence or absence of anxiety, we would likely look upon – and try to measure it – as a single dimension. However, if we wanted to know how different people experience anxiety, we might want to break down anxiety into its various components: physiological, behavioural, and cognitive symptoms. Now, anxiety would be seen as a multidimensional construct, and we would try to develop three sub-scales and have each of them unidimensional. So, the degree of unidimensionality that we want to achieve depends on the purpose of the scale; there are no ironclad rules that would obtain in all situations.

Being able to use the fit statistics to place the items along the θ continuum is useful for a number of purposes. Let's say that, after we run the program, we find that the 10 items in our scale, denoted by the letters A through J, are distributed as in Figure 25.5. What we would like to end up with are a small number of items that span the entire continuum and are about equally spread out along it. First, we see that items B and H have the same difficulty level, so we don't need both. Deciding which

Fig. 25.5 Items from a 10-item scale arranged along the θ continuum

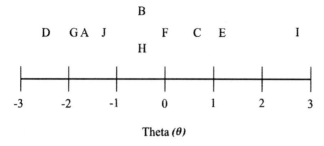

Theta (θ)

one to delete could be as simple as flipping a coin, or selecting the one that has better face validity, or (if we're using the 2PLM) choosing the one with better discriminating ability (that is, the steeper ICC). Similarly, items G and A are fairly close to one another, so we may decide one isn't necessary. Second, the scale has many items that are "easy" – that is, endorsed by people who have relatively low levels of the trait – and fewer more difficult items. Also, we also see a large gap between items E (with a level of θ just above 1) and I (just below 3). We may want to devise items with moderate difficulty levels to plug that gap and give us some more difficult ones. In this way, we can accomplish two goals: devising scales that are shorter than those derived using CTT and ensuring that the entire span of the trait is covered. By removing redundant items and those that detract from unidimensionality, IRT has been used quite successfully to shorten existing scales while still retaining – and in some cases, actually improving – their psychometric properties (e.g., Tang, Wong, Chiu, Lum, & Ungvari, 2005).

So, how many items are required to adequately cover the domain? Would you be surprised if the answer is "It all depends"? I didn't think so. How closely spaced the items should be is related to how the scale will be used. Some scales are used as screening instruments; for example, they may be given to patients in a family practitioner's office to determine if a more thorough investigation is needed, or to survey respondents to see if a section of a diagnostic questionnaire should be given. This was done with the Canadian Community Health Survey 1.2 (Gravel & Béland, 2005), for instance; those who endorsed a few key items about anxiety, depression, or substance abuse were then asked a more extensive series of questions to determine whether a disorder actually was present, while these more lengthy modules were skipped for people who did not endorse the items. In this way, people who did not have a specific disorder were spared the need to answer a long string of inapplicable questions. In this case, the screening test need have only a few items, and they would be clustered around the threshold value for 'caseness,' since this is the only region of the continuum we're interested in.

Conversely, if the scale is to be used to chart patients' improvement (or the lack of it) during treatment or as the result of some experimental intervention, we want a finer-grained tool, with the items spread out along the entire continuum. In fact, because IRT gives us the difficulty level for each item, it's a simple matter to construct different versions of the same scale by selecting items that meet our different needs.

The Uses of IRT

As mentioned, one of the most useful aspects of IRT is its ability to construct scales that are short but still reliable and valid, whether we do that *de novo* for a new scale, or by eliminating redundant items from existing ones. But there are other ways IRT is helpful. One is called *adaptive testing*. We all are accustomed to taking tests, not only in class, but also to get admitted to graduate or professional school, where we began with items that were so easy that they were laughable (at least to us) and then became so difficult that we feared for our future. The reason is that the test had to span the entire range of abilities of the test-takers, from those who have trouble filling in their name to the know-it-alls who know it all. But items that are far below or far above a person's ability level give us no useful information. The same is true for personality tests: items that tap low levels of the trait, such as introversion, are useless for people who have a lot of it, and vice versa. The most useful items are those near the middle, and these will vary from one individual to the next. In adaptive testing, the test administrator (which may be a computer) takes a guess at the person's ability level or selects an item whose θ level is near 0. If this item is passed, then it is unnecessary to give easier items; conversely, if it is failed, it would only frustrate the person to give more difficult ones. So, by choosing items judiciously, only a small proportion of all potential items need be given. Because all of the items have a value along the same θ continuum, people can be compared with one another even though each may have taken a different subset of questions. This approach is now used with individually administered tests, such as the PPVT (Dunn & Dunn, 2007), which taps receptive language in people ranging in age from 2.5 to over 90 years; with many high-stakes licensing examinations; and is being adapted for personality questionnaires (Forbey & Ben-Porath, 2007).

So Why Isn't IRT Used More?

Given all of these theoretical and practical advantages, it's fair to ask why scales are still being developed using CTT and why journals aren't replete with articles using IRT. In fact, some journals feature many such articles, but they are restricted mainly to the fields of education and personnel selection; those devoted to personality assessment have precious few that actually used IRT. The reasons for this are manifold. First, and most important, we cannot ignore one of the most powerful determinants of human behaviour – inertia. Only within the last decade have there been a significant number of people who were taught IRT in graduate school. The rest were trained in CTT, and it takes a lot of effort to change our ways. (As Max Planck may have said, "Science advances one funeral at a time.") Second, CTT is much simpler to understand than IRT; there aren't formidable-looking equations with exponentiations, Greek letters, and other arcane symbols. It's easier to comprehend one number for the SEM (even if it's wrong) than to calculate it for each individual score. Third, and equally important, all the most commonly used statistical software packages have modules that allow us to use CTT without thinking (which is the way most people seem to use them), whereas IRT requires stand-alone, and often expensive, computer programs with a fairly steep learning curve. This is much like growth curve analysis was 10 years ago. Now that it is part of readily available packages, its use has also followed a growth curve, and IRT more than likely will follow the same path.

Finally, although the 1PLM can be run with as few as 50 subjects if all the items are dichotomous, anything that complicates the model, such as using items with three or more response options or adding more parameters, increases the sample size considerably, far beyond what is needed in CTT or is available in most settings.

However, the question remains of whether IRT is really necessary in psychiatry and clinical psychology. Despite the admonition about the length of scales, in reality they are quite acceptable apart from their use in community surveys. They are not like licensing exams, which could involve hundreds of items and are ripe for shortening. Also unlike high-stakes test situations, it would be highly unusual for an examinee to bring suit against an organization because the test wasn't normed properly, so the financial incentive to use IRT isn't present in clinical testing situations. Last, our scales are at best ordinal in nature. Strictly speaking, we cannot say that a difference in 4 points at the low end is equivalent to a 4-point difference in the middle or at the upper end, and we *definitely* cannot say that a score of 10 is twice as much as one of 5. The best we can do is rank-order people on the basis of their scores – we know that a person whose BDI score is 15 is more depressed than someone whose score is 10. But we have lived with these limitations for 80 years or so, and CTT yields sufficient information about items for us to develop scales that are 'good enough.' The question remains of whether being able to devise scales that truly are interval in nature and whose psychometric properties are perhaps better described is worth the effort.

My feeling is that, now, the disincentives to adopt IRT more widely, combined with the lack of a pressing need to do so, means that we will likely not see a sudden growth in its use. But once programs become more widely available, cheaper, and easier to use, the balance will tip in the other direction and most new scales will be developed using this family of techniques.

REFERENCES

Azocar, F., Areán, P., Miranda, J., & Muñoz, R.F. (2001, Mar). Differential item functioning in a Spanish translation of the Beck Depression Inventory. *Journal of Clinical Psychology, 57*(3), 355–365. http://dx.doi.org/10.1002/jclp.1017 Medline:11241365

Beck, A.T., Steer, R.A., & Brown, G.K. (1996). *Manual for the Beck Depression Inventory-II*. San Antonio, TX: Psychological Corporation.

Birnbaum, A. (1968). Some latent trait models and their use in inferring an examinee's ability. In F.M. Lord & M.R. Novick (Eds.), *Statistical theories of mental test scores* (pp. 397–479). Reading, MA: Addison-Wesley.

Butcher, J.N., Dahlstrom, W.G., Graham, J.R., Tellegen, A., & Kaemmer, B. (1989). *Minnesota Multiphasic Personality Inventory-2: Manual for administration and scoring*. Minneapolis, MN: University of Minnesota Press.

Dunn, L.M., & Dunn, D.M. (2007). *The Peabody Picture Vocabulary Test*. (4th ed.). Bloomington, MN: NCS Pearson.

Embretson, S.E. (1996). The new rules of measurement. *Psychological Assessment, 8*(4), 341–349. http://dx.doi.org/10.1037/1040-3590.8.4.341

Forbey, J.D., & Ben-Porath, Y.S. (2007, Mar). Computerized adaptive personality testing: A review and illustration with the MMPI-2 Computerized Adaptive Version. *Psychological Assessment, 19*(1), 14–24. http://dx.doi.org/10.1037/1040-3590.19.1.14 Medline:17371120

Gravel, R., & Béland, Y. (2005, Sep). The Canadian Community Health Survey: Mental health and well-being. *Canadian Journal of Psychiatry, 50*(10), 573–579. Medline:16276847

Hambleton, S.E., & Swaminathan, H. (1985). *Item response theory: Principles and applications.* Boston: Kluwer Nijhoff.

Rasch, G. (1960). *Probabilistic models for some intelligence and attainment tests.* Copenhagen: Nielson and Lydiche.

Streiner, D.L. (1993, Mar). A checklist for evaluating the usefulness of rating scales. *Canadian Journal of Psychiatry, 38*(2), 140–148. Medline:8467441

Streiner, D.L. (2007, Jun). A shortcut to rejection: How not to write the results section of a paper. *Canadian Journal of Psychiatry, 52*(6), 385–389. Medline: 17696025

Streiner, D.L., & Norman, G.R. (2008). *Health measurement scales: A practical guide to their development and use.* (4th ed.). Oxford: Oxford University Press.

Tang, W.K., Wong, E., Chiu, H.F.K., Lum, C.M., & Ungvari, G.S. (2005, Aug). The Geriatric Depression Scale should be shortened: Results of Rasch analysis. *International Journal of Geriatric Psychiatry, 20*(8), 783–789. http://dx.doi.org/10.1002/gps.1360 Medline:16035120

TO READ FURTHER

Bond, T.G., & Fox, C.M. (2007). *Applying the Rasch model: Fundamental measurement in the human sciences.* (2nd ed.). Mahwah, NJ: Lawrence Erlbaum and Associates.

Embretson, S.E., & Reise, S.P. (2000). *Item response theory for psychologists.* Mahwah, NJ: Lawrence Erlbaum and Associates.

Streiner, D.L., & Norman, G.R. (2008). *Health measurement scales: A practical guide to their development and use.* (4th ed.). Oxford: Oxford University Press.

PART FIVE

Miscellaneous

26 Putting It All Together: Using Meta-Analysis in Psychiatric Research

DAVID L. STREINER, PH.D.

Canadian Journal of Psychiatry, 1991, 36, 357–362

This purpose of this chapter is to introduce some of the concepts of meta-analysis and to discuss a number of issues that must be addressed by those using these techniques or be considered by those who are reading the results of a meta-analysis. Glass, McGraw, and Smith (1981), who coined the term "meta-analysis," defined it as "nothing more than the attitude of data analysis applied to quantitative summaries of individual studies ... [It] is the statistical analysis of the summary findings of many empirical studies" (p. 217). Meta-analysis is not a radical departure from the usual methods of summarizing the research in a given field; rather, it is simply a more formal and, ideally, more objective way of doing so.

Reviews of any sort are necessary, since all too often the reader who is trying to make some sense of the literature is faced with the problem of having a number of studies which address the same issue but have different findings. Some articles may report a strong effect, others may indicate a much weaker one, and still others may conclude that there is either no effect or even an effect in the opposite direction. For example, Sobal and Stunkard (1989) reviewed the studies of the association between obesity and socioeconomic status (SES). Of the 27 articles using samples of men from the US, 12 articles reported an inverse correlation (that is, men of lower socio-economic status tended to weigh more), an equal number reported a direct association, and three found no relationship.

The question, then, is how to come to some conclusion regarding the weight of evidence. Traditionally, a reviewer relied on his or her subjective assessment of the various articles, placing more emphasis on some because of the reputation of the authors or the quality of the research and minimizing the importance of others because of these or other attributes of the article. Unfortunately, this approach is somewhat subjective; the results of a study may be discounted because they conflict with the existing biases of the reviewer. Needless to say, there is often disagreement over the conclusions reached by different reviewers in the same field. Oxman and Guyatt (1988), for example, pointed out that five reviews of the desirability of treating mild hypertension came to different conclusions. Similarly, Munsinger (1975) and Kamin (1978) reviewed the same group of articles on the effects of the environment on intelligence and reached opposite conclusions. Not surprisingly, their interpretations of the results coincided with beliefs they had expressed before their reviews. Despite this subjectivity, the conclusions of the "expert reviewer" are often taken as gospel and are enshrined in the annual reviews in most areas of medicine. One method of reducing subjectivity is by "vote counting," which compares the number of studies reporting results in one direction or the other. The Sobal and Stunkard review (1989) highlights one of the problems with this approach, which is simple and easy to understand: they found just as many studies reporting a positive relationship as a negative one.

There are a number of other shortcomings with this approach (Hedges & Olkin, 1980). First, vote counting does not take into account the strength of the relationship or the magnitude of the effect; one statistically significant result is assigned as much importance as another, although one could be only marginally significant and the other highly significant. It is possible that all of the studies reporting findings in one direction show a very strong association, while all of those which had results in the opposite direction may have shown only weak associations. A second problem is that vote counting may ignore important design features of the individual studies. It is generally assumed, for instance, that results from randomized controlled trials are more compelling than those from case control or cohort studies (Department of Clinical Epidemiology & Biostatistics, 1981), yet this is not taken into consideration when only the outcome is considered. A third problem is that results from studies with large samples are not given any more credence than those with small samples. As was pointed out in a previous essay in this series on research methods in psychiatry (Streiner, 1990; see Chapter 4), the absence of statistical significance can be due to an inadequate sample size. Vote counting does not differentiate between studies in which the lack of statistical significance may have been due to insufficient power and those which had sufficient power but still yielded negative results. In recent years, meta-analytic techniques have been used with increasing frequency, in the hope that its statistical approach would avoid the subjectivity of "expert reviews" and the shortcomings of vote counting. While meta-analyses were used as early as the 1930s, their popularity increased after Glass and his colleagues (Glass, 1976; Glass et al., 1981) used them to evaluate the effectiveness of psychotherapy (Smith & Glass, 1977). Since that time, literally hundreds of articles on meta-analysis have appeared in the literature in psychology, and the technique has been applied in medicine in areas ranging from the use of diuretics in pregnancy (Collins, Yusef, & Peto, 1985) to the effectiveness of anticoagulants in patients who have had myocardial infarctions (Chalmers, Matta, Smith, & Kunzler, 1977). Meta-analysis can also be used to combine the results of a number of trials which, individually, show no significant difference between treated and untreated groups and in which this lack of significance may have been due to an insufficient sample size (Streiner, 1990). Studies which have dichotomous outcomes and in which that outcome is rare (for example, death) often require well over 1,000 subjects in each group in order to detect significant differences. Many centres are unable to recruit sufficient numbers of patients. However, if most of the trials show a trend in the same direction, it is possible that combining their results may yield an overall significant result. Such was the case with 6 relatively large trials of ASA (Canner, 1983) and 13 trials of beta blockade (Peto, 1987) following a myocardial infarction.

Methods in Meta-Analysis

The Outcome

The choice of the outcome depends on whether it is continuous or dichotomous. In the case of continuous outcomes, such as the number of days in hospital or a score on a depression inventory, the results of the study can be converted to an effect size (ES; Streiner, 1990; see Chapter 4). For example, when the outcomes are the means of two groups, such as a treatment group and a control, the effect size is calculated using the formula

$$ES = \frac{\overline{X}_T - \overline{X}_C}{SD_C}. \tag{1}$$

Table 26.1 Results of a study with a dichotomous outcome

		Group treatment	Control
Outcome	Result X	A	B
	Result Y	C	D

In this formula, $\bar{X}_T$ is the mean value of the treatment group, $\bar{X}_C$ the mean of the control group, and SD_C the standard deviation of the control group. By converting all results to effect sizes, outcomes based on different scales or measured in different units can be compared. It is possible to convert other outcomes, such as proportions and correlations, to ESs: methods for doing so are explained by Glass et al. (1981).

In some studies, the outcome is dichotomous: the patient either did or did not develop side effects, was or was not readmitted to hospital, did or did not commit suicide, and so forth. In such cases, the results can be displayed in the form of a 2 × 2 table, as shown in Table 26.1. Cell A contains the number of subjects in the treatment group with outcome X, Cell B the number in the control group with outcome X, and so on. The temptation is to create one 2 × 2 summary table by simply adding the number of subjects in Cell A across all the studies and doing likewise for the remaining three cells.

However, combining results in such a manner implies that the subjects, treatments, and measurements of outcome were exactly comparable in all of the studies. We know that this is rarely, if ever, the case. For example, schizophrenics in an acute-care facility diagnosed with the aid of a structured interview like the Schedule for Affective Disorders and Schizophrenia (SADS; Endicott & Spitzer, 1978) differ in many ways from schizophrenics in a chronic hospital diagnosed after a clinical interview with a psychiatrist. Even an apparently straightforward outcome like readmission is defined differently from one facility to another, particularly if the patient had been on a leave of absence at the time he or she was readmitted. For these reasons, meta-analysis uses the results for each study and then combines them across studies. The method consists of calculating an odds ratio (OR) for each study. Using the nomenclature in Table 26.1, the OR is calculated as

$$OR = \frac{A \times D}{B \times C}. \tag{2}$$

The OR expresses how much more likely (or unlikely) an outcome is in one treatment group than another. For example, if the outcome being studied is the presence or absence of extrapyramidal side effects, an OR of 1.0 means that they are equally likely in both groups, while an OR of 2.0 indicates that the odds are 2 to 1 that they occur with treatment A than with treatment B. These ORs can now be handled like ESs; it is possible to calculate both the variance of the ORs across studies and the mean OR and to determine if this overall OR is significantly different from 1.0 (equivalent to testing whether a mean is different from zero).

Weighty Issues

However, simply using the raw ESs or ORs to calculate the mean effect size means that all of the studies contribute equally to the final result, because the sample sizes are not taken into account. That means that a study with 10 participants carries as much weight as one with 500. We solve this problem by weighting each study. It's possible to multiply each ES or OR by the sample size, but the usual approach is to use the reciprocal of the variance (Rosenthal & Rubin, 1982). Consequently, the smaller the variability and the larger the sample size for a particular study, the larger the weight and the more it contributes to the overall average.

Once this weighting is done, we can get the mean ES ($\overline{\text{ES}}$) by using the formula

$$\overline{\text{ES}} = \frac{\sum w_i \text{ES}_i}{\sum w_i},$$ [3]

which means that the ES for each study is multiplied by its weight and then everything is divided by the sum of the weights.

Looking for Differences

The next step is to calculate the variance of the ESs, giving some indication of the variability of the findings across studies (that is, the *heterogeneity*). The original statistic for this calculation is called Cochrane's Q, which is simply the squared difference between each study's ES and the overall $\overline{\text{ES}}$, again multiplied by the weight. The difficulty with Q is that it is very sensitive to the number of studies. If there are relatively few, Q won't be significant, even if the ESs differ considerably from one another. Conversely, if there are many studies, or if some of them are very large, Q may be statistically significant, even if the differences are trivial (Higgins, Thompson, Deeks, & Altman, 2003).

For these reasons, some people have advocated not bothering to do statistical tests for heterogeneity at all, but to simply quantify its extent (Thompson, 2001). We do this with the I^2 statistic, which quantifies the percentage of total variation across studies that is due to heterogeneity versus chance. A value of 0% indicates no heterogeneity, less than 25% indicates a small degree of heterogeneity, from 25% to 50% is moderate, and over 50% is large. However, I^2 has the same problem as Q in terms of low power when there are few studies (Huedo-Medina, Sánchez-Meca, Marín-Martínez, & Botella, 2006). Later, we'll discuss the implications of finding significant heterogeneity.

Explaining the Differences

If the reviewer were interested in determining the factors of the studies associated with larger or smaller ESs, he or she could proceed to the last step, which consists of computing a multiple-regression equation, using the ESs for each study as the dependent variable and various design factors of the studies as the predictor variables – a technique called *meta-regression*. For example, Smith and Glass (1977) tried to determine whether the magnitude of the effect of psychotherapy in different studies was due to the number of therapy sessions, the sample size, whether or not patients were assigned to the groups at random, and so forth; they found that none of these variables affected the magnitude of the outcome. On the other hand, Joffe, Sokolov, and Streiner (1996) found that one of the major predictors of the effectiveness of anti-depressants is how the patients were diagnosed: using a formal diagnostic framework or simply the psychiatrist's judgment. Bear in mind, though, that even when a meta-regression shows an association between some design features and the ES, the finding should be treated with caution. Like all post hoc analyses of data, meta-analysis used in this way is useful for hypothesis generation, but not for hypothesis testing.

Issues in Meta-Analysis

It may be thought that the statistical rigour introduced by meta-analytic techniques would result in a greater consensus among reviewers. However, this has not proven to be true. Abrami, Cohen and d'Apollonia (1988) found major differences among six meta-analytic reviews of the validity of student ratings of teaching effectiveness. Chalmers et al. (1987) reviewed all meta-analyses up to 1987 which included randomized controlled trials of therapeutic or diagnostic modalities and grouped them into "cohorts" of meta-analyses on the same topics. They found that 13 cohorts reached the same conclusions both statistically and clinically; 15 agreed statistically, but disagreed clinically; and 27 disagreed both clinically and statistically.

Why do these differences exist? The quality of the meta-analysis is highly dependent upon the quality of the articles reviewed and the amount of information culled from each article. In this section, we will discuss various decisions which the reviewer must make at each step of the process, based on recommendations by various authors (Abrami et al., 1988; Light & Pillemer, 1984).

Thoroughness of the Review

For the most part, the thoroughness of a review is not an issue; all relevant studies should be examined. In the following sections, we will discuss whether or not all these studies should be included in the final meta-analysis, but it is obvious that articles cannot be excluded on methodological or other grounds if they are not included in the review to begin with. The ideal starting place is a Medline search. It should be borne in mind, though, that despite popular beliefs to the contrary, two Medline searches using similar but not identical keywords may produce very different lists of articles, and it would not be surprising if neither caught more than 25% of the relevant articles (Dickersin, Hewitt, Mutch, Chalmers, & Chalmers, 1985; Haynes et al., 1985; Haynes et al., 1990). Consequently, the references cited in each article located through the searches must be checked to identify supplemental studies. It is also worthwhile to use other databases, such as Embase (with better coverage of the European literature), PsycINFO (psychological and psychiatric journals), ProQuest (theses and dissertations), and CINAHL (nursing).

However, not all studies are published, and there is considerable suspicion that articles with "negative findings" (that is, the null hypothesis is not rejected) are more common in the unpublished studies (Begg & Berlin, 1988; Greenwald, 1975; Hubbard & Armstrong, 1997). The effect of this is to overestimate the true effect size, since articles with an ES of around zero have been disproportionately excluded. One solution is to trace as many of these unpublished reports as possible. This may be feasible when there are only a few researchers in the field. Informal networks can be relied on to supply the names of most of the authors. However, it is often extremely difficult to contact all people who may have unpublished reports lying around.

A different approach has been suggested by Rosenthal (1979). He advocates calculating the number of articles with non-significant results, which would have to be tucked away in file drawers in order to make a significant summary ES no longer significant – what he calls the "file drawer problem." The fewer studies needed to achieve this result, the more questionable the results of the meta-analysis.

Similarity of Patients and Treatments

In trying to summarize the effectiveness of, for example, antidepressant medication for the treatment of panic disorders, should the review include all studies which used antidepressants or just those which used tricyclic antidepressants (TCAs)? Should the articles be limited to those which excluded patients with concomitant disorders, or should it include any study which involved patients with panic disorder, regardless of other diagnoses they may have had?

The "exclusionists" (Light, 1987; Presby, 1978) would limit the meta-analysis to studies using similar therapies with similar patients. To do otherwise, they argue, would be like comparing apples and oranges; it would be impossible to determine which treatment made the difference and on whom. Furthermore, if, for example, TCAs were effective but MAOIs were not, the negative findings might dilute the overall ES, leading to the erroneous conclusion that nothing works, or that the treatment works only marginally.

The "inclusionists," on the other hand, raise three counter arguments (Glass, 1976; Smith & Glass, 1977). First, how similar is similar? While TCAs may be more like one another than they are to MAOIs, even they differ among themselves, some are quite effective (Ballenger et al., 1988; Gorman et al., 1987), and others are totally ineffective. Even if the review were limited to studies of only one drug, these might vary with respect to the dosage and other factors. At what point do we say that the studies are close enough? Exact replicates are quite rare, and heterogeneity in treatments and patients allows the results to be generalized to a greater extent. If the results of the meta-analysis is positive, they would apply to a larger number of conditions treated in a variety of ways. The third, and possibly most cogent, argument is that it is possible to code these design features. It would then be possible to determine, through multiple-regression or some other statistical technique, whether the magnitude of the result is dependent on the type of intervention or the type of patient.

The resolution to this problem is that the "correct" approach depends on the purpose of the meta-analysis. If the purpose is to determine whether or not any medications work for patients suffering from panic disorders who may walk through a clinic's door, the scope of the review would include all treatments and all patients who receive medication in actual practice. Ideally, there would be sub-analyses to see whether some drugs were more effective than others and some patients helped more than others. However, if the aim of the review is to see whether or not there is sufficient evidence for treating non-depressed panic patients with TCAs, the articles included would have a much narrower focus.

Quality of the Research

In their meta-analysis, Smith and Glass (1977) included all articles on the effects of psychotherapy, regardless of the methodology used. They defend their position on both logical and empirical grounds (Glass, 1976). Their logical argument is that if there are 50 studies in one field, it is unlikely that all 50 are flawed in the same way: some may have problems with sampling criteria, but be strong in other respects; others may have analysed their data incorrectly, but otherwise be well done; and so on. Thus, the majority of studies will have adequate sampling strategies, data analyses and designs, and, in general, they will have met the criteria for sound methodology. Smith and Glass feel it is improbable under these circumstances that the results of the meta-analysis would have been seriously biased by the studies with poor methodologies. The empirical argument, which appears to carry more weight, is that effect sizes based only on well-designed studies differ by less than 0.1 standard deviation from that derived from all studies, regardless of the methodology used (Landman & Dawes, 1982).

Critics of this approach, who appear to be in the majority, cite the dictum of computer programmers, "garbage in, garbage out." If the individual studies are flawed, then, of necessity, the conclusions must be flawed. The critics cite numerous studies which show that the magnitude of an effect is inversely related to the rigour of the methodology; the large treatment gains reported in uncontrolled trials diminish or even disappear under the scrutiny of well-controlled studies in areas ranging from the treatment of angina (Benson & McCallie, 1979) and respiratory distress syndrome (Sinclair, 1966) to the effectiveness of creativity training programs (Mansfield & Busse, 1977). Perhaps the most extreme position is that of Slavin (1986), who argues that meta-analyses should be based only on the most reliable evidence.

Most current meta-analyses have taken one of two middle positions: relaxing strict methodological criteria while not including studies which are fatally flawed or evaluating the rigour of each study. Using systems such as that developed by Chalmers et al. (1977) for randomized controlled trials, each study could either be weighted according to its adherence to various methodological criteria (Rosenthal, 1991), or the scores could be correlated with the effect size to determine if ES goes up when standards go down.

Number of Outcomes per Study

Smith and Glass (1977) included all outcomes in their meta-analysis, even when there was more than one outcome per study. This approach has been roundly criticized by some on a number of grounds (Abrami et al., 1988; Bangert-Drowns, 1986). First, most statistical tests assume that the units of analysis are independent. This assumption is violated if some of the ESs are based on the same subjects who have undergone the same treatment. Second, it is possible that a small number of studies with many outcomes may contribute disproportionately to the final result. One review, for example, found that 73% of all ESs in one meta-analysis came from only 29% of the studies (Educational Research Service, 1980). If these studies differed in some systematic way from the majority, they could possibly have biased the overall findings.

There are a number of problems with blithely tossing out results. To begin with, unless the authors have indicated their primary outcome measures (rarely done), it is difficult to decide which one to retain. This opens the meta-analysis up to a degree of subjectivity: one reviewer may select an outcome which shows a large effect, while another reviewer of the same article, perhaps operating with a different bias, may choose another outcome which indicates a small or negative effect. Finally, many studies use more complicated factorial designs; here, each outcome may be based on different combinations of subjects who have had different mixtures of therapies. Each of the resulting outcomes is meaningful in its own right and yields different information regarding the effectiveness of treatment under varying circumstances.

The recent trend is to consider all outcomes, but to combine them in some way so that there is a global estimate for each study (Rosenthal & Rubin, 1986; Strube, 1985). The result is that no information is lost and, at the same time, all the ESs in the final analysis are independent.

Handling Significant Variance in ESs

As mentioned above, one of the first analyses usually consists of a check for homogeneity to determine whether or not all of the individual studies have similar results. The problem is what to do if the analysis shows that the individual results are heterogeneous. Some authors (e.g., Abrami et al., 1988; L'Abbé, Detsky, & O'Rourke, 1987) state that a meta-analysis should not be done under these circumstances. They hold that this variability reflects some underlying systematic difference among the studies, such as the type of treatment given or the outcome. Under such circumstances, they recommend clustering the studies into homogeneous groups and analysing each separately.

Needless to say, there is an opposing view (Bangert-Drowns, 1986; Hunter, Schmidt, & Jackson 1983). These authors feel that the behaviour of the statistics underlying meta-analysis are not well understood, especially when the number of studies is relatively small, and that the practical utility of the clustering approach is limited. This point is still being debated.

If heterogeneity does exist, the most prudent advice may be to determine its cause, using, for example, the possible reasons outlined by Oxman and Guyatt (1988): variation in study design and differences in the population, treatment, or outcome. If it is likely that the heterogeneity reflects significant and systematic differences among factors which may be important determinants of the outcome, clustering them is justified. This is especially true if the aim of the meta-analysis is data pooling – that is, combining non-significant results from many studies to see if there is an overall effect. Significant variation in the magnitude of the outcomes may indicate that the studies are looking at different treatments or patients, so that the meta-analysis would indeed be comparing apples and oranges. However, if the aim of the analysis is to arrive at some overall conclusion regarding the effectiveness of therapy based on studies with conflicting results and the variation reflects differences seen in clinical practice, it may be wise to ignore the heterogeneity and proceed directly to the meta-analysis.

Software

Recommending, or even listing, software packages that will do the heavy lifting in meta-analysis is a risky business, because companies come and go with amazing rapidity. Even doing a Web search will lead to many broken links and pages that haven't been maintained for a while. There are many dedicated, commercial programs available, and most statistical programs, such as SPSS and Stata, have modules that can be used. If you already have one of these programs, then you're set. (If you can't find the right commands, it may be because there's an additional module you must download; most are free.) If you don't have such a program, my suggestion would be to use RevMan – it's comprehensive, continuously updated by the Cochrane Collaboration (one of the leading groups that publishes meta-analyses), and, best of all, it's freely available at http://ims.cochrane.org/revman. The learning curve becomes more and more gentle with each revision, and now it can almost be described as user-friendly – almost, but not quite. However, the people who run the site are quite friendly and helpful.

Summary

Meta-analysis is a powerful set of techniques for the systematic synthesis of results from many studies. However, the methods are not well defined; decisions must be made at every step of the process, from finding and selecting the studies to determining which outcomes to include. Each of these decisions can affect both the quality of the analysis and the results obtained. The reviewer must be aware of these alternatives and sensitive to their consequences.

ACKNOWLEDGMENTS

The author wishes to thank Drs. Andrew Oxman, Gordon Guyatt, and John Hay for their extremely helpful comments on an earlier draft of this chapter.

REFERENCES

Abrami, P.C., Cohen, P.A., & d'Apollonia, S. (1988). Implementation problems in meta-analysis. *Review of Educational Research, 58*, 151–179.

Ballenger, J.C., Burrows, G.D., DuPont, R.L., Jr., Lesser, I.M., Noyes, R., Jr., Peck-
nold, J.C., ..., & Swinson, R.P. (1988, May). Alprazolam in panic disorder
and agoraphobia: Results from a multicenter trial. I. Efficacy in short-term
treatment. *Archives of General Psychiatry, 45*(5), 413–422. http://dx.doi.
org/10.1001/archpsyc.1988.01800290027004 Medline:3282478

Bangert-Drowns, R.L. (1986). Review of developments in meta-analytic
method. *Psychological Bulletin, 99*(3), 388–399. http://dx.doi.org/10.1037/
0033-2909.99.3.388

Begg, C.B., & Berlin, J.A. (1988). Publication bias: A problem in interpreting
medical data. *Journal of the Royal Statistical Society A, 151*(3), 419–463. http://
dx.doi.org/10.2307/2982993

Benson, H.L., & McCallie, D.P., Jr. (1979, Jun 21). Angina pectoris and the
placebo effect. *New England Journal of Medicine, 300*(25), 1424–1429. http://
dx.doi.org/10.1056/NEJM197906213002508 Medline:35750

Canner, P.L. (1983, May). Aspirin in coronary heart disease. Comparison of
six clinical trials. *Israel Journal of Medical Sciences, 19*(5), 413–423. Medline:
6345461

Chalmers, T.C., Berrier, J., Sacks, H.S., Levin, H., Reitman, D., & Nagalingam,
R. (1987, Oct-Nov). Meta-analysis of clinical trials as a scientific disci-
pline. II: Replicate variability and comparison of studies that agree and
disagree. *Statistics in Medicine, 6*(7), 733–744. http://dx.doi.org/10.1002/
sim.4780060704 Medline:3423497

Chalmers, T.C., Matta, R.J., Smith, H., Jr., & Kunzler, A.M. (1977, Nov 17).
Evidence favoring the use of anticoagulants in the hospital phase of acute
myocardial infarction. *New England Journal of Medicine, 297*(20), 1091–1096.
http://dx.doi.org/10.1056/NEJM197711172972004 Medline:909566

Chalmers, T.C., Smith, H., Jr., Blackburn, B., Silverman, B., Schroeder, B.,
Reitman, D., & Ambroz, A. (1981). A method for assessing the quality of a
randomized control trial. *Controlled Clinical Trials, 2*, 31–49. Medline:7261638

Collins, R., Yusuf, S., & Peto, R. (1985, Jan 5). Overview of randomised trials
of diuretics in pregnancy. *British Medical Journal, 290*(6461), 17–23. http://
dx.doi.org/10.1136/bmj.290.6461.17 Medline:3917318

Department of Clinical Epidemiology and Biostatistics. (1981, Apr 15). How to
read clinical journals: IV. To determine etiology or causation. *Canadian Medical Association Journal, 124*(8), 985–990. Medline:7260801

Dickersin, K., Hewitt, P., Mutch, L., Chalmers, I., & Chalmers, T.C. (1985).
Perusing the literature: Comparison of MEDLINE searching with a perinatal trials database. *Controlled Clinical Trials, 6*(4), 306–317. http://dx.doi.
org/10.1016/0197-2456(85)90106-0 Medline:3907973

Educational Research Service. (1980). Class size research: A critique of recent
meta-analyses. *Phi Delta Kappan, 62*, 239–241.

Endicott, J., & Spitzer, R.L. (1978, Jul). A diagnostic interview: The Schedule for Affective Disorders and Schizophrenia. *Archives of General Psychiatry*, *35*(7), 837–844. http://dx.doi.org/10.1001/archpsyc.1978.01770310043002 Medline: 678037

Glass, G.V. (1976). Primary, secondary, and meta-analysis research. *Educational Researcher*, *5*, 3–8.

Glass, G.V., McGaw, B., & Smith, M.L. (1981). *Meta-analysis in social research*. Beverley Hills, CA: Sage.

Gorman, J.M., Liebowitz, M.R., Fyer, A.J., Goetz, D., Campeas, R.B., Fyer, M.R., …, & Klein, D.F. (1987, Oct). An open trial of fluoxetine in the treatment of panic attacks. *Journal of Clinical Psychopharmacology*, *7*(5), 329–331. http://dx.doi.org/10.1097/00004714-198710000-00007 Medline:3500189

Greenwald, A. (1975). Consequences of prejudices against the null hypothesis. *Psychological Bulletin*, *82*(1), 1–20. http://dx.doi.org/10.1037/h0076157

Haynes, R.B., McKibbon, K.A., Walker, C.J., Ryan, N., Fitzgerald, D., & Ramsden, M.F. (1990, Jan 1). Online access to MEDLINE in clinical settings. A study of use and usefulness. *Annals of Internal Medicine*, *112*(1), 78–84. Medline:2403476

Haynes, R.B., McKibbon, K.A., Walker, C.J., Mousseau, J., Baker, L.M., Fitzgerald, D., …, & Norman, G.R. (1985, Nov). Computer searching of the medical literature. An evaluation of MEDLINE searching systems. *Annals of Internal Medicine*, *103*(5), 812–816. Medline:3901853

Hedges, L.V., & Olkin, I. (1980). Vote counting methods in research synthesis. *Psychological Bulletin*, *88*(2), 359–369. http://dx.doi.org/10.1037/0033-2909.88.2.359

Higgins, J.P.T., Thompson, S.G., Deeks, J.J., & Altman, D.G. (2003, Sep 6). Measuring inconsistency in meta-analyses. *BMJ (Clinical Research Ed.)*, *327*(7414), 557–560. http://dx.doi.org/10.1136/bmj.327.7414.557 Medline:12958120

Hubbard, R., & Armstrong, J.S. (1997). Publication bias against null results. *Psychological Reports*, *80*, 337–338.

Huedo-Medina, T.B., Sánchez-Meca, J., Marín-Martínez, F., & Botella, J. (2006, Jun). Assessing heterogeneity in meta-analysis: Q statistic or I^2 index? *Psychological Methods*, *11*(2), 193–206. http://dx.doi.org/10.1037/1082-989X.11.2.193 Medline:16784338

Hunter, J.E., Schmidt, F.L., & Jackson, G.B. (1983). *Meta-analysis: Cumulating research findings across studies*. Beverley Hill, CA: Sage.

Joffe, R., Sokolov, S., & Streiner, D.L. (1996). Antidepressant treatment of depression: A meta-analysis. *Canadian Journal of Psychiatry*, *41*, 613–616.

Kamin, L.J. (1978). Comment on Munsinger's review of adoption studies. *Psychological Bulletin*, *85*(1), 194–201. http://dx.doi.org/10.1037/0033-2909.85.1.194

L'Abbé, K.A., Detsky, A.S., & O'Rourke, K. (1987, Aug). Meta-analysis in clinical research. *Annals of Internal Medicine, 107*(2), 224–233. Medline:3300460

Landman, J.T., & Dawes, R.M. (1982, May). Psychotherapy outcome. Smith and Glass' conclusions stand up under scrutiny. *American Psychologist, 37*(5), 504–516. http://dx.doi.org/10.1037/0003-066X.37.5.504 Medline:7125329

Light, R.J. (1987, Apr-May). Accumulating evidence from independent studies: What we can win and what we can lose. *Statistics in Medicine, 6*(3), 221–228. http://dx.doi.org/10.1002/sim.4780060304 Medline:3303250

Light, R.J., & Pillemer, D.B. (1984). *Summing up: The science of reviewing research.* Cambridge, MA: Harvard University Press.

Mansfield, R.S., & Busse, T.V. (1977). Meta-analysis of research: A rejoinder to Glass. *Educational Researcher, 6,* 3.

Munsinger, H. (1975). The adopted child's IQ: A critical review. *Psychological Bulletin, 82*(5), 623–659. http://dx.doi.org/10.1037/0033-2909.82.5.623

Oxman, A.D., & Guyatt, G.H. (1988, Apr 15). Guidelines for reading literature reviews. *Canadian Medical Association Journal, 138*(8), 697–703. Medline:3355948

Peto, R. (1987, Apr-May). Why do we need systematic overviews of randomized trials? *Statistics in Medicine, 6*(3), 233–244. http://dx.doi.org/10.1002/sim.4780060306 Medline:3616281

Presby, S. (1978). Overly broad categories obscure important differences between therapies. *American Psychologist, 33*(5), 514–515. http://dx.doi.org/10.1037/0003-066X.33.5.514

Rosenthal, R. (1979). The "file drawer problem" and tolerance for null results. *Psychological Bulletin, 86*(3), 638–641. http://dx.doi.org/10.1037/0033-2909.86.3.638

Rosenthal, R. (1991). *Meta-analytic procedures for social research.* Beverley Hills, CA: Sage.

Rosenthal, R., & Rubin, D.B. (1982). Comparing effect sizes of independent studies. *Psychological Bulletin, 92*(2), 500–504. http://dx.doi.org/10.1037/0033-2909.92.2.500

Rosenthal, R., & Rubin, D.B. (1986). Meta-analytic procedures for combining studies with multiple effect sizes. *Psychological Bulletin, 99*(3), 400–406. http://dx.doi.org/10.1037/0033-2909.99.3.400

Sinclair, J.C. (1966, Aug). Prevention and treatment of the respiratory distress syndrome. *Pediatric Clinics of North America, 13*(3), 711–730. Medline:5949900

Slavin, R.E. (1986). Best-evidence synthesis: An alternative to meta-analytic and traditional reviews. *Educational Researcher, 15,* 5–11.

Smith, M.L., & Glass, G.V. (1977, Sep). Meta-analysis of psychotherapy outcome studies. *American Psychologist, 32*(9), 752–760. http://dx.doi.org/10.1037/0003-066X.32.9.752 Medline:921048

Sobal, J., & Stunkard, A.J. (1989, Mar). Socioeconomic status and obesity: A review of the literature. *Psychological Bulletin, 105*(2), 260–275. http://dx.doi.org/10.1037/0033-2909.105.2.260 Medline:2648443

Streiner, D.L. (1990, Oct). Sample size and power in psychiatric research. *Canadian Journal of Psychiatry, 35*(7), 616–620. Medline:2268843

Strube, M.J. (1985). Combining and comparing significance levels from non-independent hypothesis tests. *Psychological Bulletin, 97*(2), 334–341. http://dx.doi.org/10.1037/0033-2909.97.2.334

Thompson, S.G. (2001). Why and how sources of heterogeneity should be investigated. In M. Egger, G.D. Smith, & D.G. Altman (Eds.), *Systematic reviews in health care: Meta-analysis in context* (pp. 157–175). London: BMJ Publishing House. http://dx.doi.org/10.1002/9780470693926.ch9

TO READ FURTHER

Egger, M., Smith, G.D., & Altman, D.G. (Eds.). (2001). *Systematic reviews in health care: Meta-analysis in context.* London: BMJ Books. http://dx.doi.org/10.1002/9780470693926

Glass, G.V., McGaw, B., & Smith, M.L. (1981). *Meta-analysis in social research.* Beverley Hills, CA: Sage.

Hunter, J.E., Schmidt, F.L., & Jackson, G.B. (1983). *Meta-analysis: Cumulating research findings across studies.* CA: Beverley Hill.

27 "While you're up, get me a grant": A Guide to Grant Application Writing

DAVID L. STREINER, PH.D.

Canadian Journal of Psychiatry, 1996, *41*, 137–143

In the best of all possible worlds, we would have a brilliant idea that cries out for a study, we would spend a leisurely afternoon writing a brief proposal stating what we want to do, and the granting agency would then send us a cheque, asking merely that we acknowledge them in a footnote when the resulting papers are published. (Or, to plagiarize a 1970s ad for Scotch whisky, it would be as simple as saying to a friend, "While you're up, get me a Grant's.") Sad to relate, this is not the best of all possible worlds. Almost all agencies get requests for far more money than they have to disburse, and your proposal is just one among many competing for these scarce resources. Another unfortunate fact of life is that your success depends as much on how you present your ideas as on what you want to investigate. Knowing how agencies operate and what the reviewers look for will improve your chances of being among the fortunate few who get over all the hurdles. In this chapter, I will outline the general procedures that are followed by the major agencies and give some tips regarding what should and should not be in the proposal.

Standard Operating Procedures

It often seems that you rush to meet the agency's deadline, only to find that there is an interminable period when nothing happens before you get a letter telling you of the outcome. In fact, a lot does go on behind the scenes. Each agency follows a different set of procedures, but there are elements common to all of them. The first step for the larger agencies, such as the Canadian Institutes for Health Research (CIHR) or the Social Sciences and Humanities Research Council (SSHRC), is that the proposal is assigned to one of a number of review committees. This choice may be based on the judgment of the staff who read the abstracts, or you may be given the option of selecting the committee yourself (as at CIHR). Smaller agencies, which do not have a large number of grants to review, may have only one review panel.

The proposal can then be sent to two to five *external reviewers*. Although you may be asked to suggest some names, the agency is not bound to use these persons or to limit itself to the people on the list. In recent years, it has become increasing difficult to find people willing to serve as external reviewers, so this step is (sadly) sometimes omitted. However, it is still extremely important to bear in mind who these reviewers are and why they were selected. Some of them may be experts in the content area, and they are asked to comment on your grasp of the field, your knowledge of recent developments, and the importance or significance of the topic. Other external reviewers may be sent the protocol because they have expertise in research methodology, statistics, or a specific technique you are using. These people may know nothing about your content area, which has implications for the language you use, a point we will return to later.

Sometime afterwards, the committee meets as a whole. Each application will have been assigned to two or more members, who are known as the *internal reviewers*. These people are charged with the task of conducting and writing up an in-depth review of your proposal. They will see and use the reports of the external reviewers (if any, and if they have returned their reviews in time). The usual procedure is that the lead reviewer reads out his or her review. The second reviewer then comments on any additional points, following which the discussion is thrown open for the other committee members to have their say. At the end of the discussion, the two internal reviewers are requested to assign a numerical or letter grade, and then all the other members write down the score they have decided to give the proposal. In some agencies, the other members can give any score they wish; in others, they are constrained to be within a certain range of the internal reviewers' grade.

There are a number of aspects of this process that are worth noting because they can be potential traps for the unwary. First, some agencies have altered the procedure in an attempt to deal with the increasing load. The change is that the internal reviewers are asked, before reading out their critiques, what the bottom line is: fund or reject. If both reviewers say reject (the euphemism used by some agencies, such as CIHR, is "triage"), and no one else on the committee disagrees (and we'll soon see why there rarely are disagreements at this stage), then the lead reviewer gives only a brief outline of the "fatal flaws," and the committee moves on to the next proposal. So, you cannot rely on protracted deliberation by this panel of sages to recognize the worth of your ideas and rescue your proposal from oblivion; if you have not made the case strongly yourself, it will not be made by someone else.

Second, you have to bear in mind the situation of the internal reviewers. The agencies are very astute: the request for us to sit on the committee comes during slack times of the year, usually six months or so before the meeting. We are flattered by the recognition, and, unable to believe that this period of relative ease will ever end, agree to serve. Six months later, just when we are at our busiest trying to get our own grants into the mail, a delivery person arrives at our door lugging a box large enough to house two elephants, a washing machine, and a compact car. Inside are the dozen or so grant proposals for which we are the primary or secondary internal reviewer and all of the others the committee must deal with. (Nowadays, this box has been replaced by a single CD, but the workload remains identical.) We are asked to prepare written comments on "our" grant applications and to read all of the other ones so that we can honestly participate in the discussions. So, while all applicants hope that theirs is reviewed by a person who has nothing else on his or her mind except to read carefully every word in the body of the proposal and all of the appendices, in truth it will be looked at as one of a score of proposals, read at night when we would much prefer to be working on our own application or simply relaxing and watching TV.

Third, and the reason why objections to the "reject" decision are relatively infrequent, is that each reviewer barely has time to complete his or her written reviews, much less read the texts of applications assigned to other members of the committee. If the proposal is even read, most likely only the summary is looked at, which means that it may be the most important part; we'll return to this point later, when we discuss the various parts of the proposal.

Last, the internal reviews are written prior to the meeting. It sometimes happens, then, that these reviews are positive, but the ultimate decision is rejection. This can occur if the discussion around the table reveals flaws missed by the internal reviewers; although you may be disappointed by this development, don't be surprised. Indeed, in my 35+ years of serving on committees, I have found that it is often the case that good initial reviews get downgraded, but only very rarely do bad ones become more positive.

The Parts of the Grant

Before getting down to the various components of the proposal, we should discuss one aspect of it which pertains to all parts. The protocol has two purposes, one overt and one covert. The overt task of the application is to tell the reviewers what you want to do, why it is important, and how you will carry it out. The other, covert task, which is rarely acknowledged, is to convince the reviewers that you are able to carry out the research; this is particularly important for young researchers who do not have established track records they can put before the review panel in terms of previous grants they have completed or peer-reviewed papers they have published. When running a study, the issue is not whether things will go wrong, but rather how many and which ones will fail. Subjects will be lost to follow-up, forget to take the trial medication or be given it by mistake when they are in the placebo group, vials of blood will be misplaced or dropped, and results of assays will get lost in the mail. You have to demonstrate to the internal and external reviewers that these inevitable mishaps will not derail the whole project, that you and your collaborators are aware that they will happen, and that you have the expertise to account for them in the analyses.

In a similar vein, all research, especially when it uses human participants and most particularly when it uses patients, involves compromises. The ideal design may be infeasible because of logistics, the most precise assay or interview schedule may be too costly, or the best control group may be too difficult to recruit. When you are forced to make major concessions, let the reviewers know. If you do not spell out your reasoning, the reviewers may conclude that you are not aware of the problems and thus lose confidence in your ability. On the other hand, if you make your reasons clear, they may disagree with your choice, but they will be more inclined to offer suggestions about how to modify the proposal, rather than to reject it outright.

Now let's turn to the individual sections. Table 27.1 provides a "checklist" of the key elements, which are described in more detail in the text. In referring to this table, keep two things in mind. First, the elements apply primarily to quantitative research proposals; qualitative studies have different criteria. Second, not all of the elements are germane for every study; if you're doing a survey to estimate the prevalence of a disorder or to see the relationship among different variables, for example, you're not too concerned about spelling out hypotheses a priori, or you may not need control groups.

All too often, the "Summary" is written as an afterthought and at the last moment. This usually happens when the application is just about to go out the door, and the investigator suddenly realizes that there is one more box to fill in. This is a mistake of the first order; for the reasons outlined previously, the summary may be the only part of the grant that is read by all of the members of the committee, not just the reviewers. If they are going to join in the discussion and either leap to your defence or roundly criticize your ideas, it will be on the basis of reading only the summary. So put as much time and thought into the "Summary" as into the other sections.

Introduction

The "Introduction" sets the stage for everything that follows. Much has to be conveyed at both an overt and a covert level in a relatively small number of pages. The primary task is to indicate what the objectives are – what you are interested in and why. You also have to indicate why the problem is an important one; a study can be well designed, but if all it elicits in the reviewers are yawns, your chances of having it funded are not good. Simply stating that no one has looked at this issue before doesn't suffice; there may be very good reasons that nobody is interested in the question, including that no one cares what the answer is. The statement of objectives has to be buttressed by a literature review that achieves a balance between being comprehensive on the one hand, yet brief enough to allow sufficient room for the other sections of the proposal on the other. The review itself has to satisfy a number of criteria. First, it must be up to date; if the most recent publication cited is five years old, it's a sign to the reviewers that you have not been keeping up with the literature. If you are resubmitting a previously rejected proposal, be sure to update your review with any significant publications that may have appeared since the previous application. Second, the review must mention the important articles in the field; the covert message you are trying to get across is that you know the area and the key issues. It is good to mention your own publications, but not to the

Table 27.1 A checklist for writing grant applications

1. Summary
2. Introduction
   A. Are the objectives clear?
   B. Is the problem significant?
   C. Is the literature review
      i.   Up to date?
      ii. Comprehensive?
      iii. Balanced?

3. Methods
   A. Design
      i.   Is the design clearly specified?
      ii. Is the design the most rigorous one possible?
      iii. Does it adequately test the hypotheses?
      iv. Are the appropriate control or comparison groups included?
      v.   Are potential confounding variables acknowledged?
   B. Participants
      i.   Are the inclusion and exclusion criteria stated?
      ii. Are these criteria necessary and sufficient?
      iii. Are the sampling procedures described?
      iv. Will the sampling ensure representativeness?
      v.   Have you justified the sample size?
      vi. Are sufficient numbers of participants (especially patients) available?
   C. Procedure
      i.   Are the procedures described in detail?
      ii. Are the dependent variables fully described?
      iii. Do the measures relate to the hypotheses?
      iv. Is the timeline realistic?

4. Data Analysis
   A. Are the exact statistical procedures described?
   B. Does each analysis relate to a hypothesis?
   C. Are the assumptions of the tests met by the data?
   D. Are you aware of potential pitfalls, such as
      i.   Missing data
      ii. Deviations from normality

5. Relevance
   A. Have you explained the relevance of this topic?
   B. Is it relevant for this agency?

6. Budget
   A. Are monies allocated for:
      i.   Research staff plus benefits?

(Continued)

      ii. Graduate students plus benefits?
      iii. Supplies?
      iv. Printing of forms?
      v. Travel for subjects?
      vi. Payment for subjects?
      vii. Travel to conferences?
   B. Have all expenses been justified?
   C. Are all categories allowed by the agency?

7. Appendices
   A. Copies of scales and questionnaires
   B. Institutional approvals
      i. Human ethics
      ii. Animal ethics and care
      iii. Radiation protection
      iv. Biohazards
      v. Investigational drugs
   C. Support from collaborating units or labs
   D. Letters from consultants

exclusion of other players; be humble (and realistic) – you are likely not the only person to have had these brilliant insights. Third, the review must be balanced. If there are authors whose theories or findings are opposite to your own, do not pretend they do not exist. Assume that at least one of the reviewers knows the field better than you do; he or she will notice the omission and attribute it to either your stupidity or your cupidity, and you do not want either label.

The section should end with a clear and simply worded description of your hypotheses or the questions you are looking at. Statisticians like to phrase issues in terms of the null hypothesis (that is, there is no difference between treatments or groups). Do not do this in the application; state what you hope to find, not your worst fantasies.

Methods

The "Methods" portion of the grant usually has a number of subsections. A good place to start is with the "Design," where you spell out whether you will be doing a randomized controlled trial (RCT), a cohort study, a longitudinal study, a cross-sectional survey, or the like; how many groups there will be; and how often the subjects will be seen. This section need be no longer than one or two sentences, to orient the reader to the overall strategy. Some designs are more prone to biases than others (Streiner & Norman, 2009), so you should indicate that you are aware of the potential for bias, how you will try to control for it, and why the design you have chosen is the best for your purposes. Each design is a trade-off among competing pressures: an RCT controls for bias better than a cohort study, but is usually far more expensive; cohort studies allow better control of bias than case-control studies, but may be infeasible for studying disorders with a very low prevalence; cross-sectional surveys are less expensive than longitudinal studies, but do not provide good data from which you can infer causality; and so forth. Let the reviewers know, first, that you are aware of the limitations and, second, that you had sound reasons for your choice.

In the subsection "Subjects," you should spell out who they will be. If they are patients with a given diagnosis, how will the diagnosis be made, and by whom? The inclusion and exclusion criteria also have to be a balance between competing aims. On the one hand, you don't want to include people who cannot read the scales, because of either low intellectual ability or poor command of the language; subjects who may not be compliant; or those whose outcomes may be affected by co-morbid conditions. On the other hand, you do not want to limit subject selection so tightly that you cannot generalize your results beyond this narrowly defined group. Similarly, the control group or groups must be chosen carefully, and you must justify your decisions about entry criteria. This usually is not an issue in an RCT, since both groups come from the same population, but it can be quite problematic in cohort or case-control designs. For example, if you are looking at the effects of early loss on depression, with whom will you compare the depressed patients: randomly selected non-depressed people, normals with the same number of losses, patients with disorders other than depression, or some other group? A case can be made for each, and the important point is to state your case. Again, the reviewers may disagree with you, but they will be more inclined to give you the benefit of the doubt if you have shown that you have thought through the implications of select-ing certain groups but not others.

A rationale must also be given for the sample size (Streiner, 1990; see Chapter 4). You need enough subjects to show a meaningful difference, a few more to compensate for those who will inevitably be lost or drop out, and no more. By the same token, if you are looking at a relatively rare condition and are unable to recruit more than a fixed number of patients in a reasonable length of time, don't try to fool the reviewers by "fudging" the sample size calculation with a lower value for the power (the probability of finding statistical significance when, in fact, the groups differ) or a very large effect size. Be honest, and work backwards; with the number of patients who are likely to be available, you will have a given amount of power to detect a difference of this size between the groups. Again, you are letting the reviewers know you are cognizant of the potential difficulty, and then the decision is whether it is worth the risk of funding an interesting proposal with a known probability of finding nothing, rather than funding an incompetent researcher where the chances of a poor outcome are even higher. You must also show that, given the flow of patients through the unit or the number of people in the community who fit your criteria, it is feasible that a sufficient number of subjects can be found within the allotted time.

In the subsection, "Procedures," you spell out what you want to do in detail. The basic rule is that anyone else reading your proposal should be able to replicate the study: what is done to the subjects, who is doing it, how they will be trained (if necessary), and what will be measured and how. If your outcome measures are other than well-established scales or assays, you must provide information about their reliability and validity, and you should probably include copies of the scales in an appendix. Avoid the temptation to administer every scale ever developed. Not only does this increase the burden on the subjects (the tests truly become a battery), it also leads to problems in analysing the results: what will you do if Scale A shows a change but Scale B does not, and how will you handle the problem of highly correlated dependent variables? It is better to use judgment rather than a shotgun. Also, the major dependent variable should not be a scale you are currently developing, because there is too much risk that you will come up with negative findings, simply because the scale does not have sufficient reliability or validity. You should also make it plain that each measure is tied to one of the hypotheses, and that each hypothesis is linked to one or more of the dependent measures.

If the study has a number of phases or extends for any length of time, it is often worthwhile to include an illustration of the timeline of the study, such as Table 27.2. The X-axis marks off the months of the research, and there are a number of horizontal lines, one for each phase. So, for example, recruiting and training the research assistant may extend from the first through the third month, the next line down may show recruitment of subjects from months 3 through 15, another

Table 27.2 Timeline for a two-year study

	6	9	12	3	6	9	12	3	6
Recruit staff	▨								
Train staff		▨							
Recruit subjects			▨	▨					
Follow-up				▨	▨	▨	▨		
Data entry							▨	▨	
Data analysis								▨	
Writing									▨
	6	9	12	3	6	9	12	3	6
	Year 1			Year 2				Year 3	
	Month of study								

line will show the data analysis, and one will indicate when you plan to write up the results. This will show both you and the reviewers if you are being realistic in your scheduling.

Data Analysis

If you want your grant to be rejected, simply write that "the data will be analysed with appropriate parametric and non-parametric tests using SPSS/PC for Windows, Version 17.1" (or BMDP, SAS, Minitab, or whatever), and leave it at that. If you want to be more sophisticated, yet still have your proposal turned down, say only that "multivariate procedures will be used." Few phrases are as telling as these in letting the reviewers know that you do not have the foggiest idea about what you will be doing. They do not care which package, and especially which version, you will be using to analyse the data (much less to enter them); what they want to know is which tests you will be running and why. It is a good idea to start off by describing how you will screen the data for missing values, outliers, and deviations from the assumptions of the tests, such as normality or equality of variances. Then, you should indicate which statistical tests you will run for the first hypothesis, what you will look for in the results for confirmation, and so on for each of the other hypotheses. You should also state what you will do to account for missing data, lost subjects, and violations of the assumptions. If you are out of your depth, don't fake it; find a statistician who will act as a consultant or co-investigator and have him or her write this section.

Relevance

The "Relevance" section, like the "Summary," is often left to the last minute and seen as an unnecessary, bureaucratic part of the grant application. This, too, is a mistake. All agencies have terms of reference (TOR) that define the types of research they do and do not fund. A project that is seen as falling outside the TOR will not even be considered on its scientific merits. If you are lucky, this will be caught early on, and the proposal will be returned to you in enough time for you to submit it to a different agency. More often, though, it will be discovered during the review process, so you will have lost 6 to 12 months. This section is also a place where you can justify your project as important and meaningful, rather than simply well executed (the dreaded "ho-hum" review).

Budget

What you should include in the "Budget" is listed in Table 27.1 and in the manuals published by the agencies. Again, a balance is called for. You do not want to overlook or underestimate an expense that can jeopardize the execution of the project, such as long-distance telephone calls to locate subjects and remind them to come in, printing of forms, postage, and the like. On the other hand, remember that a grant is awarded in order to conduct a study, not as a way of underwriting the cost of running a clinical unit. If psychological testing is routinely done on all children seen by the service or blood is taken to determine lithium levels, then these costs should not be charged to the grant. They are allowable expenses only if they are done solely for the purpose of the study.

It is also important to justify your expenses. If you are asking for a research assistant, spell out how his or her time will be spent and how long it will take to find the subjects, enlist them in the study, test them, and enter the data into the computer. Rest assured that the reviewers will be questioning this aspect. If you are anticipating seeing 50 patients in a year, most reviewers are capable of deducing that this works out, on average, to one subject a week, so it would be hard to justify a full-time assistant, a secretary, and a graduate student. If in doubt, err on the side of including too much detail, rather than too little.

It is rare for a grant to be turned down solely on the basis of the budget, unless the reviewers feel that you are trying to pull the wool over their eyes, and an obviously padded budget could tip the balance against you. Also, remember that the reviewers have more experience than you in trying to pad a budget, so they are aware of most of the tricks.

Appendices

Some appendices are mandatory. If your study involves humans or animals as subjects, or you will be using radioactive or hazardous materials or new investigational drugs, you must include forms from the appropriate committees at your institution or the regulatory body. Because everything is always done at the last moment, it sometimes happens that you do not have the forms when it is time to send off the application. Write a covering letter indicating that they are to follow, but be sure that they arrive at the agency before the grant is reviewed.

If you are relying on units in your hospital or other organizations to refer patients or to do certain tests, append letters from them indicating their support. Similarly, any consultants to the study should send letters of support. These must be specific, saying, not simply "your idea is interesting," but something along the lines of "I look forward to working with you, and this is what I am prepared to do." As I mentioned previously, you should also include copies of any scales or questionnaires that are not widely known. If you can include any psychometric data on reliability and validity, so much the better.

As for what else you should or could include, break down and read the manual. Some agencies allow or even encourage you to include copies of previous publications in order to show what you can do; others expressly forbid this. You may have done a very thorough literature review for the "Introduction," but it is too long to include *in toto*. If the agency's rules allow, you may be able to include it as an appendix; at least some of the reviewers may be grateful to you for having saved them a lot of work for their next grant application. Some granting agencies want your full CV, while others constrain you to a form with a fixed number of pages. The moral is read the instructions (or, as emailers like to say, "RTFM" – Read the Flippin' Manual).

Getting It Together

There is more to a grant application than simply the component parts of the proposal. How you put the package and the research team together also plays a role and, as is the case in the individual sections, there are overt and covert messages.

Who Should Be on the Team

Medicine, and even psychiatry, has moved past the stage where one person has all of the requisite skills to carry out any except the simplest research project. A study often requires knowledge of the content area itself, quantitative methodology, and statistics. Moreover, if specialized techniques are required, such as brain imaging, neuropsychological testing, different forms of therapy, or qualitative research methods, it is highly unlikely that one person has mastery over all of these fields. One question all agencies ask reviewers to comment on is whether the researchers have the necessary skills to carry out the research. If your CV can leave any doubt in the reviewers' minds, and especially if your track record is limited, think seriously about having co-investigators or consultants whose areas of expertise complement your own.

The Role of Pilot Studies

The answer to the question "Is it a good or a bad idea to include pilot data?" is "yes." Pilot data indicate that you have thought about the area for more than the past week, that the methodology is feasible, and that the preliminary results (hopefully) look promising and worthy of support. On the other hand (and there is always an other hand), you want to avoid giving the impression that you were able to accomplish so much without grant support that you should be able to complete the study without any help from the agency. If you are able to achieve this balance, then on the whole, it is a good idea to provide the results of pilot studies.

The Language to Write In

Canada has two – and only two – official languages: English and French, so do not write in any other language, such as Medicalese, Psychologese, or Nursing Theory. Again, we are talking about a compromise. Specialized terms exist because they make communication easier, but only among specialists who know the jargon. Remember that not all of the reviewers who will evaluate your proposal have content expertise in your area; some are methodologists or statisticians, or, if the agency is relatively small, are content experts in other fields. (I was once the primary reviewer on a proposal about minimizing allergic reactions to bee venom, about which I have only personal knowledge.) A good model to follow is *Scientific American*, which contains articles that are aimed at intelligent but ignorant readers, that is, readers bright enough to understand what the authors are saying as long as the terms and concepts have been defined. Also, whenever possible, use terms that are used by the majority of the reviewers. To most of us, a person occupying a hospital bed is called a "patient," so don't refer to one as a "self-change agent"; you may win points for philosophy, but lose them for clarity.

Remember that not all of the reviewers are experts in your field; in smaller agencies, it will be very unlikely that the internal reviewers will be familiar with your jargon. Also, it is the internal reviewers who will speak at the meeting; they are your ambassadors, so it is worth striving to give them words they can grasp and use when they are making your case.

Neatness Does Count

Strictly speaking, your proposal should be evaluated on the basis of its scientific merit and significance, not spelling and neatness. Nevertheless, don't forget that you are trying to create an impression of being competent to carry out the research. If you cannot spell, have difficulty correctly adding the numbers in the budget, and are sloppy about packaging the proposal, then the reviewers may have doubts about your ability to look after the details of running a study and ensuring the fidelity of the data.

When All Else Fails, Read the Instructions

The importance of reading the manual cannot be emphasized too strongly. Every agency has its own rules (or quirks, depending on your perspective), and these should be followed assiduously. If you are allowed 20 pages, do not try to get away with 21; if it says to use double spacing, do not attempt to squeeze in more by using 1.5, and so on. In a similar vein, never use photo-reduction of the pages; the results are difficult to read and, even if legible, are hard work for the reader. Keep in mind the perspective of the reviewers; they are wading through a dozen or more grants and resent anything that makes their work more onerous. If they become annoyed with you, the chances of getting a positive review are lessened, so keep them happy!

Summary

Now that grant money is harder to get, competition is growing more keen. Even protocols that are seen as very worthy are not getting funded. A well-written proposal can mean the difference between acceptance and rejection, and it is just as easy to write a good one as a bad one. Following these guidelines will not guarantee funding, but it may increase your chances.

ACKNOWLEDGMENT

I would like to thank Dr. Dugal Campbell for his careful review and many helpful comments about this paper.

REFERENCES

Streiner, D.L. (1990, Oct). Sample size and power in psychiatric research. *Canadian Journal of Psychiatry, 35*(7), 616–620. Medline:2268843
Streiner, D.L., & Norman, G.R. (2009). *PDQ epidemiology.* (3rd ed.). Shelton, CT: PMPH USA.

TO READ FURTHER

Ogden, T.E., & Goldberg, I.A. (2002). *Research proposals: A guide to success.* (3rd ed.). San Diego, CA: Academic Press.
Yang, O.O. (2005). *Guide to effective grant writing: How to write a successful NIH grant application.* New York: Kluwer.

28 A Short Cut to Rejection: How Not to Write the Results Section of a Paper

DAVID L. STREINER, PH.D.

Canadian Journal of Psychiatry, 2007, 52, 385–389

Benjamin Franklin told us that the only sure things in life were death and taxes. What that proves is that he lived in the days prior to peer-reviewed publications; otherwise, he would have written, "But in this world, nothing can be certain, except death, taxes, and rejection for badly written 'Results' sections of papers." That is not to say that other sections of research articles are immune to criticism. After all, articles can be rejected for what is written, or not written, in every section of a paper. For example, the "Introduction" can present a one-sided or biased view of a controversial area; it can cite articles that are out of date; and worst of all, it can omit important ones (that is, those written by the reviewers). The "Methods" section is also a rich area for reviewers to mine for criticism. Entire books have been written about designing various types of studies, and this has several implications.

First, it illustrates just how many things must be borne in mind at every stage of a project and that therefore can (and likely will) go wrong. Second, it means that every reviewer has become a maven and feels competent, if not obligated, to comment about the design and execution of the study. The "Discussion" section is where the authors interpret their results and give their implications (concluding, needless to say, that "further research is needed"). This gives the reviewers ample opportunity to lambaste the authors on their misinterpretation of what they found and ridicule the conclusion that the world will never be the same after these results gain the recognition they so richly deserve.

However, it is in the "Results" section that authors can really excel in demonstrating their lack of understanding of research and statistics. This chapter is not a tutorial on how to correctly analyse data – no single essay can do this, and there are many books available that do a good job. Rather, it focuses on some of the more common mistakes researchers make in presenting their findings, which serve as red flags signalling to reviewers that the authors are out of their depth. Sadly, these examples are not made from whole cloth but are based on my experience reviewing papers for more than 40 journals over a span of some 40 years. It is not a comprehensive list of things that can go wrong, but is, rather, highly idiosyncratic and based solely on the criterion of what drives me up the wall. It is a tutorial about what to do to increase the chances that your article will be rejected. Sometimes, my pet peeves contradict editorial policy. In these cases, I will tell you what I think is wrong but also what you should do to keep benighted editors happy.

Give Details about Data Entry, Not Analysis

Although this is a problem seen more often in grant applications than in articles, it's not unusual to run across sentences like these: "The data were entered into Program X, Version 2.03.01 (precise reference given) and analysed with Program Y, Version 14.9b (another precise reference). Univariate and multivariate tests were used to test for differences between the groups." These two sentences give too much information about trivia and not enough regarding important issues. Some journals require you to state the statistical package and version you used, but for the life of me, I don't have the foggiest idea why. It's important if you're running highly sophisticated analyses, such as factor analysis, structural equation modelling, item response theory, or cluster analysis, because, unfortunately, different programs can give different results. However, for the vast majority of statistical tests, the program is irrelevant: they all calculate the mean or do an ANOVA in the same way and come up with identical answers. Even more meaningless is what program was used to enter the data. A 4.2 is a 4.2, whether that number was entered into a spreadsheet, into a dedicated data entry program, directly into the statistical program, or even with a word processor. Telling me which program you used is about as relevant as saying whether you used a pencil or a pen to record what the subject said.

As a reviewer, what I want to know are the details of the tests that you used. This isn't too much of an issue for the simple univariate tests because there are not many options to choose from. However, if you do have options, I want to know which ones you chose and why. For example, if you did a factor analysis, you have a choice of many different extraction methods (and the defaults in many programs are the wrong ones), a larger number of rotation methods, and different ways of determining how many factors to retain. Similarly, if you ran a stepwise regression (although about 98.34% are done for the wrong reason; Streiner, 1994; see Chapter 11), I want to know what criteria were used for entering and deleting variables. My job as a reviewer is to determine whether you did things correctly or whether you screwed up somewhere; to do so, I have to know what you did. I'm not a very trusting soul (this being the prime requisite for a reviewer, trumping even expertise); if you don't indicate what you've done, I'll assume either that you're unaware of the implications of the various options or that you're trying to hide something. At best, the article will be sent back with a request for clarification and rewriting; at worst, it will be rejected out of hand. The bottom line is that you should report the relevant details of the analyses, not the irrelevant ones.

Report p Levels of Zero

P levels of statistical tests often determine whether an article will be submitted to a journal (Sutton, Song, Gilbody, & Abrams, 2000) and, if submitted, whether or not it is accepted (Olson et al., 2002). Consequently, articles are replete with them, often reported poorly. If you truly want to demonstrate to the reviewer that you do not understand statistics, the best way is to report the p level as $p = 0.0000$. You may want to take some comfort from the fact that this is how many of the most widely used computer programs indicate highly significant results. However, it merely shows that, contrary to being "giant brains" – the name applied to the old mainframes – computers, in fact, manifest many symptoms of organic brain syndrome. They are concrete, literal, and sadly deficient in logical reasoning (although one wonders if this description should be applied to the computers or to the people who program them). The only things that have a probability of zero are those that violate one of the basic laws of nature: travel that is faster than the speed of light, perpetual-motion machines, or politicians who keep campaign promises. For everything else in the world, especially study results, probabilities may be extremely small, but they are never zero. Therefore, do not report p levels as 0.0000; they should be given as less than some value. Very often, they're written as $p < 0.0001$, but later we'll see why it's usually more accurate to say $p < 0.01$.

Report Naked p Levels

Almost as bad as p levels of zero (especially to four decimal places) are p levels that appear alone, unsullied by any association with the results of a statistical test. If you've run a t-test or an ANOVA, you must report the value of the test and the degrees of freedom in addition to the p level. For multiple regressions, the minimum necessary information is to report the standardized and unstandardized coefficients, their standard error, the t-test for each variable, and the overall multiple correlation. Simply saying that the regression was significant (even when reporting that $p = 0.0000$) is meaningless, especially when the sample size is large, because even very small multiple correlations can be statistically significant.

Other statistical tests are reported in different ways, and you should know what they are. If you're unfamiliar with reporting the results of multivariate statistics, treat yourself to a copy of Tabachnick and Fidell's (2001) excellent book. Each chapter ends with an illustration of how to do just this.

Don't Give Confidence Intervals

Until about 5 or 10 years ago, journals were quite content if articles reported the value of some parameter (for example, a mean, a proportion, or an odds ratio) and the results of any tests of significance. However, there was growing discontent with this practice, especially among statisticians, for two reasons: first, the dichotomous decision of significant (if p were equal to or less than 0.05) or not significant (if p were greater than that value); second, the recognition that neither the results of the test nor the significance level addressed the issue of the magnitude of the effect. Regarding the first point, many researchers clung (and unfortunately, in the case of drug regulatory agencies, still cling) to the naïve belief that a phenomenon doesn't exist if p is 0.051, but suddenly appears if p is 0.049 – ignoring the facts that probabilities exist along a continuum and that the criterion of 0.05 is a totally arbitrary one chosen by Sir Ronald Fisher. Nevertheless, as Rosnow and Rosenthal (1989) said, "Surely God loves the .06 nearly as much as the .05" (p. 1277). The p level reflects the probability that, if the null hypothesis is true, these results could have arisen by chance. If p is less than 0.05, they still could have arisen by chance, and, conversely, if p is greater than 0.05, the findings could be real ones. The 0.05 criterion is an agreed-upon convention, not a reflection of the way the world operates: results don't pop into and out of reality like virtual particles as the p level changes. What changes is not the results themselves but our confidence in the results.

The second point is that neither the value of a statistical test nor the associated p level says anything about the clinical importance of a finding. If you were to see that the results of an ANOVA were $F(2,128) = 3.25$, $p = 0.04$, you wouldn't know how much variance the grouping variable accounted for or whether the effect was a large or a small one. Similarly, a significant odds ratio of 2.1 could generate a lot of interest in the phenomenon if it were a good estimate of the population value, but it would elicit yawns if the estimate were only a rough approximation.

After much discussion, the American Psychological Association published guidelines for reporting the results of statistical tests (Wilkinson and the Task Force on Statistical Inference, 1999). There were two very strong recommendations: all point estimates of a parameter should be accompanied by 95% confidence intervals (CIs), and, whenever possible, statistical tests should be accompanied by an effect size. For example, a multiple correlation would report the value of R^2, an ANOVA would give the value of ε^2 (eta-squared) or ω^2 (omega-squared) in addition to F, and differences between means would be accompanied by the standardized mean difference (to find out how to calculate these, see Altman, Machin, Bryant, & Gardner, 2000; Fern & Monroe, 1996; Fleiss, 1969; Hojat & Xu, 2004; Norman & Streiner, 2008). All psychology journals and many medical journals have adopted these guidelines.

Report Negative Values of t

As long as we're on the topic of reporting results, avoid another travesty perpetrated by mindless computers: reporting negative values for the results of t-tests. The minus sign appears in the output because the program subtracts the mean of Group 2 from that of Group 1. If Group 2's mean is larger, then the result is negative. However, what is called Group 1 and what is called Group 2 are totally arbitrary. We can label the treatment group "1" and the comparison group "2," or vice versa, and nothing will change except the sign of the t-test, so the sign tells us absolutely nothing. It's even more meaningless when it's reported in a table or in the text without any indication of which group is which – so, lose the sign.

Commit Type III Errors

We are all familiar with Type I and Type II errors: the first erroneously concludes that there is a statistically significant effect when, in fact, there isn't one, and the second is the converse – falsely concluding that there is no effect when one is actually there. There is also what we (Norman & Streiner, 2008) have called a Type III error – getting the right answer to a question that no one is asking. Perhaps the most egregious (but also the most common) example of a Type III error is testing whether a reliability or a validity coefficient is significantly different from zero. There are two reasons why this is asking the wrong question. First, unless you have done something terribly wrong in the execution or analysis of the study (for example, correlating the individual's social insurance number with his or her telephone number), I guarantee that the correlation will be greater than zero: never forget Meehl's (1990) sixth law, that everything is correlated with everything else (usually around 0.30). Thus, a significant correlation by itself is no guarantee of a Nobel Prize. More important, however, is that's not what the reader needs to know. The important issue is the magnitude of the correlation, not its statistical significance. A correlation of 0.50 will be statistically significant if there are at least 16 subjects in the study, but I hope nobody would trust a scale if the test-retest reliability were that low.

People often test for a correlation that is significantly different from zero under the false impression that "null" in *null hypothesis* means "nothing." As Cohen (1994) has pointed out, however, this is actually the "nil" hypothesis; the null hypothesis is the hypothesis to be nullified. Now, in many cases, the two are the same; we want to test whether some parameter, such as a difference between means, is bigger than zero – but it needn't be so, and in the case of reliability and validity coefficients, it shouldn't be so. If I had my druthers, people wouldn't even bother to report the p levels because such reports are Type III errors. However, I doubt I'll win my battle over this one, so the most sensible course is to test not whether the correlation is greater than zero but whether it's larger than some unacceptable value, say, 0.60. Better yet, I would simply calculate a CI around the parameter and check to see that the lower bound exceeds this minimal value. This would satisfy reviewers and editors as well as the requirement that parameters be accompanied by CIs.

Say That the Test Is Reliable and Valid

While we're on the topic of reporting reliability and validity coefficients, a very nice way of demonstrating your ignorance of scales is to talk about the reliability and validity of a test, as if it were an immutable property that, once demonstrated, resides with the test forever. Actually, it's not just ignorance you're showing but also the fact that you're more than a quarter of a century out of date. Until the 1970s it was, in fact, common to talk about a test's reliability and validity and to say that validity is the determination of what a scale is measuring. However, that changed dramatically following a series of articles by Cronbach (1971) and Messick (1980), in which the focus of validity testing shifted from the test to the interaction between the test and the specific group of people completing it. As Nunnally (1970) said, "Strictly speaking, one validates not a measurement instrument but rather some use to which the instrument is put" (p. 133). For example, a scale of positive symptoms of schizophrenia may show good validity when used with English-speaking, non-Native individuals. However, it is invalid when used with those who have been raised in some traditional First Nations cultures where it is quite appropriate to hear from and speak to deceased relatives (Hoffmann, Dana, & Bolton, 1985).

Similarly, a test can show good reliability when it is used with groups that manifest a wide range of the behaviour being tapped. However, because of restriction in the range of scores, the same test will have much poorer reliability when used with more homogeneous groups of people (Streiner & Norman, 2008).

The bottom line is that reliability and validity are not inherent properties of a test. You cannot say a test is reliable or valid; you have to demonstrate that these psychometric characteristics obtain for the group in which you are using it.

Be Inaccurate with Too Much Accuracy

In the previous section, I said that reporting a highly significant result as $p < 0.01$ is more accurate than reporting it as $p < 0.0001$. This seems paradoxical, because more decimal places usually reflect a higher degree of precision. After all, 0.3333 is a closer approximation to 1/3 than is 0.3. However, the issue is whether you have enough subjects and have gathered the right information to justify a large number of digits to the right of the decimal point. Take a look at Table 28.1, which

Table 28.1 An example of a table reporting baseline differences between two groups

Variable	Group A	Group B
Number of women/men	9/11	10/10
Age (SD)	35.45 (6.00)	37.25 (5.52)
Education (SD)	13.25 (4.11)	12.50 (4.04)

is much like the first table encountered in most articles, comparing two groups in terms of their baseline characteristics. Both age and education are reported to two decimal places. Is that degree of accuracy warranted? For age, that second decimal place represents 1/100th of a year, or just under four days. If you ask an individual how old he or she is (and assuming the individual rounds to his or her nearest birthday and doesn't lie), the average response is accurate only to within plus or minus three months – that's over 90 days' worth of error! Stating that you know the average age of the study participants to within half a week is bordering on the delusional.

The situation is even worse insofar as education is concerned. Assuming that the average school year is 200 days long, the difference between 13.25 years of education and 13.26 years is two days in the classroom. Would you be willing to stand up in court and defend that degree of precision, when all you asked for is the highest grade completed? I thought not.

This problem is exacerbated when you realize that the sample size in this example is only 20 subjects per group. That means that one year of schooling for each individual changes that last digit by 0.05. Draw a new sample that is identical to the first, except that 1 individual of the 20 finished an additional year of school, and the mean increases to 13.30. Small sample sizes result in large variations from one sample to the next. With 20 subjects and an SD of 4.11, the 95% CI around the mean is plus or minus 1.8 years (that is, $1.96 \times 4.11/\sqrt{20}$). In this case, even the first decimal digit is probably accuracy overkill. Thus, the number of decimal places you report in a table should reflect sampling error.

Conclusions

I have tried to show how you can write "Results" sections in such a way as to almost guarantee that your article will be rejected. Unfortunately, it isn't a comprehensive list: it is also possible, for example, to draw graphs that are misleading or distort what is – or more often, what is not – going on (Norman & Streiner, 2008; Streiner, 1997; see Chapter 5); however, it's enough to get started.

How you report your results reflects how well you understand statistics and, by implication, whether you are aware of the possible limitations of your results. If you commit any of these, or other, errors, you will be signalling to the reviewer that something is amiss – that you simply pressed the compute button without being fully aware of what you were doing or what the results might mean. In *The Doctor's Dilemma*, Shaw had the crusty physician say, "I tell you, Colly, chloroform has done a lot of mischief. It's enabled any fool to be a surgeon" (Shaw, 2006, p. 14). In the same way, desktop computers and the ready availability of statistical packages have enabled anyone to be a statistician. Nevertheless, just as chloroform doesn't take the place of training in surgery, so computers don't obviate the need for knowledge of statistics. If you don't have it, find someone who does. Don't be afraid to ask – most statisticians are (relatively) tame and friendly.

REFERENCES

Altman, D., Machin, D., Bryant, T., & Gardner, S. (2000). *Statistics with confidence*. (2nd ed.). Toronto, ON: Wiley.

Cohen, J. (1994). The earth is round ($p < .05$). *American Psychologist, 49*(12), 997–1003. http://dx.doi.org/10.1037/0003-066X.49.12.997

Cronbach, L.J. (1971). Test validation. In R.L. Thorndike (Ed.), *Educational measurement*. (2nd ed., pp. 443–507). Washington: American Council on Education.

Fern, E.F., & Monroe, K.B. (1996). Effect size estimates: Issues and problems in interpretation. *Journal of Consumer Research, 23*(2), 89–105. http://dx.doi.org/10.1086/209469

Fleiss, J.L. (1969). Estimating the magnitude of experimental effects. *Psychological Bulletin, 72*(4), 273–276. http://dx.doi.org/10.1037/h0028022

Hoffmann, T., Dana, R.H., & Bolton, B. (1985). Measured acculturation and MMPI-168 performance of Native American adults. *Journal of Cross-Cultural Psychology, 16*(2), 243–256. http://dx.doi.org/10.1177/0022002185016002007

Hojat, M., & Xu, G. (2004). A visitor's guide to effect sizes: Statistical significance versus practical (clinical) importance of research findings. *Advances in Health Sciences Education: Theory and Practice, 9*(3), 241–249. http://dx.doi.org/10.1023/B:AHSE.0000038173.00909.f6 Medline:15316274

Meehl, P.E. (1990). Why summaries of research on psychological theories are often uninterpretable. *Psychological Reports, 66*, 195–244.

Messick, S. (1980). Test validity and the ethics of assessment. *American Psychologist, 35*(11), 1012–1027. http://dx.doi.org/10.1037/0003-066X.35.11.1012

Norman, G.R., & Streiner, D.L. (2008). *Biostatistics: The bare essentials.* (3rd ed.). Shelton, CT: PMPH USA.

Nunnally, J. (1970). *Introduction to psychological measurement.* New York, NY: McGraw-Hill.

Olson, C.M., Rennie, D., Cook, D., Dickersin, K., Flanagin, A., Hogan, J.W., …, & Pace, B. (2002, Jun 5). Publication bias in editorial decision making. *Journal of the American Medical Association, 287*(21), 2825–2828. http://dx.doi.org/10.1001/jama.287.21.2825 Medline:12038924

Rosnow, R.L., & Rosenthal, R. (1989). Statistical procedures and the justification of knowledge in psychological science. *American Psychologist, 44*(10), 1276–1284. http://dx.doi.org/10.1037/0003-066X.44.10.1276

Shaw, G.B. (2006). *The doctor's dilemma.* Lenox, MA: Hard Press. Act 1.

Streiner, D.L. (1994, May). Regression in the service of the superego: The do's and don'ts of stepwise multiple regression. *Canadian Journal of Psychiatry, 39*(4), 191–196. Medline:8044725

Streiner, D.L. (1997, May). Speaking graphically: An introduction to some newer graphing techniques. *Canadian Journal of Psychiatry, 42*(4), 388–394. Medline:9161763

Streiner, D.L., & Norman, G.R. (2008). *Health measurement scales: A practical guide to their development and use.* (4th ed.). Oxford: Oxford University Press.

Sutton, A.J., Song, F., Gilbody, S.M., & Abrams, K.R. (2000, Oct). Modelling publication bias in meta-analysis: A review. *Statistical Methods in Medical Research, 9*(5), 421–445. http://dx.doi.org/10.1191/096228000701555244 Medline:11191259

Tabachnick, B.G., & Fidell, L.S. (2001). *Using multivariate statistics.* (4th ed.). Boston, MA: Allyn and Bacon.

Wilkinson, L., & Task Force on Statistical Inference. (1999). Statistical methods in psychology journals: Guidelines and explanations. *American Psychologist, 54*(8), 594–604. http://dx.doi.org/10.1037/0003-066X.54.8.594

TO READ FURTHER

Wilkinson, L., & Task Force on Statistical Inference. (1999). Statistical methods in psychology journals: Guidelines and explanations. *American Psychologist, 54*(8), 594–604. http://dx.doi.org/10.1037/0003-066X.54.8.594

Index